Meniscus Injuries

Editors

BRETT D. OWENS
RAMIN R. TABADDOR

CLINICS IN SPORTS MEDICINE

www.sportsmed.theclinics.com

Consulting Editor
MARK D. MILLER

January 2020 • Volume 39 • Number 1

ELSEVIER

1600 John F. Kennedy Boulevard ● Suite 1800 ● Philadelphia, Pennsylvania, 19103-2899

http://www.theclinics.com

CLINICS IN SPORTS MEDICINE Volume 39, Number 1
January 2020 ISSN 0278-5919, ISBN-13: 978-0-323-75420-0

Editor: Lauren Boyle
Developmental Editor: Donald Mumford

Clinics in Sports Medicine (ISSN 0278-5919) is published quarterly by Elsevier Inc., 360 Park Avenue South, New York, NY 10010-1710. Months of issue are January, April, July, and October. Business and Editorial Offices: 1600 John F. Kennedy Blvd., Ste. 1800, Philadelphia, PA 19103-2899. Customer Service Office: 3251 Riverport Lane, Maryland Heights, MO 63043. Periodicals postage paid at New York, NY and additional mailing offices. Subscription prices are $364.00 per year (US individuals), $733.00 per year (US institutions), $100.00 per year (US students), $405.00 per year (Canadian individuals), $904.00 per year (Canadian institutions), $100.00 (Canadian students), $475.00 per year (foreign individuals), $904.00 per year (foreign institutions), and $235.00 per year (foreign students). Foreign air speed delivery is included in all *Clinics* subscription prices. All prices are subject to change without notice. **POSTMASTER:** Send address changes to *Clinics in Sports Medicine*, Elsevier Health Sciences Division, Subscription Customer Service, 3251 Riverport Lane, Maryland Heights, MO 63043. Customer Service (orders, claims, online, change of address): Elsevier Health Sciences Division, Subscription Customer Service, 3251 Riverport Lane, Maryland Heights, MO 63043. **Tel: 1-800-654-2452 (U.S. and Canada); 314-447-8871 (outside U.S. and Canada). Fax: 314-447-8029. E-mail: journalscustomerservice-usa@elsevier.com (for print support); journalsonlinesupport-usa@elsevier.com (for online support).**

Reprints. For copies of 100 or more of articles in this publication, please contact the Commercial Reprints Department, Elsevier Inc., 360 Park Avenue South, New York, NY 10010-1710. Tel.: 212-633-3874; Fax: 212-633-3820; E-mail: reprints@elsevier.com.

Clinics in Sports Medicine is covered in *MEDLINE/PubMed (Index Medicus) Current Contents/Clinical Medicine, Excerpta Medica,* and *ISI/Biomed.*

Contributors

CONSULTING EDITOR

MARK D. MILLER, MD
S. Ward Casscells Professor, Head, Department of Orthopaedic Surgery, Division of Sports Medicine, University of Virginia, Charlottesville, Virginia, USA; Team Physician, Miller Review Course, Harrisonburg, Virginia, USA

EDITORS

BRETT D. OWENS, MD
Professor, Department of Orthopedics, Brown University Alpert Medical School, Providence, Rhode Island, USA

RAMIN R. TABADDOR, MD
Assistant Professor, Department of Orthopedics, Brown University Alpert Medical School, Providence, Rhode Island, USA

AUTHORS

BJORN BARENIUS, MD
Department of Clinical Science and Education, Södersjukhuset, Karolinska Intitutet, Stockholm, Sweden

STEVEN BOKSHAN, MD
Department of Orthopedics, Brown University Alpert Medical School, Providence, Rhode Island, USA

ROBERT H. BROPHY, MD
Professor, Department of Orthopaedic Surgery, Washington University School of Medicine, Chesterfield, Missouri, USA

KENNETH L. CAMERON, PhD, MPH, ATC
John A. Feagin Jr. Sports Medicine Fellowship, Keller Army Community Hospital, West Point, New York, USA

JORGE CHAHLA, MD, PhD
Sports Medicine Fellow, Department of Orthopaedics, Midwest Orthopaedics at Rush, Chicago, Illinois, USA

PETER S. CHANG, MD
Resident, Department of Orthopaedic Surgery, Washington University School of Medicine, St Louis, Missouri, USA

BRIAN J. COLE, MD, MBA
Associate Chairman and Professor, Department of Orthopedics, Rush University, Chairman, Department of Surgery, Rush OPH, Managing Partner, Midwest Orthopaedics at Rush, Chicago, Illinois, USA

ISWADI DAMASENA, MB BS, FRACS, FAOrthA
Senior Knee Fellow, Department of Trauma and Orthopaedic Surgery, University Hospital Coventry, Coventry, Warwickshire, United Kingdom

FRANCESCA DE CARO, MD
Department of Orthopaedic Surgery, Humanitas Castelli, Bergamo, Italy

AAD DHOLLANDER, MD, PT, PhD
Department of Orthopaedic Surgery, KLINA Hospital, Brasschaat, Belgium

ZACHARY J. DiPAOLO, MD
Department of Orthopaedic Surgery, University of Missouri, Columbia, Missouri, USA

CORY EDGAR, MD, PhD
Assistant Professor, Department of Orthopedic Surgery, UConn Health, Farmington, Connecticut, USA

PAUL D. FADALE, MD
Professor, Department of Orthopedics, Brown University Alpert Medical School, Providence, Rhode Island, USA

CPT SHAWN M. GEE, MD
Tripler Army Medical Center, Honolulu, Hawaii, USA

PABLO EDUARDO GELBER, MD, PhD
ICATME-Hospital Universitari Dexeus, Hospital de la Santa Creu i Sant Pau, Universitat Autònoma de Barcelona, Barcelona, Spain

RODRIGO A. GOES, MD, MSc
Instituto Nacional de Traumatologia e Ortopedia, Rio de Janeiro, Rio de Janeiro, Brazil

TREVOR R. GULBRANDSEN, MD
Resident, Department of Orthopedic Surgery, University of Iowa Hospitals and Clinics, Iowa City, Iowa, USA

JONATHAN D. HODAX, MD, MS
Sports Medicine Fellow, Department of Orthopedic Surgery, University of California, San Francisco, San Francisco, California, USA

CHATHURAKA T. JAYASURIYA, PhD
Assistant Professor, Department of Orthopaedics, Brown University/Rhode Island Hospital, Providence, Rhode Island, USA

MITCHELL I. KENNEDY, BS
Graduate School, Georgetown University, Washington, DC, USA

ROBERT F. LaPRADE, MD, PhD
Twin Cities Orthopedics, Edina, Minnesota, USA

ROBERT LAWTON, MA, MSc, BM BCh, FRCSEd (T&O)
Senior Knee Fellow, Department of Trauma and Orthopaedic Surgery, University Hospital Coventry, Coventry, Warwickshire, United Kingdom

NICHOLAS J. LEMME, MD
Department of Orthopedics, Brown University Alpert Medical School, Providence, Rhode Island, USA

CHUNBONG BENJAMIN MA, MD
Professor, Chief of Sports Medicine and Shoulder Surgery, Department of Orthopedic Surgery, University of California, San Francisco, San Francisco, California, USA

STEPHEN MARCACCIO, MD
Department of Orthopedics, Brown University Alpert Medical School, Providence, Rhode Island, USA

ALEXANDER R. MARKES, BS
Medical Student, Department of Orthopedic Surgery, University of California, San Francisco School of Medicine, San Francisco, California, USA

NEAL B. NAVEEN, BS
Research Coordinator, Department of Orthopaedics, Midwest Orthopaedics at Rush, Chicago, Illinois, USA

LASUN O. OLADEJI, MD, MS
Department of Orthopaedic Surgery, University of Missouri, Columbia, Missouri, USA

BRETT D. OWENS, MD
Professor, Department of Orthopedics, Brown University, Providence, Rhode Island, USA

FRANCESCO PERDISA, MD
SC Chirurgia Protesica dei Reimpianti di Anca e di Ginocchio, IRCCS Istituto Ortopedica Rizzoli, Bologna, Italy

SIMONE PERELLI, MD
ICATME-Hospital Universitari Dexeus, Universitat Autònoma de Barcelona, Barcelona, Spain

LTC MATTHEW A. POSNER, MD
John A. Feagin Jr. Sports Medicine Fellowship, Keller Army Community Hospital, West Point, New York, USA

TAYLOR E. RAY, BS
Department of Orthopaedic Surgery, University of Missouri, Columbia, Missouri, USA

BARBIE M. SACHS, PT, DPT, OCS
Mizzou Therapy Services, University of Missouri, Columbia, Missouri, USA

ADNAN SAITHNA, MD
Sano Orthopedics, Kansas City, USA; Department of Specialty Medicine (Trauma and Orthopedic Surgery), Kansas City University, Kansas City, Missouri, USA

RAPHAEL SERRA CRUZ, MD
Instituto Nacional de Traumatologia e Ortopedia, Hospital São Vicente de Paulo, Instituto Brasil de Tecnologias da Saúde, Rio de Janeiro, Rio de Janeiro, Brazil

SETH L. SHERMAN, MD
Department of Orthopaedic Surgery, University of Missouri, Columbia, Missouri, USA

BERTRAND SONNERY-COTTET, MD
Centre Orthopédique Santy, FIFA Medical Centre of Excellence, Groupe Ramsay-Générale de Santé, Hôpital Privé Jean Mermoz, Lyon, France

TAYLOR M. SOUTHWORTH, BS
Research Coordinator, Department of Orthopaedics, Midwest Orthopaedics at Rush, Chicago, Illinois, USA

TIM SPALDING, MB BS, FRCS Orth
Consultant Orthopaedic Surgeon, Department of Trauma and Orthopaedic Surgery, University Hospital Coventry, Coventry, Warwickshire, United Kingdom

MARC STRAUSS, MD
Department of Orthopaedic Surgery, Oslo University Hospital, Oslo, Norway

TRACY M. TAURO, BS, BA
Research Coordinator, Department of Orthopaedics, Midwest Orthopaedics at Rush, Chicago, Illinois, USA

MAJ DAVID J. TENNENT, MD
John A. Feagin Jr. Sports Medicine Fellowship, Keller Army Community Hospital, West Point, New York, USA

JOHN TWOMEY-KOZAK, BS
Department of Orthopaedics, Brown University/Rhode Island Hospital, Providence, Rhode Island, USA

PETER VERDONK, MD, PhD
Professor of Orthopaedic Surgery, Orthoca, Antwerp, Belgium

RENE VERDONK, MD, PhD
Emeritus Professor, Department of Orthopaedic Surgery, Universite Libre de Bruxelles, Bruxelles, Belgium

THAIS DUTRA VIEIRA, MD
Centre Orthopédique Santy, FIFA Medical Centre of Excellence, Groupe Ramsay-Générale de Santé, Hôpital Privé Jean Mermoz, Lyon, France

TAYLOR J. WILEY, MD
Sports Medicine Fellow, Department of Orthopedics, Brown University Alpert Medical School, Providence, Rhode Island, USA

BRIAN R. WOLF, MD, MS
Professor, Department of Orthopedic Surgery, Director, University of Iowa Sports Medicine, John and Kim Callaghan Endowed Chair and Director of UI Sports Medicine, Professor and Vice-Chairman of Finance and Academic Affairs, Department of Orthopedics and Rehabilitation, University of Iowa Hospitals and Clinics, Head Team Physician, University of Iowa Athletics, Iowa City, Iowa, USA

Contents

The menisci are 2 fibrocartilaginous crescents anchored via bony and ligamentous attachments to surrounding structures. Their biochemical
composition and multilayered structure make them ideal for converting
compressive forces to tensile forces in addition to improving joint congruity and providing shock absorption to weight bearing. The medial
meniscus maintains more attachments at both the horns and the midbody
than the lateral meniscus, making it more susceptible to injury. Understanding of the gross anatomy, vascular anatomy, biochemical composition, and microstructure is key to understanding causes of meniscal
pathology as well as treatment options for restoring its primary functions.

Meniscus injuries affect the young and physically active population.
Although meniscus injuries are common in many sports, football, soccer,
basketball, and wrestling are associated with the greatest risk. In an occupational setting, jobs requiring kneeling, squatting, and increased physical
activity level have the greatest risk. Meniscus injury can be isolated to the
meniscus or associated with other concomitant injuries, including anterior
cruciate ligament tears and tibial plateau fractures. The frequency of meniscal repair is increasing because of a better understanding of meniscal
pathophysiology, technological advancements, and a focus on meniscal
preservation following injury to mitigate long-term consequences such
as osteoarthritis.

The meniscus plays an important, complex role in maintaining the homeostasis and health of the knee. Meniscal tears are a risk factor for early
chondral injury and eventually knee osteoarthritis. There is a growing
body of evidence about the early biological changes associated with meniscal injury that likely start the process of joint degeneration. This review
highlights the basic science, translational and clinical studies of the detrimental effects of meniscal injury and deficiency on the biology of the knee.

role of any of these procedures in terms of chondroprotection is questionable, and the overall outcomes in the long term still can be improved.

Meniscus allograft transplantation is an established surgical treatment indicated in symptomatic meniscus-deficient patients with minimal to no arthritis. Treatment decision making should be individualized after a thorough history and physical examination, with diagnostic imaging and arthroscopy to assess the status of the meniscus. The senior author prefers to use a bridge-in-slot technique, where osseous fixation of the allograft is completed through passage of a bone bridge to a tibial slot. Outcomes in meniscus allograft transplantation are favorable, with reported significant improvements in clinical outcome and low failures in short- and midterm follow-up studies.

Meniscus injuries are among the most common athletic injuries and result in functional impairment in the knee. Repair is crucial for pain relief and prevention of degenerative joint diseases like osteoarthritis. Current treatments, however, do not produce long-term improvements. Thus, recent research has been investigating new therapeutic options for regenerating injured meniscal tissue. This review comprehensively details the current methodologies being explored in the basic sciences to stimulate better meniscus injury repair. Furthermore, it describes how these preclinical strategies may improve current paradigms of how meniscal injuries are clinically treated through a unique and alternative perspective to traditional clinical methodology.

Meniscal injury potentiates a sequence of events that leads to degenerative changes and early osteoarthritis. It is therefore imperative to preserve the meniscus whenever possible. Given the expanding indications for meniscus repair, it is important to continually analyze and advance the understanding of rehabilitation and return to play following meniscal surgery. This article presents evidence-based rehabilitation and return-to-play guidelines as well as a brief review of return-to-play outcomes following isolated meniscus repair.

Meniscal injuries in athletes present a challenging problem. Surgeons must balance the needs of the healing meniscus with the desire of the athlete to

CLINICS IN SPORTS MEDICINE

SERIES OF RELATED INTERESTED

Orthopedic Clinics
Foot and Ankle Clinics
Hand Clinics
Physical Medicine and Rehabilitation Clinics
Clinics in Podiatric Medicine and Surgery

THE CLINICS ARE AVAILABLE ONLINE!
Access your subscription at:
www.theclinics.com

Foreword

Meniscal Repair: The R-Factor

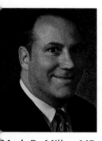

Mark D. Miller, MD
Consulting Editor

Although I am far from an expert in molecular biology, I do recall that the R-factor is named for a plasmid that codes for antibiotic resistance. The R-factor for the meniscus should be that we **R**esist any attempt to **R**emove this vital structure unless there is no other alternative. This issue of *Clinics in Sports Medicine*, expertly edited by Drs Brett Owens and Ramin Tabaddor, follows an R-factor theme of sorts. The articles begin with a discussion of the **R**ole of the meniscus and the **R**esults of **R**emoval. The issue then focuses on techniques for **R**epair and **R**eplacement. **R**emoval should always be the last option, but is sometimes unavoidable. Finally, **R**ehabilitation and **R**eturn to play are addressed.

I have been an advocate of meniscal preservation my entire career. Twenty-five years ago, we published an article that demonstrated the importance of meniscal repair in an animal model.[1] That same year, I was invited to be a Guest Editor for *Operative Techniques in Orthopaedics* and made a plea to the readers to "Save the Meniscus." Despite all that we have learned about the meniscus in the past quarter century ("ramp lesions," root tears, salvaging radial and horizontal tears, new techniques for meniscal transplantation, and so forth), I find myself once again repeating

Clin Sports Med 39 (2020) xiii–xiv
https://doi.org/10.1016/j.csm.2019.10.002
0278-5919/20/© 2019 Published by Elsevier Inc.

sportsmed.theclinics.com

this plea. **R**emember the **R**-factor: **R**epair **R**egularly, **R**esect **R**arely. *Save the Meniscus!*

Mark D. Miller, MD
Division of Sports Medicine
Department of Orthopaedic Surgery
University of Virginia
James Madison University
400 Ray C. Hunt Drive, Suite 330
Charlottesville, VA 22908-0159, USA

E-mail address:
mdm3p@virginia.edu

REFERENCE

1. Miller MD, Ritchie JR, Gomez BA, et al. Meniscal repair. An experimental study in the goat. Am J Sports Med 1995;23(1):124–8.

Preface

Meniscus Injuries in Athletes

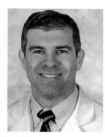 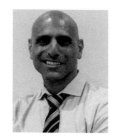

Brett D. Owens, MD   Ramin R. Tabaddor, MD
Editors

While so much of the sports medicine literature focuses on the anterior cruciate ligament (ACL), it is actually the meniscus that may be considered the critical player in the athletic knee. Much of the reasoning behind early ACL reconstruction is for preservation of the meniscus. Modern day cohorts of ACL reconstruction patients, such as the MOON cohort, continually show that it is the meniscal status that determines the athlete's overall outcome, and not all the reconstructive variables that receive so much of the surgeon's focus.

Once considered a vestigial organ, the meniscus plays a central role in knee mechanics, as both stabilizer, load distributor, and absorber. It is essential for the sports medicine clinician and knee surgeon to rule out the meniscus as a pain generator in the athlete's knee. Repair of meniscus tears remains central to the surgical treatment of athletic knee injuries. As new tear patterns become increasingly appreciated, advancing technical solutions augment the surgeon's armamentarium. Rehabilitation of these repairs has continued to advance as well, decreasing postoperative restrictions and improving active recovery. There has also been a heightened focus on return to play considerations, and this has continued to advance our field.

In this issue, we have brought together an international panel of experts on the meniscus as it relates specifically to the fields of epidemiology, cellular and tissue biology, surgical treatment, rehabilitation, and the care of athletes. We have attempted to comprehensively cover the topic of meniscus injury in athletes from epidemiology through return to play, with a large focus on surgical techniques. We added an article on basic science of meniscal repair due to its increasing relevance, given that the augmentation of repairs with biological adjuncts is becoming common. We hope you find this issue to be helpful in your care of the athletic knee, and we hope we

Clin Sports Med 39 (2020) xv–xvi
https://doi.org/10.1016/j.csm.2019.10.001
0278-5919/20/© 2019 Published by Elsevier Inc.   **sportsmed.theclinics.com**

can stimulate further dialogue and inquiry on this essential topic, because we have learned, "As goes the meniscus, goes the knee...."

Brett D. Owens, MD
Department of Orthopedics
Brown University
Providence, RI 02912, USA

1 Kettle Point Avenue
East Providence, RI 02914, USA

Ramin R. Tabaddor, MD
Department of Orthopedics
Brown University
Providence, RI 02912, USA

1 Kettle Point Avenue
East Providence, RI 02914, USA

E-mail addresses:
owensbrett@gmail.com (B.D. Owens)
rontabaddor@gmail.com (R.R. Tabaddor)

Meniscus Form and Function

Alexander R. Markes, BS*, Jonathan D. Hodax, MD, MS,
Chunbong Benjamin Ma, MD

KEYWORDS

- Meniscus • Knee • Anatomy • Function • Form • Load transmission

KEY POINTS

- Understanding of the gross anatomy, microvascular anatomy, and meniscofemoral attachments of the meniscus is vital to understanding treatment of meniscal injuries.
- The meniscus is a dense extracellular matrix comprising water and collagen, with interspersed cells, glycoproteins, and proteoglycans also contributing to its unique viscoelastic properties.
- Different meniscus injuries or tear patterns can lead to different clinical presentations.

INTRODUCTION

The menisci of the knees are 2 fibrocartilaginous discs whose unique biochemical composition and structure play a vital role in their ability to improve joint congruity, to handle load transmission, and to act as shock absorbers. Injuries to the menisci are a significant source of musculoskeletal morbidity with arthroscopic treatment of meniscal injuries accounting for 10% to 20% of all orthopedic surgeries.[1] The unique structures that allow for the various functions of the menisci also make treatment and repair challenging with long-term damage, leading to degeneration of the knee joint. Understanding these structures is vital to understanding treatment options for restoring function of the menisci after onset of injury or degeneration. This article aims to describe the underlying structure, composition, and function of the menisci and discuss current understanding of how that structure contributes to its primary functions within the knee joint.

FORM
Gross Anatomy

The menisci are 2 fibrocartilage crescents covering both the medial and lateral tibial plateaus that are anchored at the meniscal horns via bony attachments at the anterior

Disclosure Statement: All authors have no relationship with a commercial company that has a direct financial interest in subject matter or materials discussed in article or with a company making a competing product.

Department of Orthopedic Surgery, University of California San Francisco, 1500 Owens Street, San Francisco, CA 94158, USA

* Corresponding author.

E-mail address: Alexander.Markes@ucsf.edu

Clin Sports Med 39 (2020) 1–12
https://doi.org/10.1016/j.csm.2019.08.007
0278-5919/20/© 2019 Elsevier Inc. All rights reserved.

and posterior aspects of the tibial plateau (**Fig. 1** and **2**). As seen in **Fig. 1**, the lateral meniscus is C-shaped, covering 75% to 93% of the lateral tibial plateau compared with the medial meniscus that is more semicircular-shaped, covering 51% to 74% of the medial tibial plateau.[2-5]

Medial meniscus

The medial meniscus is approximately 40 mm to 45 mm long and 27 mm wide, with an anterior-posterior diameter of approximately 35 mm and a posterior region that is significantly broader than its anterior region.[3,4,6,7] The posterior horn of the medial meniscus is firmly anchored via bony attachments at the posterior intercondylar fossa directly anterior to the insertion of the posterior cruciate ligament on the tibia, as seen in **Fig. 2**.

The anterior horn attachment to the tibia is more variable, with Berlet and Fowler describing 4 different types of attachment in their classification system.[8,9] In their study of 48 cadaveric knees, they found the anterior medial meniscal horn inserted at the flat portion of the intercondylar ridge (type I) in 59% of knees, on the downward slope from the medial articular plateau to the intercondylar region (type II) in 24% of knees, and on the anterior slope of the tibial plateau (type III) in 15% of knees.[8] There was no bony insertion of the anterior horn (type IV) in 3% of knees.[8] The most common insertion site is 7 mm anterior to the anterior cruciate ligament (ACL) and is 61.4 mm^2, which is the largest insertion site of all 4 meniscal horns, the smallest of which is the posterior horn of the lateral meniscus at 28.5 mm^2.[8] The anterior medial meniscal horn is additionally connected to the anterior lateral meniscal horn via the transverse intermeniscal ligament, as seen in **Fig. 1**.

Additional attachments of the medial meniscus include the coronary ligaments and the deep medial collateral ligaments. The coronary ligaments are portions of the joint capsule that connect the inferior menisci to the tibia. The deep medial collateral ligament is a thickening of the joint capsule, which attaches to the midpoint of the meniscus.[7] Given all these attachments, the medial meniscus is considered relatively immobile.

Lateral meniscus

The lateral meniscus is C-shaped and relatively uniform in width from anterior to posterior (see **Fig. 1**). The anterior horn inserts anterior to the intercondylar eminence and

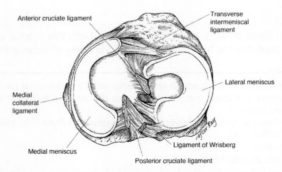

Fig. 1. Anatomy of the meniscus viewed from above. (*From* Greis PE, Bardana DD, Holmstrom MC, et al. Meniscal injury: I. Basic science and evaluation. J Am Acad Orthop Surg 2002;10(3):168-76; with permission.)

Anterior

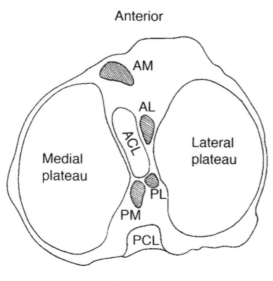

Posterior

Fig. 2. Meniscus horn insertion sites viewed from above. AL, anterior horn lateral meniscus; AM, anterior horn medial meniscus; PCL, posterior cruciate ligament; PL, posterior horn lateral meniscus; PM, posterior horn medial meniscus. (*From* Greis PE, Bardana DD, Holmstrom MC, et al. Meniscal injury: I. Basic science and evaluation. J Am Acad Orthop Surg 2002;10(3):168-76; with permission.)

lateral to the ACL attachment at the tibial spine (see **Fig. 2**). The posterior horn attaches just posterior to the lateral tibial spine and anterior to the attachment of the posterior medial meniscus.

If present, either 1 or both of the meniscofemoral ligaments additionally attaches to the lateral meniscus. These ligaments include the ligament of Humphrey and the ligament of Wrisberg (see **Fig. 1**), both of which arise from the lateral aspect of the medial femoral condyle and respectively insert just anterior or posterior to the posterior cruciate ligament. Although only 46% of people have both of these ligaments, a majority of people have at least 1 of them.[10,11] The lateral meniscus has no additional attachments to the corresponding collateral ligaments and only loose peripheral attachments to the joint capsule, which is interrupted by the popliteal tendon at the popliteal hiatus.[12] This allows for increased mobility of the lateral meniscus compared with the medial meniscus.

Vascular Anatomy

The medial and lateral middle geniculate arteries are branches of the popliteal artery responsible for providing blood supply to the meniscus. A premeniscal capillary plexus formed from branches of these arteries provides the majority of the vascular supply to the meniscus, as seen in **Fig. 3**. The adult meniscus remains a largely avascular structure, however, with only the peripheral 10% to 30% of the medial meniscus and 10% to 25% of the lateral meniscus receiving direct blood supply.[12,13] This has important implications for healing and is the basis of the 3 distinct zones of the meniscus labeled in **Fig. 3**: the peripheral vascularized red-red zone, the central avascular white-white zone, and

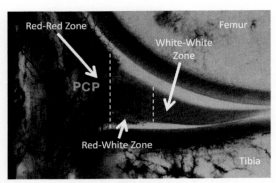

Fig. 3. Frontal section of the medial compartment of the knee following perfusion with India ink. Branching radial vessels from the perimeniscal capillary plexus (PCP) can be seen penetrating the peripheral border of the medial meniscus. Vascular red-red zone, avascular white-white zone, and in-between red-white zones are labeled. (*Adapted from* Arnoczky SP, Warren RF. Microvasculature of the human meniscus. Am J Sports Med. 1982;10:90-95; with permission.)

the intervening partially vascularized red-white zone.[13] In order to maintain their structure, it is believed the white-white and red-white zones receive more than two-thirds of their nutrition from synovial fluid via diffusion or mechanical pumping.[14,15]

Neuroanatomic Structures

The knee receives innervation from the branches of the posterior tibial nerve, obturator nerve, femoral nerve, and the common peroneal nerve, all of which penetrate the capsule and follow the same distribution as the vascular supply.[16] Thus, neural elements are most concentrated in the peripheral third of the meniscus. This was demonstrated by Dye and colleagues,[17] who found little or no pain on manual probing of the central meniscal tissue compared with slight to moderate discomfort on manual probing of the peripheral meniscal tissue in a conscious patient without intraarticular analgesia. Additionally, studies have identified 3 different mechanoreceptor subtypes that are theorized to contribute to joint proprioception and afferent sensory input.[16,18–22] Ruffini endings are unmyelinated, slowly adapting sensory fibers present that sense changes in joint deformation and pain. Pacinian corpuscles are myelinated, quickly adapting sensory fibers that respond to tension and pressure changes. Finally, Golgi tendon organs are myelinated, quickly adapting sensory fibers present that contribute to neuromuscular inhibition at terminal ranges of motion.

Microstructure and Biochemical Composition

The meniscal fibrocartilage structure is a dense extracellular matrix composed primarily of water (65%–70%), collagen (20%–25%), and proteoglycans (<1%).[12,23] This extracellular matrix is maintained by cellular components of the meniscus that vary by region. In the white-white zone, fibrochondrochytes predominate. These are anaerobic interspersed cells of the meniscus with few mitochondria, making them well suited to survive in this poorly vascularized region.[24,25] In the well-vascularized red-red zone, fibroblasts predominate and form the extracellular matrix.[26]

Collagen and microstructure

Type I collagen is predominant in the red-red zone of the meniscus, whereas type II collagen comprises the majority of the extracellular matrix of the white-white zone.[26] These collagen fibrils are arranged in an intricate 3-layer structure (**Fig. 4**), ideal for converting vertical compressive load into circumferential hoop stresses.[27] The deep layer is the most collagen dense layer and contains more type I collagen and fewer type II collagen fibers. These fibers are oriented circumferentially to resist circumferential hoop stresses.[12] Radially oriented type I collagen fibers comprise the second layer. These fibers weave themselves through the circumferential fibers, tying them together and providing further structural rigidity as well as resistance to longitudinal splitting.[28,29] The surface layer is the final layer and comprises fibers oriented parallel to the surface at various angles to provide a smooth, gliding surface.

Water, proteoglycans, and glycosoaminoglycans

In normal meniscal tissue, water comprises 65% to 70% of its total weight and predominantly resides in the posterior regions of the meniscus.[12,30] It is theorized that the hydraulic permeability of the meniscus allows for drag force generation during compressive loads. This drag may decrease the compressive strain transmitted through the meniscus and, therefore, help absorb shock and limit meniscal injury risk.[12,31] Proteoglycans are located within the interwoven layers of collagen and are formed with a core protein covalently attached to 1 or more glycosaminoglycans.[32] In healthy menisci, these negatively charged, hydrophilic molecules draw water into the meniscal tissue to allow for fluid transmission with compressive loading of the meniscus.[14,15,33]

FUNCTION

The primary functions of the meniscus include improving joint congruity and stabilization, load transmission, and shock absorption. Some investigators also theorize that the menisci play a role in proprioception and in joint lubrication. The mechanism by which the menisci carry out each of these functions is strongly rooted in their macroscopic and microscopic anatomy.

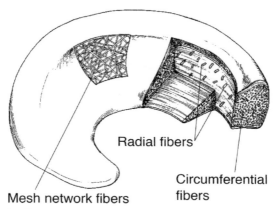

Radial fibers

Circumferential fibers

Mesh network fibers

Fig. 4. Schematic of collagen bundles and their orientation within the meniscus. (*From* Greis PE, Bardana DD, Holmstrom MC, et al. Meniscal injury: I. Basic science and evaluation. J Am Acad Orthop Surg 2002;10(3):168–76; with permission.)

Joint Congruity and Stabilization

Because there is a mismatch between the significant convexity of the medial femoral condyle and the slight concavity of the medial tibial plateau, the contact area of the medial compartment of the knee is, without a medial meniscus, focused over a small area. The wedge-shaped cross-section of the meniscus and its semicircular shape when viewed from above allow the meniscus to fill in the empty space between the plateau and condyle. The various attachments the medial meniscus has, as described previously, provide a strong stabilizing force that allows for minimal translation. This relative stability helps the medial femoral condyle remain centered over the tibial plateau, preventing translation.

On the lateral side of the knee, there is an even greater mismatch between the femoral condyle and tibial plateau, both being convex. The increased mobility of the lateral meniscus allows a greater degree of anterior and posterior translation of the femoral condyle on the tibial plateau, with the more mobile lateral meniscus maintaining its orientation around the condyle.

The role of the medial and lateral meniscus as secondary stabilizers of the knee has been shown through both biomechanical and clinical research. Absence of a functional medial meniscus in an ACL deficient knee demonstrates up to 58% increased anterior tibial translation compared with ACL tear alone,[34–36] and worsened pivot shift.[37] After meniscal transplantation or repair tibial translation is returned to premeniscectomy levels.[38]

Meniscal Tears and Load Transmission

Axial load transmitted across the knee joint is transmitted into hoop stresses by the meniscus. The wedge-shaped cross-section of the meniscus is expressed outward by compressive loads between femur and tibia, and this extrusion is resisted by the circumferential collagen fibers of the menisci and their anchor points at the anterior and posterior root.[39,40] In this way, compressive forces applied to articular cartilage are converted into tensile forces absorbed by the menisci.

Fig. 5 demonstrates the various types of meniscal tears. Horizontal tears of the meniscus (see **Fig. 5** and **6A**), also termed cleavage tears, are tears in the axial plain and are the most frequently observed tear pattern.[41] They typically are caused by sheer forces applied to the meniscus, although many patients deny awareness of an acute event.[41,42] Horizontal cleavage tears have been demonstrated to increase contact pressure in the knee joint by approximately up to 70%.[43] Débriding the inferior

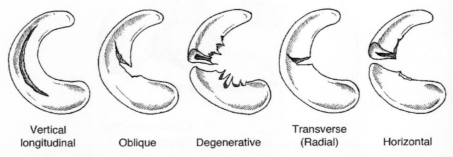

| Vertical longitudinal | Oblique | Degenerative | Transverse (Radial) | Horizontal |

Fig. 5. Different types of meniscal tears. (*From* Greis PE, Bardana DD, Holmstrom MC, et al. Meniscal injury: I. Basic science and evaluation. J Am Acad Orthop Surg 2002;10(3):168-76; with permission.)

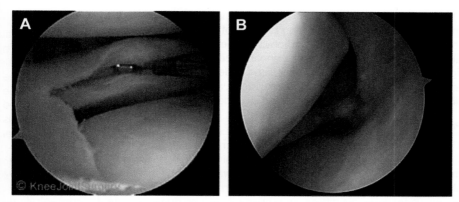

Fig. 6. (A) Horizontal meniscal tear visualized during knee arthroscopy (B) Radial meniscal root tear visualized during knee arthroscopy.

leaflet in horizontal tears leads to contact pressures 35% to 45% above baseline; however, repair may return contact pressures to within 15% of baseline.[43,44]

Radial tears of the meniscus are tears in any vertical plane originating at the central portion of the meniscus and extending toward the periphery. Radial tears of the medial meniscus increase contact pressure within the medial compartment by 70% to 110%.[45] These contact pressures approach normal after repair but significantly worsen when treated with partial meniscectomy.[45]

Meniscal root tears are a form of radial tear at the posterior attachment site of the meniscus (see **Fig. 6**B), and there has been an increase in interest and research into these tears over the past decade. Medial meniscal root tears are relatively common, presenting in 10% to 21% of arthroscopic meniscal repairs or meniscectomies, with studies suggesting magnetic resonance imaging scans may miss as many as one-third of these tears.[46–48] Medial meniscal root tears have been found essential for maintaining meniscal hoop tension and preventing meniscal extrusion.[49,50] A tear of the posterior root of the medial meniscus results in significantly decreased tibiofemoral contact area and a 25% increase in medial peak contact pressure, which is a load increase comparable to a total meniscectomy.[46,51]

In addition, Hein and colleagues[52] demonstrated an approximately 2-fold increase in medial meniscal displacement in a cadaveric knee with a medial meniscal root avulsion compared with the native knee after application of a vertical compressive force. This extrusion is thought to be partially responsible for the menisci's failure to function as a shock absorber in the degenerative knee.[53] Importantly, mean and peak compartment pressures as well as meniscal extrusion all are restored to baseline levels after root repair, which may avoid degenerative changes through restoration of normal kinematic profiles.[51–54] Precise anatomic repair is vital, however, for restoring this function. Starke and colleagues[55] elucidated this by demonstrating that a medial meniscal root repair placed nonanatomically just 3 mm medial or lateral significantly impaired the ability of the meniscus to convert axial tibiofemoral loads into hoop stresses.

Side-to-side differences also exist between tear types. Because the lateral meniscus has increased mobility, it plays less of a role of stabilization and thus receives less stress at the posterior horn than the medial meniscus.[46] Smith and Barrett[56] demonstrated in 575 meniscal tears that 75% of medial meniscal tears were in the peripheral posterior horn, compared with the lateral meniscus, which had a more even tear distribution, with 43% presenting in the peripheral posterior horn.

The location of the tear also varies with chronicity of injury, with studies showing medial meniscal tears accounting for 70% of chronic tears.[56] The consensus behind this finding is that the increased mobility of the lateral meniscus makes it more susceptible to unusual compressive and shear forces in an acute injury, such as a cruciate ligament tear.[56–59] The medial meniscus undergoes more relative strain as a secondary stabilizer with firm capsular, ligamentous, and bony attachments leaving it susceptible to chronic injury and age-related degeneration.[56]

Proprioception

The various neurologic end organs found in meniscal tissue are discussed previously. Each contributes to different functions of pain, motion, and position sensation within the knee joint. Postural stability of patients with medial and lateral meniscal tears has shown worsened balance and stability on perturbation, particularly after lateral meniscus tears.[60] This difference is suspected to be due to the greater concentration of rapidly adapting pacinian corpuscles in the lateral meniscus.[19] Magyar and colleagues[61] further demonstrated that response to a unidirectional force after meniscal injury was worsened on the injured leg compared with the noninjured leg and that the deficit in balance improved but did not return to baseline after arthroscopic partial meniscectomy.

Joint Lubrication

The menisci also function to lubricate the knee joint; however, the mechanics are not completely understood. The cartilage-meniscus interface maintains a fluid film, which varies with synovial viscosity, proteoglycan content, and compressive load of the joint.[62] Viscous synovial fluid produced by the synoviocytes is thought to dissipate sheer forces between the meniscus and articular cartilage during joint motion and weight bearing.[63] Additionally, hydrophilic mucin-like ends of proteoglycan 4, also known as lubricin, may play a role. Lubricin has been found in higher quantities specifically on the weightbearing surfaces of menisci and cartilage and is known to be up-regulated by mechanical forces.[64–66] Both the synovial fluid compression and high presence of proteoglycans lead to a dynamic friction coefficient as low as 0.015, which is lower than that of water ice, which ranges from 0.04 to 0.02.[67,68]

SUMMARY

The menisci of the knees are 2 fibrocartilaginous discs whose unique biochemical composition and structure play a vital role in its ability to improve joint congruity, to handle load transmission, and to act as a shock absorber. Capsular and ligamentous attachment differences account for the differences between chronicity and location of medial and lateral meniscal tears, with medial meniscus more susceptible to tears of the root and chronic injury. Repair of the meniscal tear, if possible, allows for adequate restoration of joint kinematics needed to limit future degeneration of the joint. Further understanding of the biochemical composition and microstructure allows for adequate understanding varying causes of meniscal pathology as well as treatment options for restoring its primary functions.

REFERENCES

1. Renstrom P, Johnson RJ. Anatomy and biomechanics of the menisci. Clin Sports Med 1990;9:523–38.

2. Arnoczky SP, Adams ME, DeHaven KE, et al. The meniscus. In: Woo SL-Y, Buckwalter J, editors. Injury and repair of musculoskeletal soft tissues. Park Ridge (IL): American Academy of Orthopaedic Surgeons; 1987. p. 487–537.
3. Clark CR, Ogden JA. Development of the menisci of the human knee joint. J Bone Joint Surg Am 1983;65:530.
4. Shaffer B, Kennedy S, Klimkiewicz J, et al. Preoperative sizing of meniscal allografts in meniscus transplantation. Am J Sports Med 2000;28:524–33.
5. Thompson WO, Thaete FL, Fu FH, et al. Tibial meniscal dynamics using three-dimensional reconstruction of magnetic resonance imaging. Am J Sports Med 1991;19:210–6.
6. McDermott ID, Sharifi F, Bull AM, et al. An anatomical study of meniscal allograft sizing. Knee Surg Sports Traumatol Arthrosc 2004;12:130–5.
7. Warren RF, Arnoczky SP, Wickiewiez TL. Anatomy of the knee. In: Nicholas JA, Hershman EB, editors. The lower extremity and spine in sports medicine. St Louis (MO): Mosby; 1986. p. 657–94.
8. Berlet GC, Fowler PJ. The anterior horn of the medial meniscus. An anatomic study of its insertion. Am J Sports Med 1998;26(4):540–3.
9. Johnson DL, Swenson TD, Harner CD. Arthroscopic meniscal transplantation: anatomic and technical considerations. Presented at: Nineteenth Annual Meeting of the American Orthopaedic Society for Sports Medicine. Sun Valley, ID, July 12–14, 1993.
10. Kusayama T, Harner CD, Carlin GJ, et al. Anatomical and biomechanical characteristics of human meniscofemoral ligaments. Knee Surg Sports Traumatol Arthrosc 1994;2:234–7.
11. Cohn AK, Mains DB. Popliteal hiatus of the lateral meniscus. Anatomy and measurement at dissection of 10 specimens. Am J Sports Med 1979;7:221–6.
12. Fox AJ, Bedi A, Rodeo SA. The basic science of human knee menisci: structure, composition, and function. Sports Health 2012;4(4):340–51.
13. Arnoczky SP, Warren RF. Microvasculature of the human meniscus. Am J Sports Med 1982;10:90–5.
14. Myers E, Zhu W, Mow V. Viscoelastic properties of articular cartilage and meniscus. In: Nimni M, editor. Collagen: chemistry, biology and biotechnology. Boca Raton (FL): CRC; 1988. p. 268–88.
15. Mow VC, Fithian DC, Kelly MA. Fundamentals of articular cartilage and meniscus biomechanics. In: Ewing JW, editor. Articular cartilage and knee joint function: basic science and arthroscopy. New York: Raven Press; 1990. p. 1–18.
16. Gardner E. The innervations of the knee joint. Anat Rec 1948;101:109–30.
17. Dye SF, Vaupel GL, Dye CC. Conscious neurosensory mapping of the internal structures of the human knee without intraarticular anesthesia. Am J Sports Med 1998;26:773–7.
18. Assimakopoulos AP, Katonis PG, Agapitos MV, et al. The innervations of the human meniscus. Clin Orthop Relat Res 1992;275:232–6.
19. Day B, Mackenzie WG, Shim SS, et al. The vascular and nerve supply of the human meniscus. Arthroscopy 1985;1:8–62.
20. Kennedy JC, Alexander IJ, Hayes KC. Nerve supply of the human knee and its functional importance. Am J Sports Med 1982;10:329–35.
21. Schutte MJ, Dabezius EJ, Zimny ML, et al. Neural anatomy of the human anterior cruciate ligament. J Bone Joint Surg Am 1987;69:243–7.
22. Zimny ML. Mechanoreceptors in articular tissues. Am J Anat 1988;64:883–8.
23. Sun Y, Mauerhan DR, Kneisl JS, et al. Histological examination of collagen and proteoglycan changes in osteoarthritic menisci. Open Rheumatol J 2012;6:24.

24. McDevitt CA, Miller RR, Sprindler KP. The cells and cell matrix interaction of the meniscus. In: Mow VC, Arnoczky SP, Jackson DW, editors. Knee meniscus: basic and clinical foundations. New York: Raven Press; 1992. p. 29–36.

25. Webber RJ, Norby DP, Malemud CJ, et al. Characterization of newly synthesized proteoglycans from rabbit menisci in organ culture. Biochem J 1984;221(3): 875–84.

26. Bryceland JK, Powell AJ, Nunn T. Knee menisci: structure, function, and management of pathology. Cartilage 2017;8(2):99–104.

27. Jones RS, Keene GC, Learmonth DJ, et al. Direct measurement of hoop strains in the intact and torn human medial meniscus. Clin Biomech (Bristol, Avon) 1996; 11:295–300.

28. Ramachandran M. Basic orthopaedic sciences: the Stanmore guide. London: Hodder Arnold; 2007. p. 80–4.

29. Bullough PG, Munuera L, Murphy J, et al. The strength of the menisci of the knee as it relates to their fine structure. J Bone Joint Surg Br 1970;52:564–7.

30. Proctor CS, Schmidt MB, Whipple RR, et al. Material properties of the normal medial bovine meniscus. J Orthop Res 1989;7:771–82.

31. Kleinhans KL, Jackson AR. Hydraulic permeability of meniscus fibrocartilage measured via direct permeation: Effects of tissue anisotropy, water volume content, and compressive strain. J Biomech 2018;72:215–21.

32. Muir H. The structure and metabolism of mucopolysaccharides (glycosaminoglycans) and the problem of the mucopolysaccharidoses. Am J Med 1969;47(5): 673–90.

33. Hascall VC. Interaction of cartilage proteoglycans with hyaluronic acid. J Supramol Struct 1977;7:101–20.

34. Greis PE, Bardana DD, Holmstrom MC, et al. Meniscal injury: I. Basic science and evaluation. J Am Acad Orthop Surg 2002;10(3):168–76.

35. Pagnani MJ, Warren RF, Arnoczky SP, et al. Anatomy of the knee. In: Nicholas JA, Hershman EB, editors. The lower extremity and spine in sports medicine. St Louis (MO): Mosby; 1995. p. 581–614.

36. Johnson DL, Swenson TM, Livesay GA, et al. Insertion-site anatomy of the human menisci: Gross, arthroscopic, and topographical anatomy as a basis for meniscal transplantation. Arthroscopy 1995;11:386–94.

37. Trojani C, Elhor H, Carles M, et al. Anterior cruciate ligament reconstruction combined with valgus high tibial osteotomy allows return to sports. Orthop Traumatol Surg Res 2014;100:209–12.

38. Spang JT, Dang AB, Mazzocca A, et al. The effect of medial meniscectomy and meniscal allograft transplantation on knee and anterior cruciate ligament biomechanics. Arthroscopy 2010;26:192–201.

39. Shrive NG, O'Connor JJ, Goodfellow JW. Load bearing in the knee joint. Clin Orthop Relat Res 1978;131:279–87.

40. Aspden RM, Yarker YE, Hukins DW. Collagen orientations in the meniscus of the knee joint. J Anat 1985;140:371–80.

41. Ferrer-Roca O, Vilalta C. Lesions of the Meniscus. Part II: Horizontal cleavages and lateral cysts. Clin Orthop Relat Res 1980;146:301–7.

42. Nguyen JC, De Smet AA, Graf BK, et al. MR imaging-based diagnosis and classification of meniscal tears. Radiographics 2014;34(4):981–99.

43. Beamer BS, Walley KC, Okajima S, et al. Changes in contact area in meniscus horizontal cleavage tears subjected to repair and resection. Arthroscopy 2017; 33(3):617–24.

44. Koh JL, Yi SJ, Ren Y, et al. Tibiofemoral contact mechanics with horizontal cleavage tear and resection of the medial meniscus in the human knee. J Bone Joint Surg Am 2016;98(21):182901836.

45. Zhang AL, Miller SL, Coughlin DG, et al. Tibiofemoral contact pressures in radial tears of the meniscus treated with all inside and inside-out repair and partial meniscectomy. Knee 2015;22(5):400–4.

46. Bhatia S, LaPrade CM, Ellman MB, et al. Meniscal root tears: significance, diagnosis, and treatment. Am J Sports Med 2014;42(12):3016–30.

47. Ozkoc G, Circi E, Gonc U, et al. Radial tears in the root of the posterior horn of the medial meniscus. Knee Surg Sports Traumatol Arthrosc 2008;16(9):849–54.

48. Bin SI, Kim JM, Shin SJ. Radial tears of the posterior horn of the medial meniscus. Arthroscopy 2004;20(4):373–8.

49. Kim JH, Chung JH, Lee DH, et al. Arthroscopic suture anchor repair versus pullout suture repair in posterior root tear of the medial meniscus: a prospective comparison study. Arthroscopy 2011;27(12):1644–53.

50. Griffith CJ, LaPrade RF, Fritts HM, et al. Posterior root avulsion fracture of the medial meniscus in an adolescent female patient with surgical reattachment. Am J Sports Med 2008;36(4):789–92.

51. Allaire R, Muriuki M, Gilbertson L, et al. Biomechanical consequences of a tear of the posterior root of the medial meniscus: similar to total meniscectomy. J Bone Joint Surg Am 2008;90(9):1922–31.

52. Hein CN, Deperio JG, Ehrensberger MT, et al. Effects of medial meniscal posterior horn avulsion and repair on meniscal displacement. Knee 2011;18(3):189–92.

53. Papalia R, Vasta S, Franceschi F, et al. Meniscal root tears: from basic science to ultimate surgery. Br Med Bull 2013;106:91–115.

54. Schillhammer CK, Werner FW, Scuderi MG, et al. Repair of lateral meniscus posterior horn detachment lesions: a biomechanical evaluation. Am J Sports Med 2012;40(11):2604–9.

55. Starke C, Kopf S, Grobel KH, et al. The effect of a nonanatomic repair of the meniscal horn attachment on meniscal tension: a biomechanical study. Arthroscopy 2010;26(3):358–65.

56. Smith JP 3rd, Barrett GR. Medial and lateral meniscal tear patterns in anterior cruciate ligament-deficient knees. A prospective analysis of 575 tears. Am J Sports Med 2001;29(4):415–9.

57. Palmer I. On the injuries to the ligaments of the knee joint: a clinical study. Acta Chir Scand 1938;81(suppl 53):1–282.

58. Thompson WO, Fu FH. The meniscus in the cruciate-deficient knee. Clin Sports Med 1993;12:771–96.

59. Warren LF, Marshall JL. The supporting structures and layers on the medial side of the knee: An anatomical analysis. J Bone Joint Surg Am 1979;61:56–62.

60. Lee JH, Heo JW, Lee DH. Comparative postural stability in patients with lateral versus medial meniscus tears. Knee 2018;25:256–61.

61. Magyar MO, Knoll Z, Kiss RM. Effect of medial meniscus tear and partial meniscectomy on balancing capacity in response to sudden unidirectional perturbation. J Electromyogr Kinesiol 2012;22:440–5.

62. Andrews SHJ, Adesida AB, Abusara Z, et al. Current concepts on structure-function relationships in the menisci. Connect Tissue Res 2017;58(3–4):271–81.

63. Arnoczky SP, Warren RF, Spivak JM. Meniscal repair using exogenous fibrin clot: an experimental study in dogs. J Bone Joint Surg Am 1988;70:1209–17.

64. Swann DA, Silver FH, Slayter HS, et al. The molecular structure and lubricating activity of lubricin isolated from bovine and human synovial fluids. Biochem J 1985;225(1):195–201.
65. MacConaill M a. The function of intraarticular fibrocartilages, with special reference to the knee and inferior radio-ulnar joints. J Anat 1932;66(Pt2):210–27.
66. Grad S, Lee CR, Gorna K, et al. Surface motion upregulates superficial zone protein and hyaluronan production in chondrocyte-seeded three-dimensional scaffolds. Tissue Eng 2005;11(1-2):249–56.
67. Galley NK, Gleghorn JP, Rodeo S, et al. Frictional properties of the meniscus improve after scaffold-augmented repair of partial meniscectomy: a pilot study. Clin Orthop Relat Res 2011;469(10):2817–23.
68. Guariguata A, Pascall MA, Gilmer MW, et al. Jamming of particles in a two-dimensional fluid-driven flow. Phys Rev E Stat Nonlin Soft Matter Phys 2012; 86(6 Pt 1):061311.

The Burden of Meniscus Injury in Young and Physically Active Populations

Shawn M. Gee, MD[a],*, David J. Tennent, MD[b],
Kenneth L. Cameron, PhD, MPH, ATC[b], Matthew A. Posner, MD[b]

KEYWORDS

- Meniscus • Epidemiology • Prevalence • Incidence • Athlete • Occupational
- Risk factors

KEY POINTS

- The incidence of meniscus injury ranges from 0.61 to 0.70 per 1000 person-years in the United States, and is common in the young and physically active population.
- The medial meniscus is 2 to 3 times more likely to be injured than the lateral meniscus.
- Radial and vertical tears are most prevalent with acute traumatic knee joint injuries, whereas horizontal and complex tears of the meniscus are most commonly associated with degenerative joint disease and osteoarthritis.
- Modifiable risk factors include activity level and body mass index, whereas nonmodifiable risk factors include age, gender, and anatomic factors, to include posterior tibial slope, medial meniscal slope, a biconcave medial tibial plateau, and knee malalignment.
- Football, soccer, basketball, and wrestling have the greatest incidence of meniscus injuries. Concomitant knee joint injuries, such as anterior cruciate ligament tears and tibial plateau fractures, are associated with high rates of meniscus injury.

INTRODUCTION
Historical Perspective

The first description of meniscus injury came in the late eighteenth century. Between 1782 and 1803, British surgeon William Hey published several articles describing "internal derangement" of the knee as being caused by "semilunar displacement."[1] The first detailed anatomic description of the meniscus came from the brothers Weber and Weber[2] in 1836, in their book *Mechanik der menschlichen Gehwerkzeuge*. From the original description, the menisci were referred to as internal and external semilunar

Disclosures: None.
[a] Tripler Army Medical Center, 1 Jarrett White Road, Honolulu, HI 96859, USA; [b] John A. Feagin Jr. Sports Medicine Fellowship, Keller Army Community Hospital, 900 Washington Road, West Point, NY 10996, USA
* Corresponding author.
E-mail address: shawn.m.gee.mil@mail.mil

Clin Sports Med 39 (2020) 13–27
https://doi.org/10.1016/j.csm.2019.08.008
0278-5919/20/Published by Elsevier Inc.

cartilage. Their anatomy and function were further examined by John Goodsir, Professor of Anatomy at the University of Edinburgh, in his anatomic memoirs in 1868. Goodsir and Lonsdale[3] described the menisci as a "curved, yielding, but elastic railway" that moves with flexion and extension of the knee.

During the nineteenth century, the semilunar cartilage was a well-known cause of internal derangements of the knee. In 1889, British surgeon Herbert Allingham[4] described the internal and external semilunar cartilages as the "most generally recognized causes of internal derangements of the knee-joint." He stated that the knee may be "thrown out of gear, and from a cartilage moving too quickly or too slowly, or a condyle moving too slowly or too quickly, great damage may arise."[4] He also stated that meniscus injuries are "virtually neglected, and have failed to receive from most of the profession that consideration which they really deserve."[4] Up until 1885, meniscus injuries were treated by closed means, as originally described by William Hey, through closed reduction with flexion followed by extension of the knee and casting.[1] Meniscal injuries are now frequently treated surgically.

Incidence and Prevalence of Meniscal Tears

The incidence of meniscus injury ranges from 0.61 to 0.70 per 1000 person-years in the general population in the United States to as high as 8.27 per 1000 person-years in young and physically active populations.[5–7] Meniscal disorder ranges from the discoid meniscus in the pediatric population to traumatic tears in athletes. Asymptomatic, degenerative tears are common in older adults. In high school athletes, for whom most of the epidemiologic data exist, meniscus tears occur at a rate of 0.51 per 10,000 athlete exposures (AEs), accounting for approximately 10% to 20% of all knee injuries.[8–10] Meniscus injuries occur in a variety of sports but are most frequent in football, soccer, basketball, and wrestling.[8] Pathologic conditions, such as anterior cruciate ligament (ACL) tears and tibial plateau fractures, are associated with meniscus injury.

Not all tears are symptomatic and require treatment. With the advancement of MRI, meniscus tears are becoming easier to identify. In a study of patients aged 18 to 39 years, the prevalence of asymptomatic meniscus tears was 5.6%.[11] In asymptomatic individuals, there is an increased prevalence of meniscal abnormalities on MRI with increasing age.[11,12] In the elderly population, aged 50 to 90 years, the prevalence of meniscus tears is 31%.[13] These tears tend to be horizontal and complex.

Epidemiology of Tear Types

Location (medial vs lateral)
When discussing the incidence of medial versus lateral meniscus injury, several factors come into play, to include mechanism, acuity of injury, and age. Despite these factors, the medial meniscus is consistently 2 to 3 times more likely to be injured compared with the lateral meniscus. In 1889, Allingham[4] had 19 medial meniscus injuries, with only 6 lateral meniscus injuries, giving a ratio of 3:1. In 1948, Fairbank's[14] original study included 80 total medial meniscectomies and 27 lateral meniscectomies, producing a ratio of 3:1 medial to lateral meniscus injury. Over the years, this proportion has been documented in athletes,[15] military service members,[7] asymptomatic adults (aged 18–39 years),[11] and symptomatic adults with knee osteoarthritis.[13,16]

A few exceptions to the 3:1 rule exist. In acute and chronic ACL tears, the proportion of lateral meniscus injury is higher, producing a ratio closer to 1:1, medial to lateral meniscus tears.[17–19] Tibial plateau fractures also have a higher proportion of lateral meniscus injuries.[20,21] In contrast, in occupations requiring kneeling, a higher proportion of medial meniscus tears are present, up to 20:1 in a study of miners.[22]

Type

Meniscus tears are categorized by type and location. Horizontal, complex, radial (and flap tears), vertical (longitudinal and bucket-handle tears), root tears, and ramp lesions are frequently described. Horizontal and complex tears are most common and typically exist on the osteoarthritis spectrum. Radial and vertical tears are common in acute injuries, whereas root tears and ramp lesions are typically higher-energy injuries associated with ACL tears. Unlike horizontal and complex tears, radial and vertical tears are typically seen in a younger population.[23] These tear types are discussed here in their order of prevalence.

Horizontal tears run parallel to the tibial plateau. They are the most common tear type, encompassing 24% to 40% of all tears.[13,24] Although most common, they exist on the spectrum of degenerative disease. Complex tears also exist on this spectrum. In a study of patients aged 50 to 90 years (Framingham study), the prevalence of meniscus tear was 31%.[13] Most tears involved the posterior horns, and were horizontal (40%) and complex (37%). Ninety percent of patients with severe osteoarthritis had meniscal damage.[13] In another study by Bergkvist and colleagues[25] (all ages included), horizontal and complex tears encompassed 68% of all tears. In general, horizontal and complex tears are considered degenerative tears.

Radial tears are oriented perpendicular to the tibial plateau and the meniscal axis. They disrupt the longitudinal collagen bundles and hoop strength of the meniscus, resulting in increased meniscal extrusion and greater cartilage damage compared with horizontal tears.[23] In the Framingham study (ages 50–90 years), radial tears accounted for 15% of all tears,[13] compared with 7% in the study by Bergkvist and colleagues[25] (all ages). Lateral radial tears are more common in younger patients and are associated with ACL injury. In the study by Bergkvist and colleagues,[25] 36% of lateral radial tears had an associated ACL injury, compared with 8% with medial radial tears.

Vertical (longitudinal and bucket-handle) tears extend perpendicular to the tibial plateau and parallel to the meniscal axis. Similar to radial tears, they occur in a younger population.[23,25] In the Framingham study, 7% of patients had a longitudinal tear,[13] versus 25% in the study by Bergkvist and colleagues.[25] The average age was 36 years for vertical tears. Vertical tears are also associated with ACL injury. Forty-five percent of ACL injuries present with vertical tears (including bucket-handle tears) to the medial meniscus, whereas only 28% occur on the lateral side.[25]

Meniscal root tears occur within 1 cm of the bony tibial attachment and lead to significant meniscus extrusion, accelerating the development of arthritis.[23] Compared with other tear types, they occur infrequently, at a rate of 1%.[13] In degenerative arthritis, posterior root tears often occur on the medial side and are present in up to 6% of patients with osteoarthritis.[26] Although root tears are not traditionally thought of as degenerative tears, medial meniscus posterior root tears (MMPRTs) occur with increased age, higher body mass index (BMI), increased varus, and lower sports activity level compared with other tear types.[27] In the acute setting, meniscal root tears have been reported in multiligamentous knee injuries and in cases of hyperflexion and squatting.[28]

Ramp lesions are meniscocapsular lesions in the posterior horn of the medial meniscus, often disrupting the meniscotibial ligamentous attachment.[29] They occur frequently with ACL injury, occurring in 9% to 17% of all ACL tears.[30,31] The MRI sensitivity of ramp lesions is only 48%, making the arthroscopic examination the gold standard.[28] If ramp lesions are not recognized and treated, they can result in continued pain, dysfunction, and instability caused by altered knee joint kinematics.[32]

Risk Factors

Modifiable risk factors

Both modifiable and nonmodifiable risk factors exist for meniscus injury (**Table 1**). Increased activity level and BMI are considered the most significant modifiable risk factors. Meniscus injuries occur in a variety of sports but are most frequent in football, soccer, basketball, and wrestling.[8] These activities require cutting, pivoting, and quick and unanticipated direction changes, which are associated with the mechanism of acute traumatic meniscus injury. Concomitant injuries to the knee joint, such as ACL tears and tibial plateau fractures, are also associated with meniscus injury. A more thorough discussion of modifiable and nonmodifiable risk factors for meniscal injuries is provided later.

Activity level Increased activity level is a recognizable risk factor for meniscus injury. This finding is evident from numerous studies in athletes, showing increased rates of meniscus injury compared with the general population. A good example of this comes from the military population, in which the incidence of meniscus injury is 8.27 per 1000 person-years.[7] In the civilian population, the rate is 0.61 to 0.70 per 1000 person-years.[5,6] This effect is magnified in cases of knee instability, such as ACL tear, in which cases of recurrent instability result in increased rates of meniscal damage.[33–35]

Although increased activity level has been linked with most meniscus tears, lower sports activity level has been associated with MMPRT.[27] Note that this factor may be confounded by increased BMI as a result of a sedentary lifestyle. Ultimately, in some instances of MMPRT, increased activity level may be protective against meniscus injury.

Body mass index In athletes and nonathletes, BMI has been identified as a factor associated with meniscus injury. In a recent biomechanical study by Achtnich and colleagues,[36] BMI correlated positively to medial meniscus extrusion. With meniscal

Table 1
Modifiable and nonmodifiable risk factors for meniscus injury

Risk Factor	Description
Modifiable	
Activity level	Increased activity level for most tears; decreased activity level for MMPRT
BMI	BMI>25 kg/m^2
Nonmodifiable	
Age	Increased age; younger age may be protective, especially in cases of delayed ACL reconstruction
Gender	Men at increased risk; among gender-comparable sports, women may be at greater risk; women at risk for MMPRT
Anatomy	
PTS	PTS>13° may increase risk in ACL-deficient knees
MMS	MMS>3.5° may increase risk of ramp lesion in ACL deficiency
Biconcave medial tibial plateau	Biconcave plateau may increase risk of complex medial meniscus tears
Knee malalignment	<178° or >182°; higher risk of meniscal extrusion with valgus knees

Abbreviations: MMS, medial meniscal slope; PTS, posterior tibial slope.

extrusion, the normal function of the meniscus is impaired, leading to altered loading conditions within the knee.[37] In a study of the general population, the probability of having meniscus surgery increased with a BMI greater than 27.5 kg/m^2 in men and 25 kg/m^2 in women. Patients with a BMI greater than 40 kg/m^2 had 15 times greater odds of having meniscus surgery. In a study of middle-aged individuals, meniscus lesions were found nearly twice as often in overweight and obese individuals.[38] Of various meniscus injuries, MMPRT may have the greatest association with BMI, with a 4.9-fold increase with BMI greater than 30 kg/m^2.[27]

In athletes, this risk remains relevant. In a study of National Basketball Association (NBA) players, BMI was a significant predictor of meniscus injury risk. For players with a BMI greater than 25 kg/m^2, the risk of meniscus injury increased from 1.6 to 2.2 injuries per 100 athlete-seasons.[39] In a study of ACL reconstructed patients, increased BMI (>25 kg/m^2) was associated with a greater number of medial and lateral meniscus tears.[40] Although this association exists in many studies, some studies have not shown an association between meniscus injury and BMI in athletes[35,41]; however, these studies may be underpowered for BMI given their homogenous patient populations.

Nonmodifiable risk factors

Age Similar to rotator cuff tears, the prevalence of meniscus tears increases with age. In a population aged 50 to 90 years, the prevalence of meniscus tears was 31%,[13] whereas, in a younger, asymptomatic population aged 18 to 39 years, the prevalence was 5.6%.[11] In asymptomatic individuals, there is an increased prevalence of meniscal abnormalities and degenerative tears on MRI with increasing age.[11,12] Although the prevalence increases with age, the incidence of acute, traumatic tears decreases with age.[15,42] In boys and men, the peak incidence occurs between 12 and 30 years of age, compared with 11 to 20 years in women.[15,42] This finding is likely caused by decreased activity level with increasing age. In contrast, in young, active populations with similar activity requirements, the incidence of meniscus tear seems to increase with increasing age. In a recent study, military service members more than 40 years of age experienced 4 times as many meniscus injuries as those less than 20 years old.[7]

In cases of ACL injury, advancing age increases the risk of chondral damage and meniscus injuries. There is evidence to suggest that, in patients age 22 years and younger, there is a lower rate of meniscus injury in cases of delayed ACL reconstruction.[35,43,44] As a result, younger age may have a protective effect on meniscus injury in cases of ACL injury.

Gender The incidence of meniscus injury differs among male and female individuals. At the high school level, across multiple studies, there is a higher prevalence of meniscus injuries in boys than in girls.[8,9,17,45] However, among gender-comparable sports, injury rates may be higher in girls.[9] A recent study analyzed sex differences among high school and collegiate sports. Overall, the injury rates were slightly higher for male athletes at 0.68 per 10,000 AEs versus 0.53 per 10,000 AEs for female athletes.[45] In the military, men are 20% more likely to sustain a meniscus injury.[7] In patients undergoing ACL reconstruction, male sex is associated with more meniscus injuries than female sex at the time of surgery.[17,28,31,40,45,46]

Although male athletes may be at greater risk for meniscus injuries than female athletes, adult women are at greater risk for MMPRT.[27,47] In 1 study, female sex was associated with a 5.9-fold increase in risk for MMPRT, even higher than BMI greater than 30 kg/m^2, which had a 4.9-fold increase in risk.[27]

Anatomy Anatomic factors may increase the risk of medial meniscus injury. These factors include posterior tibial slope (PTS), medial meniscal slope (MMS), a biconcave medial tibial plateau, and knee malalignment. The discoid meniscus as a risk factor is discussed later. In theory, the shape of the tibial plateau and meniscus affects force transmission across the menisci, especially in cases of ACL deficiency.

Posterior tibial slope and medial meniscal slope In cases of ACL deficiency, every 10° increase in PTS leads to an additional 6 mm of anterior tibial translation.[48] In turn, increased PTS has been associated with an increased incidence of posterior horn medial meniscus tears.[49,50] In 1 study, PTS greater than 13° was a risk factor for secondary meniscus tears in ACL-deficient knees.[50] At present, PTS remains a controversial risk factor for meniscus injury, partially because of the challenges associated with measuring PTS, which lead to substantial variability. Similarly, medial meniscal slope may also be associated with an increased risk for meniscus tears in combination with ACL injury.[41] Patients with an ACL injury and ramp lesion had an MMS of 3.5°, which was larger than that of patients with an isolated ACL tear (2°). This effect was greater in cases of delayed ACL reconstruction (>6 months from injury). There was no association between increased PTS and ramp lesion.[41] It is hypothesized that an increased MMS may predispose the posterior horn of the medial meniscus to higher stress, increasing its risk for injury.[41]

Biconcave medial tibial plateau A biconcave medial tibial plateau is characterized by a coronal plane tibial plateau ridge separating the anterior and posterior portions of the tibial plateau.[51] The biconcavity can either be cartilaginous or bony. In a study by Barber and colleagues,[51] patients with biconcave medial tibia plateaus had more complex medial meniscus tears (69%) than those without biconcavity (53%). The group with biconcave plateaus had a lower average BMI, making confounding unlikely. Given the paucity of literature on this topic, more research is needed to confirm these findings.

Knee malalignment Knee malalignment increases load transmission in the medial or lateral tibiofemoral compartment, resulting in increased meniscal extrusion with greater malalignment. Meniscal extrusion increases the risk for meniscus injury. In the Multicenter Osteoarthritis Study, both varus and valgus malalignment (<178° or >182°) was associated with meniscal extrusion. Valgus malalignment was associated with a higher risk of meniscal extrusion than varus malalignment.[52] Moreover, there was a strong association with increasing malalignment and progressive meniscal damage, especially in valgus knees.[53] Some studies have found that mild malalignment (<3° from neutral) does not increase meniscal extrusion[54]; however, these studies do not apply to cases of moderate to severe malalignment.

Activities Associated with Meniscus Injury

Sports
High school sports In high school sports, the rate of knee injuries is 2.98 injuries per 10,000 AEs.[9] Meniscus tears occur at a rate of 0.51 per 10,000 AEs,[8,9] accounting for approximately 10% to 20% of all knee injuries.[8–10] They occur more frequently in competition and during player-on-player contact.[8,9] In a large study of more than 21 million AEs, boys' football, girls' soccer, girls' basketball, and boys' wrestling had the greatest incidence of meniscus injuries (**Table 2**). Cheerleading, track and field, and swimming had the lowest incidence of injuries.[8] Although the incidence of meniscus injury was greater in boys, among gender-comparable sports, the incidence

Table 2	
Sports associated with meniscus injury	
Level of Risk	Sports (Highest to Lowest Risk)
High	Football>soccer>basketball>wrestling
Moderate	Gymnastics>lacrosse>ice hockey>field hockey>baseball/softball
Low	Track and field>swimming>cheerleading

was higher in girls. In girls' soccer, basketball, softball, lacrosse, and track and field, meniscus injury risk was twice that of their male counterparts.[8]

Collegiate sports In collegiate sports, limited data exist for meniscus injury. In 1 study, the rate of meniscus injury in college sports was similar among men and women.[45] Similar to high school, soccer and basketball had higher rates of meniscus injury compared with lacrosse, softball/baseball, and ice hockey, but other sports were not included in the study.[45] In a study of West Point cadets with ACL tears, football, rugby, wrestling, basketball, and soccer accounted for the greatest number of meniscus injuries.[17]

In a study of division I National Collegiate Athletic Association football players, meniscus injury was the second leading cause of surgery after shoulder labral injury, and accounted for 13% of all surgeries.[55] Although 30 partial meniscectomies were performed, no meniscal repairs were performed. More than twice as many lateral meniscectomies were performed than medial meniscectomies.[55] Presently, limited data exist on college athletes and meniscus injury.

Professional sports In the NBA, the rate of meniscus injury is 1.58 per 10,000 AEs.[39] Lateral meniscus tears account for 58% to 60% of all meniscus tears, and result in a similar amount of lost playing time (40–50 days) compared with medial meniscus tears.[39,56] At the Women's National Basketball Association combine, meniscus surgery was the second most common surgical procedure, with 11% of all athletes having had a previous meniscus surgery.

In the National Football League (NFL), epidemiologic studies are lacking. In 1 study of NFL combine players from 2009 to 2015, 51% of all players had sustained a prior knee injury. Knee injuries were less frequent than ankle (53%) and shoulder (52%) injuries. Twelve percent of players reported a prior meniscus injury.[57] Similar to the NBA, most meniscus tears (66%) involved the lateral meniscus. In another study of NFL combine participants, athletes with a prior meniscectomy performed significantly worse in their first 2 seasons in the NFL.[58]

In Major League Baseball (MLB), a significant number of injuries occur during sliding, accounting for 4263 missed playing days per season from 2011 to 2015.[59] Meniscus injury accounted for 9% of these sliding injuries. Similar to the NFL, epidemiologic data on injuries in general, and meniscus injuries specifically, are limited in MLB players. However, for other professional sports, such as soccer, rugby, and ice hockey, epidemiologic data are sparse and should be a topic of further research.

Other sports Other sports that have been identified as having a high risk of meniscus injuries include off-road motorcycling (20% of all injuries)[60] and skiing (10%–20% of all injuries).[61] Interestingly, long distance runners (marathon runners) have a similar prevalence of meniscus tears and degeneration to sedentary persons, who are at lower risk.[62]

Occupations

Occupations at high risk of meniscus injury include occupations that require prolonged squatting and occupations that have fitness requirements (**Box 1**). Squatting particularly increases the incidence of meniscus tears. A recent biomechanical study showed increased frontal plane motion during squatting, which is known to increase the risk of meniscus tears and subsequent knee osteoarthritis.[63] Miners, carpet/floor layers, and construction workers are at particularly high risk. In a systematic review of 19 articles, the investigators showed excess risk of meniscus injury in occupations requiring kneeling, to include mining and carpet/floor laying.[64]

Occupations with increased activity levels and fitness requirements, including the military, are also at significantly higher risk than the general population. In the military, the incidence of meniscus injury is 8.27 per 1000 person-years[7] compared with a rate of 0.61 to 0.70 per 1000 person-years in the civilian population.[5,6] Within the military, the Army and Marine Corps have higher rates than the Air Force and Navy. Junior enlisted service members have the highest rate, followed by senior enlisted, senior officers, and junior officers.[7]

Conditions Associated with Meniscus Injury

Anterior cruciate ligament tears

In patients with traumatic hemarthroses, meniscus tears have been reported in 73% of cases, whereas ACL tears are identified in 88% of cases (**Table 3**).[65] In patients with acute ACL tears, meniscus tears have been reported in 40% to 82% of cases.[17,35,66,67] In a large prospective study of more than 10,000 cadets, meniscus tears were identified in 40% of patients with ACL tears.[17] Although most studies show a preponderance of lateral meniscus injuries (56%) versus medial meniscus injuries (46%),[35,66,68] other studies show a larger proportion of medial meniscus tears (53%) versus lateral (47%).[17] As previously discussed, ramp lesions occur in 9% to 17% of all ACL tears.[30,31]

When discussing timing of ACL surgery, many studies show an increased rate of medial meniscus injury cases of delayed ACL reconstruction and chronic ACL tears.[35,44,69–72] Because the medial meniscus serves as a secondary stabilizer in ACL deficiency, it is at increased risk of injury. A recent systematic review showed an increased number of medial meniscus lesions in chronic ACL tears with recurrent instability episodes, although these findings were a result of low-level evidence.[34] Other large studies show similar rates of meniscus injuries in acute and chronic ACL tears.[17] In cases of revision ACL reconstruction, meniscus injury is noted in 70% to 75% of patients, occurring more frequently in the medial meniscus.[18,19,73]

Fractures

In tibial plateau fractures, 57% to 80% of patients have meniscus tears.[20,21] For displaced tibial plateau fractures, approximately 30% have lateral meniscus tears requiring repair.[74] Of the fracture types, split depression fractures have the highest

---

Box 1
Occupations at highest risk for meniscus injury

Occupations requiring kneeling
  Miners, carpet/floor layers, construction workers, and so forth

Occupations with increased activity and/or fitness requirements
  Military, law enforcement, firefighters, and so forth

Table 3 Conditions associated with meniscus injury	
Condition	Rate of Meniscus Injury
Primary ACL reconstruction	40%–82%; most commonly affecting lateral meniscus; higher rate of medial meniscus injury in delayed ACL reconstruction; 9%–17% of ACL tears have ramp lesions
Revision ACL reconstruction	70%–75%; most frequently affecting the medial meniscus
Tibial plateau fractures	57%–80%; 30% require repair, most often in split depression–type fractures

incidence of lateral meniscus tears requiring repair (45%).[74] Ultimately, although the prevalence remains high, not all meniscus tears require operative repair.

Pediatric Meniscus Injury and Discoid Meniscus

The estimated prevalence of discoid meniscus is 3% to 5% in the United States and as high as 15% in the Japanese population.[75,76] The exact prevalence is largely unknown, because asymptomatic patients do not present for evaluation. Although most patients are asymptomatic, a large proportion of lateral meniscus disorder in adolescents involves the discoid meniscus. In a study of adolescents (14–16 years old) undergoing knee arthroscopy for lateral meniscus disorder, 75% were discoid.[77] All patients less than 10 years old with lateral meniscus disorder had a discoid meniscus on arthroscopy.[77] In another study, 25% of all children had discoid meniscus tears; however, medial meniscus disorder was included in this study.[78] Despite the high prevalence of discoid lateral meniscus tears, other tear types, such as complex and vertical tears, are more common.[78] Overall, the prevalence of discoid lateral meniscus tears is noteworthy, and should be taken into consideration when evaluating lateral meniscus disorders in young adult and pediatric populations.

Epidemiologic Considerations

Advancement of imaging

With the advancement of imaging, the likelihood of identifying asymptomatic tears has increased. In a study of patients aged 18 to 39 years, the prevalence of asymptomatic meniscus tears was 5.6%.[11] Interestingly, 3.7% were identified in the lateral meniscus, whereas 1.9% were found in the medial meniscus. In asymptomatic individuals, there is an increased prevalence of meniscal abnormalities on MRI with increasing age.[11,12] Because of the high prevalence of asymptomatic meniscus tears, history and physical examination remain of utmost importance when interpreting MRI results and evaluating meniscus tears.

Long-term consequences of meniscal injury

In 1948, Fairbank[14] published "Knee Joint Changes after Meniscectomy." He described ridge formation, narrowing of the joint space, and flattening of the femoral condyle caused by meniscectomy. This article was the first published evidence to suggest that the meniscus plays a role in osteoarthritis development. Further studies elaborated on Fairbank's[14] original work, showing increased radiographic osteoarthritis in cases of total meniscectomy compared with partial meniscectomy.[79,80] Recently, meniscal injury alone (without surgery) has been identified as a strong risk factor. In the Multicenter Osteoarthritis Study (MOST), meniscal tear without surgery was identified as a significant risk factor for the development of osteoarthrtis.[81] Notably, although a meniscal tear can lead to knee osteoarthritis, knee osteoarthritis can also lead to meniscal tears.[80] As mentioned earlier, there is an increased prevalence of meniscal abnormalities and degenerative tears on MRI with increasing age.[11,12] In discussing treatment, biomechanical studies show that meniscus function can be reestablished with meniscus repair.[82,83] Recently, because of a better understanding of osteoarthritis progression and improved technology, meniscal repair has become the standard of care when achievable.[84]

Treatment trends
With the advent of new meniscal repair technology and the morbidity of postmeniscectomy osteoarthritis, meniscal repair is increasingly common. In 1990, in a large database study of more than 6000 meniscus tears, the rate of meniscus repair was 24.5% for the medial meniscus and 21.2% for the lateral meniscus.[15] In the United States, from 2004 to 2012, the rate of repair increased from 11% to 17%. Per surgeon, the rate increased 37%, from 1.6 to 2.2 cases per surgeon.[85] Similarly, in Japan, the proportion of patients undergoing meniscus repair increased from 7% in 2007 to 26% in 2014.[84]

SUMMARY

Meniscus injuries are common in pediatric and adult populations. Although tears are more often symptomatic in young and physically active patients, they are more prevalent in older adults, affecting around 31% of the elderly population. Horizontal and complex tears are most common and exist on the osteoarthritis spectrum. Radial and vertical tears are common in acute injuries, whereas root tears and ramp lesions are typically higher-energy injuries and occur in association with ACL tears. Epidemiologic data in high school and college athletes show that football, soccer, basketball, and wrestling have the greatest incidence of meniscus injury. Among professional sports, quality epidemiologic data on meniscal injuries are lacking but show a large association between meniscus injury and degrading athletic performance. Although meniscal repair is now gaining significant traction, more focus should be placed on primary injury prevention, particularly given the long-term consequences of meniscal injury. It is hoped that future epidemiologic studies will provide further insight into the primary, secondary, and tertiary injury prevention of meniscal injuries in both athletes and individuals in high-risk occupations.

REFERENCES

1. Lipscomb PR, Henderson MS. Internal derangements of the knee. J Am Med Assoc 1947;135(13):827–31.
2. Weber W, Weber E. Mechanik der menschlichen Gehwerkzeuge. Göttingen; 1836.
3. Goodsir J, Lonsdale H. The anatomical memoirs of John Goodsir, Vol. 2. Edinburgh: A. and C. Black; 1868.
4. Allingham HW. The treatment of internal derangements of the knee-joint by operation. Churchill; 1889.
5. Baker BE, Peckham AC, Pupparo F, et al. Review of meniscal injury and associated sports. Am J Sports Med 1985;13(1):1–4.
6. Nielsen AB, Yde J. Epidemiology of acute knee injuries: a prospective hospital investigation. J Trauma 1991;31(12):1644–8.
7. Jones JC, Burks R, Owens BD, et al. Incidence and risk factors associated with meniscal injuries among active-duty US Military service members. J Athl Train 2012;47(1):67–73.

8. Mitchell J, Graham W, Best TM, et al. Epidemiology of meniscal injuries in US high school athletes between 2007 and 2013. Knee Surg Sports Traumatol Arthrosc 2016;24(3):715–22.

9. Flanigan C, Fields SK, Comstock RD. Epidemiology of Knee Injuries among US High School Athletes, 2005/06–2010/11. Med Sci Sports Exerc 2013;45(3):462–9.

10. Majewski M, Susanne H, Klaus S. Epidemiology of athletic knee injuries: a 10-year study. Knee 2006;13(3):184–8.

11. Laprade RF, Quinter BM, Veenstra MA, et al. The prevalence of abnormal magnetic resonance imaging findings in asymptomatic knees. Am J Sports Med 1994;22(6):739–45.

12. Fukuta S, Masaki K, Korai F. Prevalence of abnormal findings in magnetic resonance images of asymptomatic knees. J Orthop Sci 2002;7(3):287–91.   .

13. Englund M, Guermazi A, Gale D, et al. Incidental meniscal findings on knee MRI in middle-aged and elderly persons. N Engl J Med 2008;359(11):1108–15.

14. Fairbank TJ. Knee joint changes after meniscectomy. J Bone Joint Surg Br 1948; 30B(4):664–70.

15. Poehling GG, Ruch DS, Chabon SJ. The landscape of meniscal injuries. Clin Sports Med 1990;9(3):539–49.

16. Kumm J, Roemer FW, Guermazi A, et al. Natural history of intrameniscal signal intensity on knee MR images: six years of data from the osteoarthritis initiative. Radiology 2016;278(1):164–71.

17. Kilcoyne KG, Dickens JF, Haniuk E, et al. Epidemiology of meniscal injury associated with ACL tears in young athletes. Orthopedics 2012;35(3):208–12.

18. Wright RW, Huston LJ, Spindler KP, et al. Descriptive epidemiology of the multicenter ACL revision study (MARS) cohort. Am J Sports Med 2010;38(10): 1979–86.

19. Widener DB, Wilson DJ, Galvin JW, et al. The prevalence of meniscal tears in young athletes undergoing revision anterior cruciate ligament reconstruction. Arthroscopy 2015;31(4):680–3.

20. Shepherd L, Abdollahi K, Lee J, et al. The prevalence of soft tissue injuries in nonoperative tibial plateau fractures as determined by magnetic resonance imaging. J Orthop Trauma 2002;16(9):628–31.

21. Abdel-Hamid MZ, Chang CH, Chan YS, et al. Arthroscopic evaluation of soft tissue injuries in tibial plateau fractures: retrospective analysis of 98 cases. Arthroscopy 2006;22(6):669–75.

22. Ricklin P, Ruttiman A, Del Buono M. Meniscus lesions: practical problems of clinical diagnosis. Grune & Stratton; 1971.

23. Jarraya M, Roemer FW, Englund M, et al. Meniscus morphology: Does tear type matter? A narrative review with focus on relevance for osteoarthritis research. Semin Arthritis Rheum 2017;46(5):552–61.

24. Henry S, Mascarenhas R, Kowalchuk D, et al. Medial meniscus tear morphology and chondral degeneration of the knee: Is there a relationship? Arthroscopy 2012;28(8):1124–34.

25. Bergkvist D, Dahlberg LE, Neuman P, et al. Knee arthroscopies: Who gets them, what does the radiologist report, and what does the surgeon find? Acta Orthop 2016;87(1):12–6.

26. Guermazi A, Hayashi D, Jarraya M, et al. Medial posterior meniscal root tears are associated with development or worsening of medial tibiofemoral cartilage damage: the multicenter osteoarthritis study. Radiology 2013;268(3):814–21.

27. Hwang BY, Kim SJ, Lee SW, et al. Risk factors for medial meniscus posterior root tear. Am J Sports Med 2012;40(7):1606–10.

28. DePhillipo NN, Cinque ME, Chahla J, et al. Incidence and detection of meniscal ramp lesions on magnetic resonance imaging in patients with anterior cruciate ligament reconstruction. Am J Sports Med 2017;45(10):2233–7.
29. Chahla J, Dean CS, Moatshe G, et al. Meniscal ramp lesions: anatomy, incidence, diagnosis, and treatment. Orthop J Sports Med 2016;4(7):1–7.
30. Bollen SR. Posteromedial meniscocapsular injury associated with rupture of the anterior cruciate ligament: a previously unrecognised association. J Bone Joint Surg Br 2010;92(2):222–3.
31. Liu X, Feng H, Zhang H, et al. Arthroscopic prevalence of ramp lesion in 868 patients with anterior cruciate ligament injury. Am J Sports Med 2011;39(4):832–7.
32. Sonnery-Cottet B, Conteduca J, Thaunat M, et al. Hidden lesions of the posterior horn of the medial meniscus: a systematic arthroscopic exploration of the concealed portion of the knee. Am J Sports Med 2014;42(4):921–6.
33. Chen G, Tang X, Li Q, et al. The evaluation of patient-specific factors associated with meniscal and chondral injuries accompanying ACL rupture in young adult patients. Knee Surg Sports Traumatol Arthrosc 2015;23(3):792–8.
34. Sommerfeldt M, Raheem A, Whittaker J, et al. Recurrent instability episodes and meniscal or cartilage damage after anterior cruciate ligament injury: a systematic review. Orthop J Sports Med 2018;6(7):1–9.
35. Kluczynski MA, Marzo JM, Bisson LJ. Factors associated with meniscal tears and chondral lesions in patients undergoing anterior cruciate ligament reconstruction: a prospective study. Am J Sports Med 2013;41(12):2759–65.
36. Achtnich A, Petersen W, Willinger L, et al. Medial meniscus extrusion increases with age and BMI and is depending on different loading conditions. Knee Surg Sports Traumatol Arthrosc 2018;26(8):2282–8.
37. Allaire R, Muriuki M, Gilbertson L, et al. Biomechanical consequences of a tear of the posterior root of the medial meniscus. Similar to total meniscectomy. J Bone Joint Surg Am 2008;90(9):1922–31.
38. Laberge MA, Baum T, Virayavanich W, et al. Obesity increases the prevalence and severity of focal knee abnormalities diagnosed using 3T MRI in middle-aged subjects–data from the osteoarthritis initiative. Skeletal Radiol 2012;41(6):633–41.
39. Yeh PC, Starkey C, Lombardo S, et al. Epidemiology of isolated meniscal injury and its effect on performance in athletes from the National Basketball Association. Am J Sports Med 2012;40(3):589–94.
40. Brambilla L, Pulici L, Carimati G, et al. Prevalence of associated lesions in anterior cruciate ligament reconstruction. Am J Sports Med 2015;43(12):2966–73.
41. Song GY, Liu X, Zhang H, et al. Increased medial meniscal slope is associated with greater risk of ramp lesion in noncontact anterior cruciate ligament injury. Am J Sports Med 2016;44(8):2039–46.
42. Clayton RAE, Court-Brown CM. The epidemiology of musculoskeletal tendinous and ligamentous injuries. Injury 2008;39(12):1338–44.
43. Granan L-P, Bahr R, Lie SA, et al. Timing of anterior cruciate ligament reconstructive surgery and risk of cartilage lesions and meniscal tears: a cohort study based on the Norwegian National Knee Ligament Registry. Am J Sports Med 2009;37(5):955–61.
44. Magnussen RA, Pedroza AD, Donaldson CT, et al. Time from ACL injury to reconstruction and the prevalence of additional intra-articular pathology: is patient age an important factor? Knee Surg Sports Traumatol Arthrosc 2013;21(9):2029–34.
45. Stanley LE, Kerr ZY, Dompier TP, et al. Sex differences in the incidence of anterior cruciate ligament, medial collateral ligament, and meniscal injuries in collegiate

and high school sports: 2009-2010 through 2013-2014. Am J Sports Med 2016; 44(6):1565–72.

46. Moksnes H, Engebretsen L, Risberg MA. Prevalence and incidence of new meniscus and cartilage injuries after a nonoperative treatment algorithm for ACL tears in skeletally immature children: a prospective MRI study. Am J Sports Med 2013;41(8):1771–9.

47. Bhatia S, Laprade CM, Ellman MB, et al. Meniscal root tears: Significance, diagnosis, and treatment. Am J Sports Med 2014;42(12):3016–30.

48. Dejour H, Bonnin M. Tibial translation after anterior cruciate ligament rupture. Two radiological tests compared. J Bone Joint Surg Br 1994;76(5):745–9.

49. Alici T, Esenyel CZ, Esenyel M, et al. Relationship between meniscal tears and tibial slope on the tibial plateau. Eurasian J Med 2011;43(3):146–51.

50. Lee J-J, Choi Y-J, Shin K-Y, et al. Medial meniscal tears in anterior cruciate ligament-deficient knees: effects of posterior tibial slope on medial meniscal tear. Knee Surg Relat Res 2011;23(4):227–30.

51. Barber FA, Getelman MH, Berry KL. Complex medial meniscus tears are associated with a biconcave medial tibial plateau. Arthroscopy 2017;33(4):783–9.

52. Crema MD, Roemer FW, Felson DT, et al. Factors associated with meniscal extrusion in knees with or at risk for osteoarthritis: the multicenter osteoarthritis study. Radiology 2012;264(2):494–503.

53. Felson DT, Niu J, Gross KD, et al. Valgus malalignment is a risk factor for lateral knee osteoarthritis incidence and progression: findings from the Multicenter Osteoarthritis Study and the osteoarthritis initiative. Arthritis Rheum 2013;65(2): 355–62.

54. Erquicia J, Gelber PE, Cardona-Muñoz JI, et al. There is no relation between mild malalignment and meniscal extrusion in trauma emergency patients. Injury 2012; 43(Suppl 2):S68–72.

55. Mehran N, Photopoulos CD, Narvy SJ, et al. Epidemiology of operative procedures in an NCAA division i football team over 10 seasons. Orthop J Sports Med 2016;4(7):1–6.

56. Krinsky MB, Abdenour TE, Starkey C, et al. Incidence of lateral meniscus injury in professional basketball players. Am J Sports Med 1992;20(1):17–9.

57. Beaulieu-Jones BR, Rossy WH, Sanchez G, et al. Epidemiology of injuries identified at the NFL scouting combine and their impact on performance in the national football league: evaluation of 2203 athletes from 2009 to 2015. Orthop J Sports Med 2017;5(7):1–11.

58. Chahla J, Cinque ME, Godin JA, et al. Meniscectomy and resultant articular cartilage lesions of the knee among prospective national football league players: an imaging and performance analysis. Am J Sports Med 2018;46(1):200–7.

59. Camp CL, Curriero FC, Pollack KM, et al. The epidemiology and effect of sliding injuries in major and minor league baseball players. Am J Sports Med 2017; 45(10):2372–8.

60. Sanders MS, Cates RA, Baker MD, et al. Knee injuries and the use of prophylactic knee bracing in off-road motorcycling: results of a large-scale epidemiological study. Am J Sports Med 2011;39(7):1395–400.

61. Paletta GA Jr, Levine DS, O'Brien SJ, et al. Patterns of meniscal injury associated with acute anterior cruciate ligament injury in skiers. Am J Sports Med 1992;20(5): 542–7.

62. Shellock FG, Deutsch AL, Mink JH, et al. Do asymptomatic marathon runners have an increased prevalence of meniscal abnormalities? An MR study of the knee in 23 volunteers. Am J Roentgenol 1991;157(6):1239–41.

63. Tennant LM, Chong HC, Acker SM. The effects of a simulated occupational kneeling exposure on squat mechanics and knee joint load during gait. Ergonomics 2018;61(6):839–52.

64. McMillan G, Nichols L. Osteoarthritis and meniscus disorders of the knee as occupational diseases of miners. Occup Environ Med 2005;62(8):567–75.

65. Adalberth T, Roos H. Magnetic resonance imaging, scintigraphy, and arthroscopic evaluation of traumatic hemarthrosis of the knee. Am J Sports Med 1997;25(2):231–7.

66. Bellabarba C, Bush-Joseph CA, Bach BR. Patterns of meniscal injury in the anterior cruciate-deficient knee: a review of the literature. Am J Orthop (Belle Mead NJ) 1997;26(1):18–23.

67. Warren RF, Levy IM. Meniscal lesions associated with anterior cruciate ligament injury. Clin Orthop Relat Res 1983;172:32–7.

68. Thompson WO, Fu FH. The meniscus in the cruciate-deficient knee. Clin Sports Med 1993;12(4):771–96.

69. Anderson AF, Anderson CN. Correlation of meniscal and articular cartilage injuries in children and adolescents with timing of anterior cruciate ligament reconstruction. Am J Sports Med 2015;43(2):275–81.

70. Spindler KP, Schils JP, Bergfeld JA, et al. Prospective study of osseous, articular, and meniscal lesions in recent anterior cruciate ligament tears by magnetic resonance imaging and arthroscopy. Am J Sports Med 1993;21(4):551–7.

71. Piasecki DP, Spindler KP, Warren TA, et al. Intraarticular injuries associated with anterior cruciate ligament tear: findings at ligament reconstruction in high school and recreational athletes. An analysis of sex-based differences. Am J Sports Med 2003;31(4):601–5.

72. Mok YR, Wong KL, Panjwani T, et al. Anterior cruciate ligament reconstruction performed within 12 months of the index injury is associated with a lower rate of medial meniscus tears. Knee Surg Sports Traumatol Arthrosc 2019;27(1):117–23.

73. Wyatt RWB, Inacio MCS, Liddle KD, et al. Prevalence and incidence of cartilage injuries and meniscus tears in patients who underwent both primary and revision anterior cruciate ligament reconstructions. Am J Sports Med 2014;42(8):1841–6.

74. Stahl D, Serrano-Riera R, Collin K, et al. Operatively treated meniscal tears associated with tibial plateau fractures: a report on 661 patients. J Orthop Trauma 2015;29(7):322–4.

75. Jordan MR. Lateral meniscal variants: evaluation and treatment. J Am Acad Orthop Surg 1996;4(4):191–200.

76. Kocher MS, Logan CA, Kramer DE. Discoid lateral meniscus in children: Diagnosis, management, and outcomes. J Am Acad Orthop Surg 2017;25(11):736–43.

77. Ellis HB, Wise K, LaMont L, et al. Prevalence of discoid meniscus during arthroscopy for isolated lateral meniscal pathology in the pediatric population. J Pediatr Orthop 2017;37(4):285–92.

78. Shieh A, Bastrom T, Roocroft J, et al. Meniscus tear patterns in relation to skeletal immaturity: children versus adolescents. Am J Sports Med 2013;41(12):2779–83.

79. Englund M, Lohmander LS. Risk factors for symptomatic knee osteoarthritis fifteen to twenty-two years after meniscectomy. Arthritis Rheum 2004;50(9):2811–9.

80. Englund M, Guermazi A, Lohmander SL. The role of the meniscus in knee osteoarthritis: a cause or consequence? Radiol Clin North Am 2009;47(4):703–12.

81. Englund M, Guermazi A, Roemer FW, et al. Meniscal tear in knees without surgery and the development of radiographic osteoarthritis among middle-aged and elderly persons: the multicenter osteoarthritis study. Arthritis Rheum 2009;60(3): 831–9.
82. Beamer BS, Masoudi A, Walley KC, et al. Analysis of a New all-inside versus inside-out technique for repairing radial meniscal tears. Arthroscopy 2015; 31(2):293–8.
83. Alentorn-Geli E, Choi J, Stuart J, et al. Inside-out or outside-in suturing should not be considered the standard repair method for radial tears of the midbody of the lateral meniscus: a systematic review and meta-analysis of biomechanical studies. J Knee Surg 2015;29(07):604–12.
84. Annandale T. Excision of the internal semilunar cartilage, resulting in perfect restoration of the joint-movements. Br Med J 1889;1(1467):291–2.
85. Parker BR, Hurwitz S, Spang J, et al. Surgical trends in the treatment of meniscal tears. Am J Sports Med 2016;44(7):1717–23.

As Goes the Meniscus Goes the Knee

Early, Intermediate, and Late Evidence for the Detrimental Effect of Meniscus Tears

Peter S. Chang, MD[a], Robert H. Brophy, MD[b],*

KEYWORDS

- Meniscus • Meniscal injury • Meniscal tears • Osteoarthritis • Knee biology

KEY POINTS

- Meniscal injury has a negative effect on the biology of the knee within a very short period of time.
- In patients with meniscus injuries, degenerative changes of the articular cartilage become apparent within a decade.
- Over the long run, meniscal injury and deficiency increases the likelihood of severe osteoarthritis necessitating total knee arthroplasty, and these patients undergo total knee arthroplasty at a younger age compared with patients with an intact meniscus.

INTRODUCTION

Historically, the meniscus was thought of as vestigial remnant, with relatively little importance for the knee joint.[1] In the mid-twentieth century, injuries to the meniscus were often treated with surgical resection of the entire meniscus.[2] Later, intermediate and long-term follow-up studies demonstrated a high rate of osteoarthritis in these patients, suggesting the meniscus did have an important role in the knee.[1,3] Subsequent studies have demonstrated that the meniscus plays an important, complex role in maintaining the homeostasis and health of the entire knee. Meniscal injury and deficiency can have a significant negative impact on knee mechanics and biology, often initiating a turn toward joint degeneration and ultimately knee osteoarthritis (OA).

The impact of meniscal injury on the biomechanics of the knee is well established.[4,5] The purpose of this review is to highlight the basic science, translational and clinical

[a] Department of Orthopaedic Surgery, Washington University School of Medicine, 1 Barnes Jewish Hospital Plaza, St Louis, MO 63110, USA; [b] Department of Orthopaedic Surgery, Washington University School of Medicine, 14532 South Outer Forty Drive, Chesterfield, MO 63017, USA
* Corresponding author.
E-mail address: brophyrh@wustl.edu

Clin Sports Med 39 (2020) 29–36
https://doi.org/10.1016/j.csm.2019.08.001
0278-5919/20/© 2019 Elsevier Inc. All rights reserved.

studies emphasizing the detrimental effects of meniscal injury and deficiency on the biology of the knee. One important distinction is that this review focuses on meniscus tears rather than intrasubstance degeneration, which may be a distinct pathologic state as a precursor to further changes[6] or an "incidental" finding with little or no clinical relevance.[7–9]

MENISCAL BIOLOGY

The biology of the injured meniscus has been shown to be affected by several variables. Meniscal tears have traditionally been classified as traumatic, associated with longitudinal, bucket handle and radial patterns; or degenerative, associated with transverse, flap, and complex patterns.[10,11] The cellularity of the injured meniscus is negatively affected by older age, more time from injury, and degenerative and radial tear types.[12] A recent study demonstrated differential gene expression between traumatic and degenerative meniscus tears with higher expression of chemokines and matrix metalloproteinases (MMPs) and lower expression of COL1A1 in traumatic tears.[13] Patient age seems to play an important role on the biological response of the meniscus to injury, whereas the relative significance of the other factors are unknown. Although degenerative tears have been associated with more diffuse and severe knee pathology,[14–19] a recent review concluded that there is a lack of data on how tear morphology relates to OA both cross-sectionally and longitudinally.[20]

EARLY CHANGES

A meniscus tear can affect the knee within a couple of years. A study by Biswal and colleagues[21] reviewed baseline and follow-up MRIs comparing patients with meniscus tears with those with intact menisci at a mean follow-up of 1.8 years. They found that patients with meniscal tears had a higher average rate of progression of cartilage loss than those with intact menisci (22% vs 14.9% progression of cartilage loss). They concluded that meniscal tears tended to accelerate the natural course of cartilage loss. It has been previously demonstrated that meniscal abnormalities alter articular forces and ultimately lead to enhanced chondromalacia.[22,23]

It is known that injury to the meniscus, as well as subsequent surgery, is associated with an increased risk for OA.[3] In a study by Rangger and colleagues,[24] at an average follow-up of 4.5 years, degenerative changes were reported in 38% of patients after arthroscopic partial medial meniscectomy and in 24% of patients after arthroscopic partial lateral meniscectomy. The relationship between meniscal injury and development of chondral injury and OA has also been studied in a young cohort of National Football League (NFL) athletes. In a study by Nepple and colleagues,[25] a large group of largely asymptomatic elite football players at the NFL combined with a mean age of 22.7 years underwent an MRI. It was found that a previous partial meniscectomy was associated with full-thickness cartilage lesions. It was also found that partial meniscectomies in the lateral compartment were associated with a higher rate of articular cartilage defects in the respective compartment (25%) compared with medial meniscectomies, suggesting that the lateral compartment may be more predisposed to chondral damage after partial meniscectomy. A separate analysis of the same NFL cohort demonstrated that meniscal surgery is also associated with an increased rate of knee OA in these athletes.[26] This follow-up study looked at early evidence for OA rather than full-thickness cartilage defects. The rate of early OA after medial and lateral partial meniscectomies was similar between the 2 compartments (26% and 24% respectively), suggesting that meniscectomy in the medial compartment may be more likely to lead to OA than full-thickness cartilage defects. A case-control study showed that a history of a partial meniscectomy in elite college athletes is associated with a shorter career in professional football.[27]

In a systematic review by Salata and colleagues,[28] there was a significant increase in the development of OA with preexisting chondral damage. In addition, studies have reported worse patient outcomes after meniscectomy in patients with preexisting chondral damage.[28,29] Another study examining patient-reported outcomes measurement information system (PROMIS) scores in the early postoperative period after partial meniscectomy found that patients with high-grade articular cartilage lesions did not have as much clinical improvement at 6 weeks post-op as measured by PROMIS physical function and pain interference as those with no or low-grade articular lesions.[29] A study by Hunter and colleagues[30] evaluated baseline and follow-up MRIs of patients with OA and determined that a substantial portion of the variance in joint space narrowing was associated with the position and degeneration of the meniscus. A study of the same cohort demonstrated that meniscal malposition and damage was associated with increased risk of cartilage loss; overall in this study each aspect of meniscal abnormality had a major effect on cartilage loss.[19]

The association of meniscal injury in the setting of anterior cruciate ligament (ACL) reconstruction has been well studied. In a Multicenter ACL Revision Study (MARS) cohort of 725 knees undergoing revision ACL reconstruction, it was found that knees that had undergone previous partial meniscectomy were significantly more likely to have chondrosis than knees with previous meniscal repair or no history of meniscal surgery.[31] The study concludes that at the time of ACL reconstruction it is preferable if possible to repair the meniscus when meniscal pathology is encountered. A 2016 study of the same cohort showed that previous medial and lateral meniscal pathology and treatment were found to be significantly associated with poorer patient reported outcomes at 2-year follow-up following revision ACL reconstruction.[32] A study by Westermann in 2017 of the multicenter orthopedic outcomes (MOON) cohort, which evaluated outcomes 2 years after ACL reconstruction associated with meniscus surgery, showed that medial meniscectomy was associated with worse patient-reported outcomes and the greatest degree of joint space narrowing after surgery.[32] Finally, in an MARS cohort of patients undergoing revision ACL reconstruction it was found that patients with intact meniscus had a 64% to 84% decrease odds of having chondrosis compared with those with meniscal injury.[33] A study by Michalitsis and colleagues[34] examining the articular cartilage 2 years after arthroscopic ACL reconstruction with MRI showed that patients who underwent medial meniscus surgery at the time of ACL reconstruction were found to have statically significant deterioration of cartilage lesions in the lateral and medial femoral condyles. A similar study by Li and colleagues[35] found that at follow-up times ranging from 2 to 4.2 years ACL-associated meniscus injury treated with either partial meniscectomy or repair was associated with significantly higher T2 scores on MRI, which suggests cartilage degeneration.

Recent studies have also examined the biological impact of meniscal injury on synovial fluid and articular cartilage. One study demonstrated elevated MMP activity and prostaglandin E2 (PGE2) in the synovial fluid of patients with meniscus tears.[36] These biomarkers are proinflammatory and may play a role in joint degeneration. MMP and PGE2 were found to be elevated nearly 25- and 290-fold in knees with meniscus tears compared with controls. Specifically, levels of MMP-2, MMP-3, sulfate glycosaminoglycan (sGAG), cartilage oligomeric matrix protein, interleukin 6 (IL-6), and PGE2 were higher in the synovial fluid than in the serum of the meniscus patients in this cohort. Complex meniscus tears were associated with higher levels of MMP-10 and lower levels of serum tumor necrosis factor alpha (TNF-α) and IL-8 compared with other tear patterns. A previous study from the same group demonstrated that total MMP activity in synovial fluid is positively correlated with increased cartilage strain at maximum knee flexion in patients with meniscus tears,[37] suggesting the MMP levels are a biological marker for the mechanical effects of the meniscus tear on the joint. These markers are likely poor prognostic indicators both in terms of the healing potential of the injured meniscus as well as the initiation of changes that lead to the development of OA. Another study demonstrated elevated synovial fluid cytokines IL-1, IL-8, and TNF-α consistent with a proinflammatory state that last for several months following meniscal injury.[38] Although these levels would likely contribute to the initiation and acceleration of degenerative change in the articular cartilage, this study did not find any association between the level of synovial fluid cytokines and the degree of chondral damage in the knee at the time of meniscectomy.

In contrast to the finding with regard to synovial fluid, there is some evidence for an association between gene expression in meniscus tears and the condition of the articular cartilage at the time of partial meniscectomy surgery.[39,40] In one study, the torn menisci from knees with early degenerative changes on radiograph demonstrated higher expression of resistin compared with knees without any degenerative change.[41] A couple of studies have demonstrated negative effects of resistin on the meniscus.[42,43] Resistin has been shown to stimulate rapid and extensive catabolism of meniscus tissue, similar to IL-1, but not of articular cartilage.[42] Another study demonstrated that resistin had the most significant negative effect out of several tested adipokines on the meniscus, inducing sGAG release and depleting sGAG content.[43]

A study by Rai and colleagues[20] demonstrated that macroscopically normal articular cartilage of patients undergoing partial meniscectomy demonstrated distinct patterns of gene expression exhibiting molecular signatures that reflect OA. Patients could be segregated by genetic risk alleles or by OA-associated gene transcripts, both of which identified subsets of patients with biological evidence for OA in the absence of macroscopic cartilage changes. The presence of a meniscus tear has been shown to alter the gene expression in ACL tear remnants.[44] The combined injury pattern modulates genes and pathways that reflect a diminished healing capacity and elevated neurogenic signal compared with isolated ACL tears, demonstrating yet another biological effect of the injured meniscus on the rest of the knee.

LATE CHANGES

The natural history of meniscal injury eventually leads to late changes of OA. A study by Roos and colleagues[19] established that open meniscectomy results in a high prevalence of OA at 21-year follow-up with a 14-fold increased risk for developing OA compared with age- and sex-matched controls. It has been shown that there is an inverse relationship between function of the knee and the amount of meniscal tissue resected.[1] In a long-term follow-up study, 80% of knees demonstrated degenerative changes in patients who had undergone a partial lateral meniscectomy at a follow-up of 12.3 years.[45] A study by Lohmander and colleagues[46] showed that after meniscectomy about 50% of patients developed OA within 10 to 20 years. A study by Englund and Lohmander examined a cohort of 317 patients who had undergone a meniscal resection 15 to 22 years previously and determined that risk factors for progression of OA after meniscal injury was similar to risk factors for OA overall, including obesity, female gender, and preexisting early stage OA.[18] They also found that after meniscectomy there was an increased risk of OA in patients with a body mass index of greater than 30 kg/m². A 2017 meta-analysis demonstrated a 3.54-fold increase risk factor for developing OA after ACL reconstruction in patients who underwent partial meniscectomy compared with patients who did not.[47] A systematic review by Paxton and colleagues[48] showed that at long-term clinical follow-up meniscal injury treated with meniscal repair was associated with higher Lysholm scores and less radiographic deterioration than partial meniscectomies. However, at both short- and long-term follow-up, partial meniscectomies had a lower reoperation rate than meniscal repair.

Recent studies have shown an association between meniscal surgery and total knee arthroplasty (TKA). A 2014 study examining prevalence of TKA after previous knee surgery showed that after meniscectomy, men and women underwent TKA, 9.6 and 8.2 years younger, respectively, than patients without any history of knee surgery.[49] After meniscectomy, patients underwent a TKA at an average interval of 12.6 years after meniscectomy. In addition, as many as 14% of patients underwent TKA within 1 year after meniscectomy. A matched case-control study of all TKAs in the United Kingdom from 1990 to 2011 by Khan and colleagues[50] showed that patients with previous meniscal injury underwent TKA at 65.08 years compared with controls who underwent arthroplasty at 70.83 years. The adjusted odds ratio of TKA after a meniscal injury compared with patients without meniscal injury was 15.24.

SUMMARY

Meniscal tears are known to be associated with a higher risk for knee OA. There is a growing body of evidence regarding the early biological changes associated with meniscal injury strongly implicating it as a cause of joint degeneration. Similarly, there are more studies demonstrating the intermediate and long-term clinical sequelae of meniscal injury in terms of chondral damage and ultimately OA.

REFERENCES

1. Hede A, Larsen E, Sandberg H. The long term outcome of open total and partial meniscectomy related to the quantity and site of the meniscus removed. Int Orthop 1992;16(2):122–5.
2. McMurray TP. The semilunar cartilages. Br J Surg 1942;29:407–14.
3. McDermott ID, Amis AA. The consequences of meniscectomy. J Bone Joint Surg Br 2006;88(12):1549–56.
4. Allaire R, Muriuki M, Gilbertson L, et al. Biomechanical consequences of a tear of the posterior root of the medial meniscus. Similar to total meniscectomy. J Bone Joint Surg Am 2008;90(9):1922–31.
5. Ding C, Martel-Pelletier J, Pelletier JP, et al. Knee meniscal extrusion in a largely non-osteoarthritic cohort: association with greater loss of cartilage volume. Arthritis Res Ther 2007;9(2):R21.
6. Rai MF, Patra D, Sandell LJ, et al. Relationship of gene expression in the injured human meniscus to body mass index: a biologic connection between obesity and osteoarthritis. Arthritis Rheumatol 2014;66(8):2152–64.
7. Englund M, Roemer FW, Hayashi D, et al. Meniscus pathology, osteoarthritis and the treatment controversy. Nat Rev Rheumatol 2012;8(7):412–9.
8. Crema MD, Guermazi A, Li L, et al. The association of prevalent medial meniscal pathology with cartilage loss in the medial tibiofemoral compartment over a 2-year period. Osteoarthritis Cartilage 2010;18(3):336–43.
9. Crema MD, Hunter DJ, Burstein D, et al. Delayed gadolinium-enhanced magnetic resonance imaging of medial tibiofemoral cartilage and its relationship with meniscal pathology: a longitudinal study using 3.0T magnetic resonance imaging. Arthritis Rheumatol 2014;66(6):1517–24.

10. Lecouvet F, Van Haver T. Acid S, et al. Magnetic resonance imaging (MRI) of the knee: identification of difficult-to-diagnose meniscal lesions. Diagn Interv Imaging 2018;99(2):55–64.

11. Makris EA, Hadidi P, Athanasiou KA. The knee meniscus: structure-function, pathophysiology, current repair techniques, and prospects for regeneration. Biomaterials 2011;32(30):7411–31.

12. Mesiha M, Zurakowski D, Soriano J, et al. Pathologic characteristics of the torn human meniscus. Am J Sports Med 2007;35(1):103–12.

13. Brophy RH, Sandell LJ, Rai MF. Traumatic and degenerative meniscus tears have different gene expression signatures. Am J Sports Med 2017;45(1):114–20.

14. Lange AK, Fiatarone Singh MA, Smith RM, et al. Degenerative meniscus tears and mobility impairment in women with knee osteoarthritis. Osteoarthritis Cartilage 2007;15(6):701–8.

15. Christoforakis J, Pradhan R, Sanchez-Ballester J, et al. Is there an association between articular cartilage changes and degenerative meniscus tears? Arthroscopy 2005;21(11):1366–9.

16. Terzidis IP, Christodoulou A, Ploumis A, et al. Meniscal tear characteristics in young athletes with a stable knee: arthroscopic evaluation. Am J Sports Med 2006;34(7):1170–5.

17. Englund M, Roos EM, Roos HP, et al. Patient-relevant outcomes fourteen years after meniscectomy: influence of type of meniscal tear and size of resection. Rheumatology (Oxford) 2001;40(6):631–9.

18. Englund M, Lohmander LS. Risk factors for symptomatic knee osteoarthritis fifteen to twenty-two years after meniscectomy. Arthritis Rheum 2004;50(9):2811–9.

19. Roos H, Lauren M, Adalberth T, et al. Knee osteoarthritis after meniscectomy: prevalence of radiographic changes after twenty-one years, compared with matched controls. Arthritis Rheum 1998;41(4):687–93.

20. Rai MF, Sandell LJ, Zhang B, et al. RNA microarray analysis of macroscopically normal articular cartilage from knees undergoing partial medial meniscectomy: potential prediction of the risk for developing osteoarthritis. PLoS One 2016;11(5):e0155373.

21. Biswal S, Hastie T, Andriacchi TP, et al. Risk factors for progressive cartilage loss in the knee: a longitudinal magnetic resonance imaging study in forty- three patients. Arthritis Rheum 2002;46(11):2884–92.

22. Dandy DJ, Jackson RW. Meniscectomy and chondromalacia of the femoral condyle. J Bone Joint Surg Am 1975;57:1116–9.

23. Frankel VH, Burstein AH, Brooks DB. Biomechanics of internal derangement of the knee: pathomechanics as determined by analysis of the instant centers of motion. J Bone Joint Surg Am 1971;53:945–62.

24. Rangger C, Klestil T, Gloetzer W, et al. Osteoarthritis after arthroscopic partial meniscectomy. Am J Sports Med 1995;23(2):240–4.

25. Nepple JJ, Wright RW, Matava MJ, et al. Full-thickness knee articular cartilage defects in national football league combine athletes undergoing magnetic resonance imaging: prevalence, location, and association with previous surgery. Arthroscopy 2012;28(6):798–806.

26. Smith MV, Nepple JJ, Wright RW, et al. Knee osteoarthritis is associated with previous meniscus and anterior cruciate ligament surgery among elite college american football athletes. Sports Health 2017;9(3):247–51.

27. Brophy RH, Gill CS, Lyman S, et al. Effect of anterior cruciate ligament reconstruction and meniscectomy on length of career in National Football League athletes: a case control study. Am J Sports Med 2009;37:2102–7.
28. Salata MJ, Gibbs AE, Sekiya JK. A systematic review of clinical outcomes in patients undergoing meniscectomy. Am J Sports Med 2010;38(9):1907–16.
29. Bernholt D, Wright RW, Matava MJ, et al. Patient reported outcomes measurement information system scores are responsive to early changes in patient outcomes following arthroscopic partial meniscectomy. Arthroscopy 2018;34(4): 1113–7.
30. Hunter DJ, Zhang YQ, Tu X, et al. Change in joint space width: hyaline articular cartilage loss or alteration in meniscus? Arthritis Rheum 2006;54(8):2488–95.
31. Brophy RH, Wright RW, David TS, et al. Association between previous meniscal surgery and the incidence of chondral lesions at revision anterior cruciate ligament reconstruction. Am J Sports Med 2012;40(4):808–14.
32. Westermann RW, Jones M, Wasserstein D, et al. Clinical and radiographic outcomes of meniscus surgery and future targets for biologic intervention: a review of data from the MOON Group. Connect Tissue Res 2017;58(3–4):366–72.
33. Brophy RH, Haas AK, Huston LJ, et al. Association of meniscal status, lower extremity alignment, and body mass index with chondrosis at revision anterior cruciate ligament reconstruction. Am J Sports Med 2015;43(7):1616–22.
34. Michalitsis S, Hantes M, Thriskos P, et al. Articular cartilage status 2 years after arthroscopic ACL reconstruction in patients with or without concomitant meniscal surgery: evaluation with 3.0T MR imaging. Knee Surg Sports Traumatol Arthrosc 2017;25(2):437–44.
35. Li H, Chen S, Tao H, et al. Quantitative MRI T2 relaxation time evaluation of knee cartilage: comparison of meniscus-intact and -injured knees after anterior cruciate ligament reconstruction. Am J Sports Med 2015;43(4):865–72.
36. Liu B, Goode AP, Carter TE, et al. Matrix metalloproteinase activity and prostaglandin E2 are elevated in the synovial fluid of meniscus tear patients. Connect Tissue Res 2017;58:305–16.
37. Carter TE, Taylor KA, Spritzer CE, et al. In vivo cartilage strain increases following medial meniscal tear and correlates with synovial fluid matrix metalloproteinase activity. J Biomech 2015;48(8):1461–8.
38. Bigoni M, Turati M, Sacerdote P, et al. Characterization of synovial fluid cytokine profiles in chronic meniscal tear of the knee. J Orthop Res 2017;35:340–6.
39. Rai MF, Patra D, Sandell LJ, et al. Transcriptome analysis of injured human meniscus reveals a distinct phenotype of meniscus degeneration with aging. Arthritis Rheum 2013;65(8):2090–101.
40. Brophy RH, Zhang B, Cai L, et al. Transcriptome comparison of meniscus from patients with and without osteoarthritis. Osteoarthritis Cartilage 2018;26(3): 422–32.
41. Lee JH, Ort T, Ma K, et al. Resistin is elevated following traumatic joint injury and causes matrix degradation and release of inflammatory cytokines from articular cartilage in vitro. Osteoarthritis Cartilage 2009;17:613–20.
42. Nishimuta JF, Levenston ME. Adipokines induce catabolism of newly synthesized matrix in cartilage and meniscus tissues. Connect Tissue Res 2017;58(3–4): 246–58.
43. Nishimuta JF, Levenston ME. Meniscus is more susceptible than cartilage to catabolic and anti-anabolic effects of adipokines. Osteoarthritis Cartilage 2015;23(9): 1551–62.

44. Brophy RH, Rothermich MA, Tycksen ED, et al. Presence of meniscus tear alters gene expression profile of anterior cruciate ligament tears. J Orthop Res 2018; 36(10):2612–21.
45. Scheller G, Sobau C, Bulow JU. Arthroscopic partial lateral meniscectomy in an otherwise normal knee: clinical, functional, and radiographic results of a long-term follow-up study. Arthroscopy 2001;17(9):946–52.
46. Lohmander LS, Englund PM, Dahl LL, et al. The long-term consequence of anterior cruciate ligament and meniscus in- juries: osteoarthritis. Am J Sports Med 2007;35:1756–69.
47. Ruano JS, Sitler MR, Driban JB. Prevalence of radiographic knee osteoarthritis after anterior cruciate ligament reconstruction, with or without meniscectomy: an evidence-based practice article. J Athl Train 2017;52(6):606–9.
48. Paxton ES, Stock MV, Brophy RH. Meniscal repair versus partial meniscectomy: a systematic review comparing reoperation rates and clinical outcomes. Arthroscopy 2011;27(9):1275–88.
49. Brophy RH, Gray BL, Nunley RM, et al. Total knee arthroplasty after previous knee surgery: expected interval and the effect on patient age. J Bone Joint Surg Am 2014;96(10):801–5.
50. Khan T, Alvand A, Prieto-Alhambra D, et al. ACL and meniscal injuries increase the risk of primary total knee replacement for osteoarthritis: a matched case-control study using the clinical practice research datalink (CPRD). Br J Sports Med 2019;53(15):965–8.

Meniscal Repair Techniques

Tim Spalding, MB BS, FRCS Orth*, Iswadi Damasena, MB BS, FRACS, FAOrthA,
Robert Lawton, MA, MSc, BM BCh, FRCSEd (T&O)

KEYWORDS

- Knee • Meniscus • Meniscal repair • Meniscus transplantation • Bucket-handle tear
- Meniscal root-tear

KEY POINTS

- The menisci have a primary role of improving congruency between the convex surface of the distal femur and the surfaces of the proximal tibia.
- The menisci play a vital role in knee joint stability, load distribution, and lubrication, protecting the joint surfaces from degenerative change.
- Meniscal repair protects the joint from increased loading and when successful reduces progression of osteoarthritis.
- Successful repair involves accurate surgical techniques and guarded postoperative rehabilitation An integrated approach to meniscal surgery is required as part of an overall strategy to preserve and restore knee function, preserving meniscal tissue whenever possible.

 Video content accompanies this article at http://www.sportsmed.theclinics. com.

INTRODUCTION

Meniscal tears are common, with a yearly incidence of 60 to 70 per 100,000 population.[1] Loss of meniscal tissue predisposes the knee joint to degenerative change and symptoms of activity related knee pain that can develop over a variable length of time. Repair is an important option for meniscal tears with the intention of improving symptoms and reducing the risk of subsequent arthritis. Sutures or devices to repair the meniscus can be delivered via inside-out, outside-in, or all-inside techniques. The tear location and orientation determine the optimal technique for suture placement. This article reviews current techniques for meniscal repair specifically focusing on all-inside, inside-out, and outside-in techniques. Repair of ramp lesions and root tears are not addressed in this review.

Department of Trauma and Orthopaedic Surgery, University Hospital Coventry, Clifford Bridge Road, Coventry, CV2 2DX, UK
* Corresponding author.
E-mail address: tim.spalding@uhcw.nhs.uk

Clin Sports Med 39 (2020) 37–56
https://doi.org/10.1016/j.csm.2019.08.012
0278-5919/20/© 2019 Elsevier Inc. All rights reserved.
sportsmed.theclinics.com

CONSEQUENCES OF MENISCAL DEFICIENCY

Long-term follow-up of meniscal deficient patients after partial or total meniscectomy has demonstrated increased risk of osteoarthritis (OA). In a systematic review of risk factors for OA, Papalia and colleagues[2] reported a 7 times increase in the radiologic diagnosis of OA at 5 to 30 years of follow-up after surgical management of meniscal tears. The incidence was 40% in the operated knee and 6% in the contralateral/control knee, with a higher incidence following lateral compared with medial meniscal surgery and with total compared with partial meniscectomy. In a single cohort follow-up study of adolescents who underwent total meniscectomy at a mean age of 16 years, Pengas and colleagues[3] reported a 132-fold increase in the incidence of knee arthroplasty at mean 40 years follow-up compared with geographic- and age-matched controls.[3]

Menisci have a primary role of improving congruency between the convex surface of the distal femur and the surfaces of the proximal tibia. They enhance stability and help to distribute load evenly across the knee, reducing load on the articular cartilage, effectively being load distributors while also contributing to proprioception, cartilage nutrition, and lubrication.

RELEVANT ANATOMY WHEN CONSIDERING MENISCAL REPAIR

The medial meniscus has a slightly asymmetrical C-shaped structure with larger posterior than anterior horn (**Fig. 1**). It covers 50% ± 6% of the medial plateau and is firmly attached to the periphery via the deep medial collateral ligament, which has both meniscofemoral and meniscotibial attachments.[4] This makes it relatively immobile with only about 5 mm anterior–posterior translation during knee flexion–extension.[5]

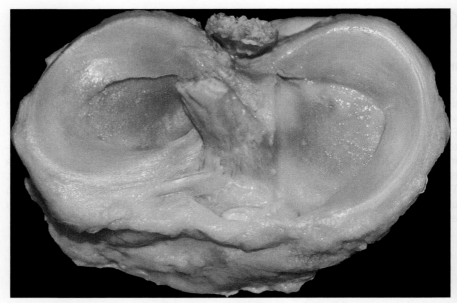

Fig. 1. Superior view of a cadaveric right tibial plateau showing meniscal anatomy and attachments. Posterior aspect at top of picture. ACL, anterior cruciate ligament; PCL, posterior cruciate ligament. (*Courtesy of* Charles H. Brown Jr., MD, International Knee & Joint Centre, Abu Dhabi, United Arab Emirates.)

The lateral meniscus is more symmetric and a tighter C shape. It is similar in volume to the medial meniscus but covers a relatively larger proportion of the lateral tibial plateau—59% ± 7%.[4] Being less firmly attached to the periphery, it is more mobile with approximately 11 mm posterior translation during knee flexion.[5] The medial meniscus bears about 50% of load, whereas the lateral meniscus bears up to 70% through its respective compartment.[6]

The predominantly circumferential arrangement of the collagen fibers is vital to meniscal function, resisting extrusion on compression. Weight bearing after repair therefore compresses the healing area while flexion under load applies a shear force to the repairing area. At full extension, the femur has a large contact area with the tibial plateaus pressing anteriorly on the meniscal horns. As the knee flexes, tibial internal rotation occurs and contact moves posteriorly toward the posterior meniscal horns owing to femoral roll-back. Contact area with the tibial plateau is decreased as the lesser radii of curvature of the femoral condyles sequentially come into contact. The center of contact on the medial side remains relatively constant, whereas the lateral condyle rolls posteriorly toward the posterior horn of the mobile lateral meniscus and thus tibial rotation occurs mainly about a medial axis, with the center of rotation medial to the knee joint in the axial plane (**Fig. 2**).[7] The result is that meniscal load increases in flexion to as much as 85% and without a meniscus the tibiofemoral contact area is decreased by 50% to 75% and the peak contact pressure is increased by 200% to 300%.[8,9]

Meniscal vascularity is crucial to the chances of a repair being successful. The lateral meniscus is vascularized in only the outer 10% to 25% of its width and the medial meniscus in the outer 10% to 30% in adults, although this percentage is higher in less than 12 years of age.[10]

ASSESSMENT OF MENISCAL TEARS WHEN CONSIDERING REPAIR

The European Society of Sports Traumatology, Knee Surgery and Arthroscopy (ESSKA) and the International Society of Arthroscopy, Knee Surgery and Orthopaedic Sports Medicine (ISAKOS) Classification (2006) is based on tear depth (full/partial thickness), residual rim width (<3 mm, 3-5 mm, >5 mm), and location (posterior, mid-body, anterior). Residual rim width is a proxy for meniscal function, because lesions with less than 3 mm of rim remaining compromise the circumferential fibers

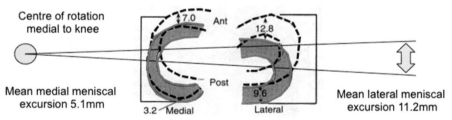

Centre of rotation medial to knee

Mean medial meniscal excursion 5.1mm

Mean lateral meniscal excursion 11.2mm

Fig. 2. Diagram of meniscal excursion. Mean meniscal excursion from anterior (Ant) to posterior (Post) is shown as the knee moves from extension (meniscal position in extension shown by *black dotted line*) to 120° flexion (meniscal position in 120° flexion shown by *red line* and shaded meniscus). The mean lateral meniscal excursion is greater than the mean medial meniscal excursion (11.2 mm vs 5.1 mm), such that in the axial plane the center of rotation of the knee lies medial to the knee joint. (*From* Thompson, WO, Thaete, FL, Fu FH, Dye SF. Tibial meniscal dynamics using three-dimensional reconstruction of magnetic resonance images. Am. J. Sports Med. 1991;19:210–216; with permission.)

and the ability of the meniscus to resist hoop stress, effectively defunctioning the meniscus. Tear classifications are summarized in **Figs. 3** and **4**.

MENISCAL VASCULARITY

Understanding meniscal vascularity has led to the mainstay of assessment. Red–red tears, as popularized after the anatomic description by Arnoczky and Warren,[10] are in the peripheral vascularized area (0-3 mm from the rim) and have the best chance of healing. White–white tears in the inner avascular zone (5-7 mm from the rim) have the lowest healing potential and tears in the intermediate zone (3-5 mm from the rim) are termed red–white, and have intermediate potential for healing, being more favorable in the younger patient.

Tear Orientation and Fiber Disruption

Vertical tears can be longitudinal, producing a bucket handle type tear or a flap, or radial in direction disrupting the circumferential fibers (see **Fig. 4**). Vertical oblique tears disrupt a mixture of both radial and circumferential fibers.

Horizontal tears (see **Fig. 4H**) occur in the plane of the meniscus parallel to the articular surface and in general do not disrupt the radial or circumferential fibers. Such tears are associated with meniscal degeneration and with parameniscal cyst development. Contact surface area and contact pressures are not altered and pain probably arises from peripheral capsule irritation. Removal of the inferior leaf reduces contact area by 59% and produces peak pressures similar to dual leaflet resection.[11]

Complex tears (see **Fig. 4I**) include a mixture of horizontal and vertical components and are most commonly degenerate in etiology, resulting from repetitive physiologic forces leading to gradual attrition of the menisci. Such tears are often accompanied by OA.

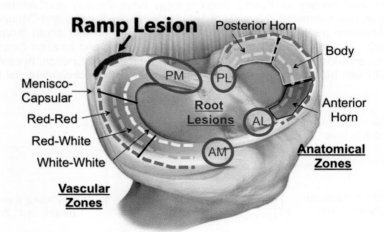

Fig. 3. Anatomic classifications of meniscal tear location. Vascular zones: meniscocapsular (peripheral), red–red (0–3 mm from the periphery), red–white (3–5 mm from the periphery), white–white (5–7 mm from the periphery). Anatomic zones: posterior horn, body and anterior horn. Meniscal root tear locations: AL, anterolateral; AM, anteromedial; PL, posterolateral; PM, posteromedial. (*From* Chahla J, Dean CS, Moatshe G, Mitchell JJ, Cram TR, Yacuzzi C, LaPrade RF. Meniscal Ramp Lesions: Anatomy, Incidence, Diagnosis, and Treatment. Orthop J Sports Med. 2016 Jul 26;4(7); with permission.)

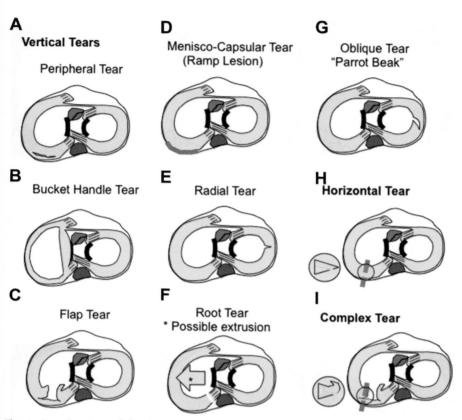

Fig. 4. Superior view of the descriptive classification of meniscal tears based on tear orientation and meniscal fiber disruption. Anterior cruciate ligament (ACL) insertion shown in *red*. Posterior cruciate ligament (PCL) insertion shown in blue. MM, medial meniscus (*left*); LM, lateral meniscus (*right*). Tear types: (*A*) vertical longitudinal peripheral tear (posterior horn of MM); (*B*) vertical longitudinal displaced "bucket handle" tear (of MM); (*C*) vertical longitudinal flap tear (posterior horn of MM); (*D*) vertical longitudinal meniscocapsular tear (of MM); (*E*) vertical radial tear (body of LM); (*F*) meniscal root tear (posterior root of MM); (*G*) vertical oblique "parrot beak" tear (body of LM); (*H*) horizontal tear (posterior horn MM), with the horizontal component shown on the inset sagittal image; (*I*) complex tear (posterior horn of MM) with the vertical flap component shown on the superior view and the horizontal component shown on the inset sagittal view.

TEAR REPAIRABILITY

Repairability of a tear depends on several factors and these are all taken into account when considering technique and repair.

Vertical Longitudinal Tears

Acute, peripheral, vertical longitudinal tears demonstrate good capacity for healing (72% to 94% reported).[12] Repaired tears in the red–red or red–white zones lead to good and excellent clinical midterm results. As a rough guide, such repairable tears include those less then 4 mm from the meniscal rim. Tears less than 10 mm long can be left unrepaired because they have good healing potential.[13] **Fig. 5**

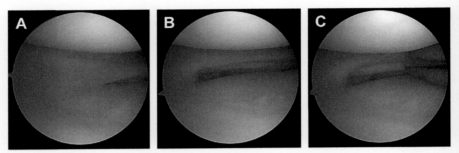

Fig. 5. Stable lateral meniscal undersurface tear not needing repair or resection. (*A*) Intact superior surface. (*B*) Initial view of undersurface tear. (*C*) Probing and confirmation tear length and stability such that no treatment was required.

demonstrates a stable undersurface tear of the lateral meniscus not needing resection or repair while **Fig. 6** shows an unstable lateral meniscal tear requiring repair and closure if the anterior aspect of the popliteofibular hiatus.

Radial Tears

Radial tears extending to the peripheral zone cause complete loss of meniscal function. Because the periphery is vascular these tears can be repaired, but specific suture

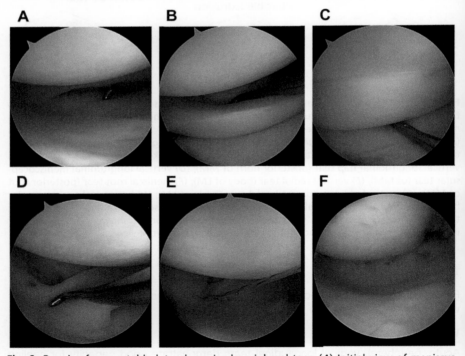

Fig. 6. Repair of an unstable lateral meniscal peripheral tear. (*A*) Initial view of meniscus, appearing normal. (*B*) Identification of the tear. (*C*) Traction on the undersurface shows that it can be displaced under the femoral condyle, explaining the locking sensation. (*D*) Probing the anterior end of tear showing a widened popliteal hiatus. (*E*) Stabilization and closing of the anterior end. (*E*) Final result after repair of tear with all-inside devices.

or anchor techniques are required to tolerate the high forces in the rim. The authors prefer the method using tie-grip sutures as a vertical configuration before placing horizontal sutures to draw the edges together, and in this way the sutures do not pull out through the circumferential fibers of the meniscus (**Figs. 7** and **8**).

Horizontal Tears

These tears were once thought to have minimal healing capacity, because they are associated with degenerative changes and OA. In young patients, however, healing similar to other tear patterns has been observed, with a healing rate of 78% reported in a systematic review of 9 studies.[14] Preliminary results are encouraging, demonstrating better results in terms of functional scores and secondary meniscectomy.[15] Although complex, this treatment has to be compared with resection, which will inevitably expose the joint to increased risk of early OA. **Fig. 9** demonstrates use of vertical suture loops in closing a horizontal tear in a young patient.

Age of the Tear

It is difficult to define or quantify repairability in terms of age of the tear but there is clinical dogma that fresh tears have a higher chance of healing after repair. A figure of 4 weeks is often quoted, but a tear in the peripheral red zone where the fragment has not been damaged should still be considered for repair even after several months. This notion is supported by Van der Wal and colleagues[16] who studied 238 meniscal repairs and found that the interval between trauma and meniscal repair had no influence on the failure rate.

Age of the Patient

It has been suggested that the older the patient the less the intrinsic healing capability of the meniscus owing to decreased cellularity and reduced healing response.[17] Eggli and colleagues[18] in their series of 56 arthroscopic meniscal repairs found patients aged less than 30 had better healing potential at an average 7.5 years follow-up. More recently, however, investigators have not found age to be a significant factor in the failure of the meniscus to heal.[19] Contemporary attitudes toward meniscal repair seem to place more importance on the macroscopic appearance, location, size, and orientation of the tear, and less so on the chronicity of the tear or the age of the patient.

ALL-INSIDE MENISCAL REPAIR TECHNIQUE

All-inside meniscal repair involves insertion of a suture through the meniscus and fixation inside the knee without involving perforation through the skin. Techniques

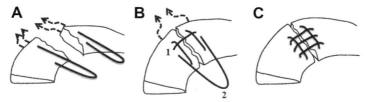

Fig. 7. Tie grip configuration for repair of lateral meniscal radial tear, showing vertical loop sutures inserted first (*A*) before horizontal sutures on superior and inferior surface of the meniscus (*B* and *C*). (*From* Tsujii A, et al., Second look arthroscopic evaluation of repaired radial/oblique tears of the midbody of the lateral meniscus in stable knees, Journal of Orthopaedic Science (2017), https://doi.org/10.1016/j.jos.2017.09.023; with permission.)

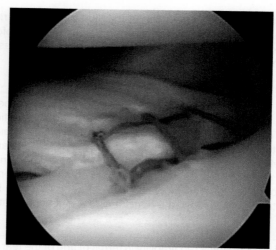

Fig. 8. Radial tear repair using tie grip method suture configuration. Two or 3 further horizontal loop in to out sutures are inserted on the underside.

involving manual tying of knots inside the joint have evolved into use of fixation devices that implant anchor devices in the peripheral tissue with a self-tying slipknot in-between. There are now several commercial variations available and the range has been grouped in **Table 1**.

The principles for most of the techniques are the same. **Fig. 10** illustrates the principles of the technique and the detail is shown in Video 1, using the medial meniscus as an example for repair.

1. The meniscal tear is identified and prepared using a mechanical rasp or pic to stimulate vascular response for enhancing healing.
2. Planning is made for targeting access for the suture fixation, choosing appropriate portal.
3. A slotted cannula device is inserted through the appropriate portal enabling access for the fixation device, and manipulation of the Meniscus (**Fig. 11**).
4. The first fixation device is then inserted along the cannula guide and deployed across the meniscus tear followed by the second fixation device.
5. The intended pattern should be a vertical or oblique fixation.
6. A knot pusher and cutter device in inserted to tighten the preplaced knot, avoiding over-tension.
7. Additional sutures are then inserted to create a vertical stacked mattress type of pattern.

INSIDE-OUT MENISCAL REPAIR TECHNIQUE

This technique involves passing sutures from inside the knee through to the outside, using long needles either with preattached sutures or separate needles with an eye on the end when using free sutures. Sutures are passed with the aid of a curved delivery system and examples of the several commercially available devices available are shown in **Table 2**. In outline the stages of performing inside-out repair are as follows.

1. The meniscal tear is identified and prepared with a rasp or microfracture pic.
2. Appropriate planning for the direction of the sutures is made, considering the use of an opposite side portal.

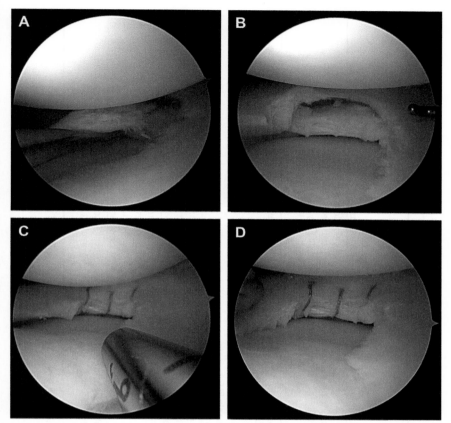

Fig. 9. Vertical suture repair of horizontal tear in lateral meniscus in an 18 year old man. (*A*) Identification of tear showing a posterior based flap and horizontal split in periphery of meniscus, which if resected would defunction the lateral meniscus. (*B*) After resection of the flap component the full nature of the tear is apparent. (*C*) Three vertical loops of in to out sutures are inserted to close the gap. (*D*) Final appearance after tying sutures over the capsule demonstrating maintaining meniscal height.

3. The curved cannula is inserted.
4. The long needle is passed through the cannula.
5. Once 2 to 3 mm of needle is exposed, it is positioned and passed across the meniscal tear, and retrieved through the skin or through a preplaced incision
6. A second needle on the other end of the suture is then passed creating a vertical or oblique loop on the meniscus.
7. The ends of the suture outside of the knee are tied over the capsule. Care is taken to dissect down to the medial collateral ligament medially or the iliotibial band laterally, retracting soft tissue to avoid injury to the saphenous nerve branches medially and the cutaneous nerves laterally.

In this technique a decision is made as to how best to pass the sutures, and there are 3 options.

a. The surgeon holds the arthroscope and the curved guide, while the assistant passes the needle through the guide 1 to 2 cm at a time, to avoid any buckling

Table 1
All-inside meniscal repair techniques

Device	Curve	Material/Absorption	Strength (Load to Failure)	Comments	
Meniscal cinch (Arthrex)	Linear 0°	2.0 fiber-wire nonabsorbable PEEK anchors	98 N	2 preloaded anchors deployed with needle delivery system. Pretied sliding knot for tensioning.	www.arthrex.com
Truespan (Depuy-Mitek)	0°, 12°, 14° curved needles	Orthocord suture (partially absorbable) nonabsorbable PEEK anchors, or partially absorbable PLGA implants	105.8 N	Needle delivery system.	www.depuysynthes.com
Fast-fix 360 (Smith and nephew)	Curved or reverse curved	PLLA or polyacetal implant and ultra braid 2.0 nonabsorbable suture	75.9 N	Needle spring-loaded implant delivery system.	www.smith-nephew.com
Novostitch plus (Ceterix Plus)	Straight lower jaw, curved upper jaw	0 or 2.0 braided USP suture	Not tested	Circumferential compression, all suture implant. Avoids excessive capsular entrapment.	www.smith-nephew.com
Rapidloc (Depuy Mitek)	0°, 12°, 27° curved needles	PDS implant 2.0 absorbable or nonabsorbable	Not tested	Small absorbable backstop implant connected to tophat.	www.depuysynthes.com

Abbreviations: PDS, polydioxanone; PLGA, poly-lactic-co-glycolic acid; PLLA, poly-L-lactide acid.

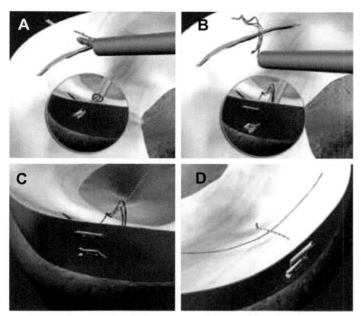

Fig. 10. All-inside device configuration. (A) Needle passed across meniscus tear and first implant deployed. (B) Needle withdrawn and passed second time across the tear inserting anchor in vertical configuration. (C) Slip knot tightened using know pusher device. (D) Final view showing anchors and suture configuration. (*From* Smith and Nephew FastFix 360 technique overview; is http://www.smith-nephew.com/uk/products/sports-medicine/knee-repair/fast-fix-360-meniscal-repair/; with permission.)

of the long needle. The same or additional assistant can retrieve the suture from outside the knee.
b. An assistant holds the arthroscope while the surgeon manipulates the curved guide and passes the suture. The surgeon or another assistant can assist by retrieving the suture.

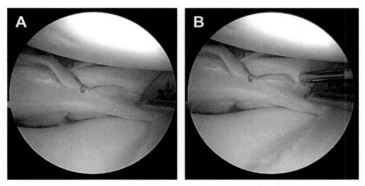

Fig. 11. Use of cannula to assist positioning of fixation suture. (A) Slotted cannula device inserted to hold superior aspect of meniscus. (B) All-inside fixation device carefully steered into place, directed by the slotted cannula device.

Table 2
Inside-out meniscal repair technique

Device	Curve/Bendable	Suture	Deployment	Comments	
Zone specific II (Conmed)	Rigid - 6 different angles R/L anterior, R/L middle, R/L posterior	Double arm meniscal repair needles 2/ 0 braided suture	Manual	6 prebent cannulas with fluid venting	www.conmed.com
Meniscal Stitcher (Smith & Nephew)	Curved up L/R, straight R/ L, curved down, R/L bendable, tool	2/0 Ticron suture	Manual	10 needles	www.smith-nephew.com
Sharp Shooter (Stryker)	Rigid delivery R/L posterior, middle, anterior	2-0 ultrahigh molecular weight polyethylene suture 2-0 polyester braided suture	Mechanical trigger (incremental needle delivery)	Single-handed delivery, less requirement for assistant	www.stryker.com
Protector (Arthrex)	Malleable nitinol needles with memory	2-0 FibreWire suture lasso (needle each end)	Manual deployment with needle pusher	Joystick - optional extra for improved placement control	www.arthrex.com

c. An assistant holds the arthroscope while the surgeon both passes the needle through the meniscus and retrieves on the opposite side.

The choice depends on surgical preference and availability of additional assistants. It is often difficult holding the arthroscope in an appropriate position and the authors' preference is the first technique.

OUTSIDE-IN MENISCAL REPAIR TECHNIQUE

Outside-in meniscal repair techniques involve the insertion of a needle or suture delivery device from outside to inside the joint with subsequent retrieval of the suture through the meniscus, leaving a loop on the inside. The sutures are tied on the outside of the joint, over the capsule. In early versions of the technique, a knot was tied on the suture inside the knee rather than passing through the meniscus. This technique resulted in a prominent knot, potentially causing secondary damage on the articular cartilage and is now an uncommon technique.

There are different variations of this technique that have been described and these are shown in detail in Video 2.

Two Needle System: Straight and Curved

In the Meniscal Mender system by Smith & Nephew (Meniscus Mender II; Smith and Nephew, Andover, MA), straight and curved spinal type needles are available along with a wire snare for retrieving suture. In the simplest form the technique is shown in **Fig. 12**.

1. The fixation suture is preplaced in the curved needle and the snare wire in the straight needle.
2. First the straight needle is inserted from outside across the meniscus tear, often helped by using the arthroscopy probe to stabilize the meniscus tear.

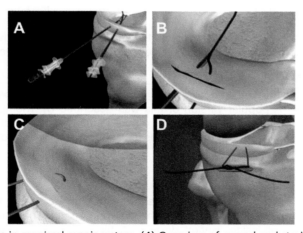

Fig. 12. Outside-in meniscal repair system. (A) Overview of curved and straight spinal needles. (B) Insertion of suture through curved needle captured by wire snare in straight needle. (C) Loop of suture on meniscus. (D) Suture tied over the capsule. (From Smith and Nephew FastFix Meniscal Mender overview; is http://www.smith-nephew.com/uk/products/sports-medicine/knee-repair/meniscus-mender-ii/; with permission.)

3. The obturator is removed, and the wire snare inserted.
4. The curved needle is inserted across the meniscus tear and the obturator is removed.
5. The repair suture is passed out of the curved needle through the snare on the straight needle, and the snared end is pulled out through the meniscus leaving a loop on the meniscus tissue (see Video 2 for more detail).

Single Straight Spinal Needle Technique

A variation of the procedure using the Meniscal mender system was described by Menge and associates[20] as a technique for anterior horn repair, using the straight spinal needle and the loop suture retriever. With the arthroscope in the opposite portal to the tear, the vertical arthroscopy portal on the affected side is extended to expose joint capsule. The straight spinal needle is inserted from outside-in, traversing the tear and a No. 1 polydioxanone suture (Ethicon, Somerville, NJ) is passed into the joint and held by arthroscopic grasper. The straight spinal needle is removed and reinserted through the meniscus and a looped suture retriever from the system passed into the joint to capture the free end of the polydioxanone suture, subsequently pulling it through the meniscus creating a mattress configuration.

Two Spinal Techniques Passing Sutures Outside of Joint

In this technique, 2 straight spinal needles are used, and the advantage is that there is no fiddly passage of suture through a loop system inside the joint. The important aspect is to avoid any catching on a soft tissue bridge.

1. The first spinal needle is loaded with a monofilament suture, pulling one-half the suture length outside the needle to act as a retrievable loop.
2. The needle loop is passed through the meniscus leaving a loop inside the knee, which is retrieved out through the access portal using a grasper.
3. A second spinal needle with definitive meniscus suture as a free end is passed from outside in, through the meniscus tear and the free end is retrieved, pulling it outside the joint.
4. The free end is passed through the suture loop—outside of the knee joint, avoiding any difficulty inside the knee.
5. The suture loop is pulled back through the knee leaving the definitive suture as a loop on the meniscus with 2 ends outside the joint ready for tying over the capsule.

Single Needle System

A neat variation of the fixation device using a single short needle has been described in various forms. A popular version of this was described by Thompson and colleagues[21] and involves keeping the same suture in the needle and creating a loop once the free end is inserted in the joint. This technique is best understood by viewing Video 2.

HYBRID TECHNIQUES

For longitudinal tears that extend from the posterior third to anterior third, such as a large displaced and mobile bucket handle tear, it can be impractical and expensive to use all-inside fixation devices. Achieving fixation points every 4 to 5 mm may involve a large number of implants at high expense. In this situation meniscal repair involves the use of all-inside fixation devices for the posterior third and inside-out techniques for mid and anterior thirds. This method allows for the placement of a high numbers of sutures to obtain optimal hold on bucket handle type tears.

Video 3 shows repair of a chronic displaced Lat bucket handle, using all-inside devices for posterior third and inside-out for anterior component. Open exposure for suture of posterior third is avoided by the use of all-inside fixation sutures, but can be used if necessary. The technique for exposure of the posteromedial and posterolateral corner is outside the scope of this article but is described and illustrated in the excellent paper by Noyes and Barber-Westin.[22]

ABSORBABLE OR NONABSORBABLE SUTURES

Meniscus healing takes several months and traditionally nonabsorbable sutures have been used. If absorbable sutures are used, then these should be chosen to last at least 3 months. Polydioxanone type sutures are therefore more appropriate than absorbable Vicryl sutures.

INDICATIONS FOR REPAIR

There a few published guides that give clear definitive indication for repair and, more important, when not to attempt repair.[23] As a rough guide, repairable tears include those less than 4 mm from the meniscal rim, ideally within 4 weeks of injury, in patients who are in their 40s or younger, and who will comply with the necessary rehabilitation avoiding sport for 4 months minimum (a personal rule of 4s from the authors). There are, however, no definitive criteria for repairability.

Four factors should be considered by the surgeon and patient in the decision-making process for repair of a meniscal tear.

1. Vascular versus nonvascular
   - Best healing potential seen in peripheral one-third. Those tears within 2 mm and up to 4 mm from the meniscocapsular junction being identified as the tears most likely to heal.
   - Good results have also been reported for tears in the avascular zones in both young (<20) and older (>45) patients with midterm follow-up.[24,25]
2. Pattern and location
   - Vertical longitudinal tears being more peripheral show better healing potential.
   - Radial, oblique, and horizontal cleavage tears are typically found more central and are devoid of blood supply resulting in poor healing potential.
3. Isolated versus combined with ligament reconstruction
   - Concurrent anterior cruciate ligament reconstruction is thought to be beneficial to a repaired meniscus. The release of pluripotent stem cells and growth factors during tunnel drilling create an environment conducive to healing. Cannon and Vittori[26] found that 91% of meniscal tears healed when they were combined with an anterior cruciate ligament reconstruction, as opposed to 51% of those repaired in isolation.
4. Traumatic versus degenerative
   - Traumatic tears result from supraphysiologic stress on an otherwise normal meniscus, whereas degenerative tears result from wear and tear over a period of time and are often associated with nonrepairable horizontal cleavage or complex tears in the avascular zone.

REPAIR METHODS FOR DIFFERENT TYPES OF TEARS

In general, the different types of tear have optimal fixation methods to ensure a high healing rate. These are grouped into vertical longitudinal tears, radial tears, and horizontal tears.

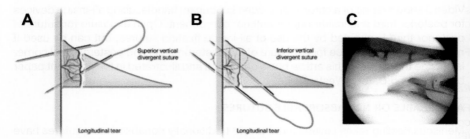

Fig. 13. Double-stacked inside-out vertical suture technique performed in the repair of a vertical longitudinal meniscal tear. (*A*) The superior sutures are placed first to close the superior gap and to reduce the meniscus to its bed. (*B*) Then, the inferior suture is placed through the tear to close the inferior gap. (*C*) Arthroscopic photograph of a vertical longitudinal meniscal repair performed using an inside-out suture technique. (*From* Noyes FR, Barber-Westin SD. Meniscus tears: diagnosis, repair techniques, and clinical outcomes. In: Noyes FR, Barber-Westin SD, eds. Noyes' Knee Disorders: Surgery, Rehabilitation, Clinical Outcomes. Philadelphia: Saunders; 2009:733-771; with permission.)

Vertical Longitudinal Tears

Biomechanically, a stacked vertical mattress suture configuration (**Figs. 13** and **14**) using in to out sutures or all-inside techniques every 3 to 5 mm has been shown to provide superiority over horizontal mattress.[27,28] Both inside-out

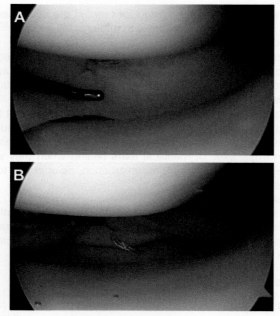

Fig. 14. Repair using all-inside devices achieving vertical mattress configuration on superior surface (*A*) and inferior surface (*B*).

and all-inside techniques have been reported to have equal healing rates, complications, and functional outcomes, according to a recent systematic review by Fillingham and colleagues.[29] Tears less than 10 mm can be left alone[13] (see **Fig. 5**).

Radial Tears

Radial tears within the inner 60% of the meniscus, with an intact periphery, do not compromise overall function and can be resected, removing unstable edges (**Fig. 15**). Radial tears extending to the peripheral zone should be repaired to restore the integrity of the rim. Repair can be performed using inside-out and anchor-based all-inside techniques with horizontal mattress suture configurations on the superior and inferior surfaces to generate tension against the periphery of the meniscus or capsule (see **Figs. 7** and **8**). Video 4 shows the tiegrip technique for repair in greater detail.

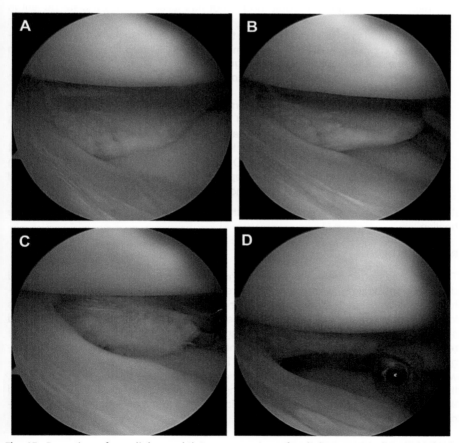

Fig. 15. Resection of a radial tear. (*A*) Demonstration of radial tear extending two-thirds of the meniscus. (*B*) Resection with combination punch and shaver. (*C*) Further resection to leave smooth rim. (*D*) Final appearance of saucerized meniscus with stable rim remaining.

Horizontal Tear Repair

Peripheral horizontal tears that do not communicate with the joint can be repaired using an open technique as described by Pujol and colleagues.[30] Horizontal tears that are apparent on arthroscopy affecting the free margin and body of the meniscus can be repaired using vertical sutures augmented by use of blood clots.[14]

REPAIR ENHANCEMENT: USE OF BIOLOGICS

Several methods have been proposed to enhance healing of the meniscus. The conclusion can be summarized from a recent comprehensive review by Woodmass and colleagues[31]

- Marrow venting procedures aim to replicate the biological environment created by anterior cruciate ligament tunnel drilling and have been shown to be effective in a goat model, but at the 2-year follow-up no clinical benefit in humans has been observed.
- Mechanical stimulation (synovial rasping and abrasion of tear surfaces) promotes neovascularization in a rabbit model, but has failed to show a clear benefit in humans.
- Trephination to create channels from the vascular to avascular areas has demonstrated improved healing in a goat model and 90% good to excellent results in humans, but without a comparison group.
- Fibrin clot has also shown high success ,rates but it is a difficult technique to perform.
- Bone marrow aspirate injection in combination with all-inside repairs in the avascular zone have shown 86% clinical improvement and 76% nonhomogeneous MRI with no evidence of a tear, but again without a comparison group.[32]
- Platelet-rich plasma has been investigated by 2 human trails, which have not shown a difference in outcomes. One study has reported good results with platelet-rich plasma injection after repair for the specific indication of horizontal cleavages in athletes, but again without a comparison group.[33]

It is clear that more work is required in this field, to evaluate strategies to improve healing.

REHABILITATION

Tear patterns determine postoperative rehabilitation. Vertical tears are compressed during weight bearing, whereas radial tears are distracted. Radial tear repairs therefore should be protected from weight bearing, usually for 6 weeks. For vertical tears loading is appropriate, but loading and sheer forces are increased in flexion beyond 40°. There is little evidence to favor a free regime without restriction versus a restrictive regimen incorporating a brace.[23] The authors of this review prefer a restrictive program allowing immediate weight bearing in a splint locked in extension with non-weight bearing flexion allowed to 90°, unlocking the brace hinges. From 4 weeks, the splint is removed, and full weight bearing allowed from 0 to 90°. Squatting beyond 90°, pivoting, twisting, and cutting are avoided until 3 months. Return to sport is typically at 4 to 6 months.

SUMMARY OF REPAIR STRATEGIES

Meniscal repair is an important surgical skill with high level evidence of effectiveness. This paper has reviewed the indications for repair and the key surgical techniques. Inside-out remains the primary method of meniscal repair with sutures passed using a curved cannula through the meniscus and subsequently tied over the capsule.

Inside-out techniques are particularly useful for longer tears (>3 cm) or bucket handle tears. With this technique, the middle third and most of the anterior third can be reached. All-inside fixation devices are particularly useful for posterior third tears, decreasing the risk of neurovascular injury from outside-in needles. They can also be used in middle third tears. All-inside and inside-out techniques have been shown to have equal healing rates, functional outcomes and complications.[29] Outside-in techniques can be useful for anterior third tears that are difficult to reach.

SUPPLEMENTARY DATA

Supplementary data related to this article can be found online at https://doi.org/10.1016/j.csm.2019.08.012.

REFERENCES

1. Fox AJ, Wanivenhaus F, Burge AJ, et al. The human meniscus: a review of anatomy, function, injury and advances in treatment. Clin Anat 2015;28:269–87.
2. Papalia R, Del Buono A, Osti L, et al. Meniscectomy as a risk factor for knee osteoarthritis: a systematic review. Br Med Bull 2011;99:89–106.
3. Pengas IP, Assiotis A, Nash W, et al. Total meniscectomy in adolescents. J Bone Joint Surg Br 2012;94-B:1649–54.
4. Bloecker K, Wirth W, Hudelmaier M, et al. Morphometric differences between the medial and lateral meniscus in healthy men - a three-dimensional analysis using magnetic resonance imaging. Cells Tissues Organs 2012;195:353–64.
5. Thompson WO, Thaete FL, Fu FH, et al. Tibial meniscal dynamics using three-dimensional reconstruction of magnetic resonance images. Am J Sports Med 1991;19:210–6.
6. Walker PS, Erkman MJ. The role of the menisci in force transmission across the knee. Clin Orthop Relat Res 1975;(109):184–92.
7. Williams A, Logan M. Understanding tibio-femoral motion. Knee 2004;11:81–8.
8. Ahmed AM, Burke DL. In-vitro measurement of static pressure distribution in synovial joints–part I: tibial surface of the knee. J Biomech Eng 1983;105:216–25.
9. Paletta GA, Manning T, Snell E, et al. The effect of allograft meniscal replacement on intraarticular contact area and pressures in the human knee. Am J Sports Med 1997;25:692–8.
10. Arnoczky SP, Warren RF. Microvasculature of The human meniscus. Am J Sports Med 1982;10:90–5.
11. Haemer JM, Wang J, Carter DR, et al. Benefit of single-leaf resection for horizontal meniscus tear. Clin Orthop Relat Res 2007;457:194–202.
12. Pujol N, Lorbach O. Meniscal repair: results. In: Hulet C, Pereira H, Peretti G, et al, editors. Surgery of the meniscus. Berlin: Springer Verlag; 2016. p. 343–55.
13. Vaguero-Picado A, Rodriguez-Merchan E. Arthroscopic repair of the meniscus; surgical management and clinical outcomes. EFORT Open Rev 2018. https://doi.org/10.1302/2058-5241.3.170059.
14. Kurzweil PR, Lynch NM, Coleman S, et al. Repair of horizontal meniscus tears: a systematic review. Arthroscopy 2014;30:1513–9.
15. Pujol N, Bohu Y, Boisrenoult P, et al. Clinical outcomes of open meniscal repair of horizontal meniscal tears in young patients. Knee Surg Sports Traumatol Arthrosc 2013;21:1530–3.

16. Van der Wal RJ, Thomassen BJ, Swen JW, et al. Time interval between trauma and arthroscopic meniscal repair has no influence on clinical survival. J Knee Surg 2016;29(5):436–42.

17. Mesiha M, Zurakowski D, Soriano J, et al. Pathologic characteristics of the torn human meniscus. Am J Sports Med 2007;35:103–12.

18. Eggli S, Wegmuller H, Kosinia J, et al. Long-term results of arthroscopic meniscal repair. An analysis of isolated tears. Am J Sports Med 1995;23(6):715–20.

19. Everhart JS, Higgins JD, Poland SG, et al. Meniscal repair in patients age 40years and older: a systematic review of 11 studies and 148 patients. Knee 2018;25(6):1142–50.

20. Menge TJ, Dean CS, Chahla J, et al. Anterior horn meniscal repair using an outside-in suture technique. Arthrosc Tech 2016;5(5):e1111–6.

21. Thompson SM, Spalding T, Church S. A novel and cheap method of outside-in meniscal repair for anterior horn tears. Arthrosc Tech 2014;3(2):e233–5.

22. Noyes FR, Barber-Westin SD. Meniscus tears: diagnosis, repair techniques, and clinical outcomes. In: Noyes FR, Barber-Westin SD, editors. Noyes' knee disorders: surgery, rehabilitation, clinical outcomes. Philadelphia: Saunders; 2009. p. 733–71.

23. Beaufils P, Becker R, Kopf S, et al. The knee meniscus: management of traumatic tears and degenerative lesions. EFORT Open Rev 2017;2(5):195–203.

24. Noyes FR, Barber-Westin SD. Arthroscopic repair of meniscus tears extending into the avascular zone with or without anterior cruciate ligament reconstruction in patients 40 years of age and older. Arthroscopy 2000;16(8):822–9.

25. Noyes FR, Barber-Westin SD. Arthroscopic repair of meniscal tears extending into the avascular zone in patients younger than twenty years of age. Am J Sports Med 2002;30(4):589–600.

26. Cannon WD Jr, Vittori JM. The incidence of healing in arthroscopic meniscal repairs in anterior cruciate ligament-reconstructed knees versus stable knees. Am J Sports Med 1992;20(2):176–81.

27. Ranki CC, Lintner DM, Noble PC, et al. Biomechanical analysis of meniscal repair techniques. Am J Sports Med 2002;30:492–7.

28. Noyes FR, Chen RC, Barber-Westin SD, et al. Greater than 10-year results of red-white longitudinal meniscal repairs in patients 20 years of age or younger. Am J Sports Med 2011;39:1008–17.

29. Fillingham YA, Riboh JC, Erickson BJ, et al. Inside-out versus all-inside repair of isolated meniscal tears. Am J Sports Med 2017;45(1):234–42.

30. Pujol N, Beaufils P. During ACL reconstruction, small asymptomatic lesions can be left untreated. A systematic review. J ISAKOS 2016;1:135–40.

31. Woodmass JM, Laprade RF, Sgaglione NA, et al. Meniscal repair reconsidering indications, techniques, and biologic augmentation. J Bone Joint Surg Am 2017;99:1222–53.

32. Cotter EJ, Wang KC, Yanke AB, et al. Bone marrow aspirate concentrate for cartilage defects of the knee: from bench to bedside evidence. Cartilage 2018;9(2):161–70.

33. Pujol N, Salle De Chou E, Boisrenoult P, et al. Platelet-rich plasma for open meniscal repair in young patients: any benefit? Knee Surg Sports Traumatol Arthrosc 2015;23:51–8.

Injury of the Meniscus Root

Mitchell I. Kennedy, BS[a], Marc Strauss, MD[b],
Robert F. LaPrade, MD, PhD[c],*

KEYWORDS

- Meniscus root • Radial root tear • Transtibial pull-out repair • Ghost sign

KEY POINTS

- Medial meniscus root tears are biomechanically equivalent to a subtotal medial meniscectomy.
- Lateral meniscus root tears provide both an important joint loading function and also result in increased anterior tibial translation and internal rotation in the anterior cruciate ligament–deficient knee.
- Anatomic root repairs restore joint loading and knee stability.
- Meniscal root repairs in patients with no to mild osteoarthritis yield significantly improved patient outcomes and stall the progression of osteoarthritis.

INTRODUCTION

Within the knee joint, the meniscus provides shock absorption and stability by generating circumferential stresses as load bearing occurs.[1–3] This is enabled by the root attachments of the meniscus to the tibia, preventing meniscus extrusion and a subsequent alteration of the transmitted hoop stresses.[4–6] Meniscus root tears lead to an increase of peak tibiofemoral contact pressure[7] and tibiofemoral contact area,[8] which has been shown to lead to altered biomechanics and an acceleration of degenerative changes of the knee joint.[9–15] The treatment method for meniscus injuries now primarily focuses on preservation[16] and anatomic restoration, because nonoperative and meniscectomy treatments are associated with poorer clinical outcomes and a higher rate of conversion to total knee arthroplasty.[17–19] Not only have root repairs demonstrated a restoration of tibiofemoral joint mechanics,[20,21] but comparison studies have ultimately shown the outperformance of root repair procedures relative to nonoperative and meniscectomy procedures in delaying progression of osteoarthritis.[17,22,23] In this review, we detail

Disclosures: R.F. LaPrade is a consultant and receives royalties from Arthrex, Ossur, and Smith and Nephew.
a Graduate School, Georgetown University, Washington, DC, USA; b Department of Orthopaedic Surgery, Oslo University Hospital, Oslo, Norway; c Twin Cities Orthopedics, 4060 West 65th Street, Edina, MN 55435, USA
* Corresponding author.
E-mail address: laprademdphd@gmail.com

the function and etiology of meniscus root injuries by the anatomic and biomechanical features of the root attachments, along with the validated treatment procedures currently detailed in the literature.

MENISCAL ROOT FEATURES
Anatomy of the Meniscal Roots

Generally, the medial meniscal root attachments are greater in area than those of the lateral meniscus,[24] with the anterior horn of the medial meniscus being the largest[24–27] and strongest[28] footprint of all. The fan-shaped[27] anterior horn of the medial meniscus inserts broadly onto the anterior intercondylar crest,[26,27] with its posterior aspect measuring roughly 11.5 mm anterior to the center of the anterior cruciate ligament (ACL) tibial insertion[29] and a reported area of 61.4 mm^2,[24] 139.0 mm^2,[27] and 101.7 mm^2.[28] Berlet and Fowler[30] reported various insertions within close proximity of each other in this area, while supporting a potential fibrous link with the ACL.[16,27]

The anterior horn attachment of the lateral meniscus is smaller than the anterior root attachment of the medial meniscus, with early estimates reporting an attachment area of 44.5 mm^2[24] and 93 mm^2,[27] and more recent data reporting 99.5 mm^2.[28] This attachment appears directly anterior to the lateral tibial eminence and laterally adjacent to the tibial insertion of the ACL.[24] Ziegler and colleagues[31] reported a lateral distance of 7.5 mm to the center of the ACL tibial attachment and supported earlier reports of attachment between the anterior horn of the lateral meniscus to the bundles of the ACL.[24,27]

The posterior root attachment of the medial meniscus is known to insert anteromedial to the posterior cruciate ligament (PCL) tibial attachment,[24,25,27,32] appearing 9.6 mm posterior and 0.7 mm lateral to the medial tibial eminence, while being 3.5 mm lateral from the articular cartilage inflection point of the medial tibial plateau

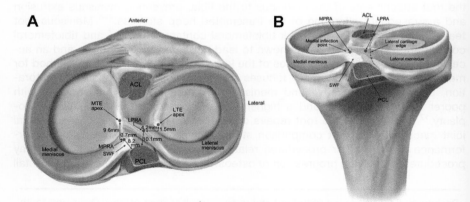

Fig. 1. The medial and lateral meniscal posterior root attachments and relevant arthroscopically pertinent anatomy (right knee). (*A*) Superior view and (*B*) posterior view. ACL, anterior cruciate ligament bundle attachments; LPRA, lateral meniscus posterior root attachment; LTE, lateral tibial eminence; MPRA, medial meniscus posterior root attachment; MTE, medial tibial eminence; PCL, posterior cruciate ligament bundle attachments; SWF, shiny white fibers of posterior horn of medial meniscus. (*From* Johannsen AM, Civitarese DM, Padalecki JR, Goldsmith MT, Wijdicks CA, LaPrade RF. Qualitative and quantitative anatomic analysis of the posterior root attachments of the medial and lateral menisci. *Am J Sports Med.* 2012;40(10):2342-2347; with permission.)

(Fig. 1).[32] Early approximations reported attachment areas of 47.2 mm[224] and 80 mm[2],[27] but more recent studies report areas of 30.4 mm[232] and 68.0 mm[2].[28] Johannsen and colleagues[32] attribute this reduction in approximated area to excluding the transverse shiny white fibers when measuring the medial root attachment; on inclusion, the total root attachment area increased to 69.6 mm[2].

Early in the literature, the posterior horn of the lateral meniscus was typically known as the smallest of the root attachments, with early studies reporting 28.5 mm[224] and 115 mm[2],[27] and more recent studies reporting 39.2 mm[232] and 83.1 mm[228]; recent studies suggest the posterior root of the medial meniscus may be the smallest on exclusion of the transverse shiny white fibers. This posterior lateral meniscus insertion appears just anterior to the insertion of the posterior attachment of the medial meniscus.[24,25] Directly 12.7 mm anterior from the PCL tibial attachment[32] and 10.8 mm posterior to the posteromedial bundle of the ACL,[31] the posterior root of the lateral meniscus inserts 1.5 mm posterior and 4.2 mm medial to the lateral tibial eminence apex, while being 4.3 mm medial from the lateral articular cartilage edge (**Fig. 2**).

Structural Properties of the Root Attachments

During ultimate failure testing, Ellman and colleagues[28] reported the failure mechanism of meniscus root injuries to exclusively consist of small bony avulsions of the meniscal root. The anterior roots sustain greater force before failure relative to the posterior roots,[28,33] with the anterior medial and anterior lateral roots failing at strengths of 655.5 N and 652.8 N, respectively and the posterior medial and posterior lateral roots falling at 513.8 N and 509.0 N, respectively. Literature suggests the ability of the anterior roots to sustain greater force may be derived from the features of greater thickness and uncalcified fibrocartilage relative to the posterior roots.[34]

As previously stated, the inclusion or exclusion of the shiny white fibers within the posterior medial meniscal root attachment can affect the properties of the attachment. Once sectioned, ultimate failure strength lessened to 245.9 N from 513.8 N, suggesting the shiny white fibers account for 47.8% of the native root strength.[28] A similar decrease, but less profound, was reported with sectioning of the surrounding fibers of the posterior lateral and anterior medial roots.

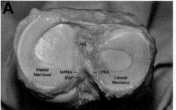
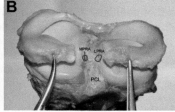

Fig. 2. Medial and lateral meniscal posterior root attachments and relevant arthroscopically pertinent anatomy. (*A*) Superior view and (*B*) posterior view. ACL, anterior cruciate ligament bundle attachments; LPRA, lateral meniscus posterior root attachment; LTE, lateral tibial eminence; MPRA, medial meniscus posterior root attachment; MTE, medial tibial eminence; PCL, posterior cruciate ligament bundle attachments; SWF, shiny white fibers of posterior horn of medial meniscus. (*From* Johannsen AM, Civitarese DM, Padalecki JR, Goldsmith MT, Wijdicks CA, LaPrade RF. Qualitative and quantitative anatomic analysis of the posterior root attachments of the medial and lateral menisci. *Am J Sports Med.* 2012;40(10):2342-2347; with permission.)

ETIOLOGY OF MENISCUS ROOT TEARS

The meniscus is responsible for distributing tibiofemoral loads, joint stabilization, and congruency.[35–39] These abilities stem from both the intrinsic material properties and gross anatomic structure and attachments,[2] with the root insertions enabling transformation of axial tibiofemoral stress into circumferential hoop stresses.[40,41] Root tears are reported to have been encountered/diagnosed in 4.3% of all arthroscopic surgeries, with posterior medial and posterior lateral root tears accounting for 52% and 41% of all meniscal root tears, respectively.[42] Increased mobility of the anterior attachments is thought to account for the higher failure strength and, ultimately, fewer failures, relative to the posterior roots.[34] Disruption of these root attachments often leads to extrusion and a subsequent failure of load distribution accompanied by increased contact pressures and stress concentration,[43] resulting in greater vulnerability of underlying cartilage degeneration.[42,44–46] This resultant biomechanical condition mirrors that of an absent meniscus.[7,8]

Long-term outcomes of lateral root disruption has been shown to significantly affect the lateral compartment,[47–49] due to the function of the lateral meniscus in transmitting 70% of lateral compartment load,[50] and the posterior root transmitting 50% to 85% between extension and 90° of flexion, respectively.[39] Disruption also may affect the conditions of neighboring structures within the knee, because the lateral meniscus posterior root contributes to stabilization of anterior tibial translation at lower flexion angles and internal rotation at higher flexion angles[51]; absence of the posterior lateral meniscus root attachment results in greater strain placed on the ACL, which also supports anterior tibial translation[52] and internal rotation.[53]

The posterior root of the medial meniscus carries a greater load than its anterior root,[54] making medial menisucs posterior root injuries more likely to induce disruptions to contact pressures and load distribution.[7] Significant correlations exist between posterior root tears of the medial meniscus and spontaneous osteonecrosis of the knee,[15,55–58] likely resulting from reduced medial meniscus mobility from its robust attachment to the medial tibial plateau[16,59] coupled with the medial compartment enduring significantly greater loads during weightbearing.[60]

DIAGNOSIS OF MENISCAL ROOT TEARS

Root tears can be challenging to diagnose with simple clinical evaluation because no clinical test or deliberate sign for a definitive diagnosis exists. Patients may describe a sudden onset of pain after a small twisting injury or deep knee flexion, resulting in a recurrent effusion, joint line pain, loss of flexion, or deep knee flexion pain.[61] Other times, the patient may experience popping or locking of the knee. Meniscal tests, like the McMurray and Apley tests, may be positive but not necessary with a mechanical click.[62] Various techniques for evaluation have been described, one being the valgus/varus test in the fully extended knee.[62] This test will be positive due to extrusion or lack of residual hoop strain of the meniscus when compressing the ipsilateral joint space. Important risk factors to identify include concomitant injuries, osteoarthritis (OA), alignment, and high body mass index (BMI).[63]

A thorough history, physical examination, and MRI will need to be performed to assess potential root pathology.[64] Choi and colleagues[65] reported a positive predictive value of 100% for detection of medial root tears and a 93% sensitivity and 100% specificity on a 3T MRI scanner. De Smet and Mukherjee[64] reported an MRI specificity of 88% for lateral meniscus tears and 86% for medial meniscus tears and a sensitivity of 83% for lateral meniscus root tears and 97% for medial meniscus tears using a 1.5T MRI scanner. Lee and colleagues[66] reported that the use of

T2-weighted sequences increases diagnostic specificity and sensitivity when diagnosing meniscus root tears. Other signs of meniscus root tear to look for on the MRI are meniscus extrusion, subchondral bone marrow edema, and the "ghost" sign. It has been reported that medial meniscus extrusion 3 mm or greater at the level of the medial collateral ligament shows a strong correlation with a meniscus root tear, but should not be used as the only diagnostic criterion.[6,67] Subchondral edema can be an indirect expression for a dysfunctional meniscus and is often seen when a root tear is present.

The "ghost sign" (shown in **Fig. 3**) is a characteristic finding for meniscus root tear and is radiologically defined as a sudden absence of a well-defined meniscus structure in the sagittal plane on the MRI.[6,13,66]

OUTCOMES OF MENISCUS ROOT REPAIRS

Treatment of meniscal root tears has transitioned into the favoring of preservation[16] of the meniscus by various root repair techniques,[68] as opposed to treatment by meniscectomy. Although meniscectomy procedures have been shown to significantly improve from preoperative conditions in both the International Knee Documentation Committee (IKDC) and Lysholm, these subjective measures were superior with repairs, in addition to lesser joint space narrowing and progression of OA.[23,69] Furthermore, although root repair surgeries do not avert OA progression entirely, similar OA grades compared with preoperative conditions have been reported following repair techniques,[70] in addition to slower progression of OA determined by decelerative OA changes[17] and lesser joint space narrowing[23] in relation to meniscectomy procedures. Lateral posterior root techniques vary from no treatment,[14] all-inside repair,[71–73] and transtibial pull-out repair,[74,75] whereas medial posterior root techniques mainly consist of various transtibial pull-out[76] and all-inside techniques.[70,77–80] This review highlights the anatomic transtibial pull-out repair technique, which is supported by restoration of tibiofemoral joint mechanics in biomechanical models,[20,21] in addition to displaying significant improvements in

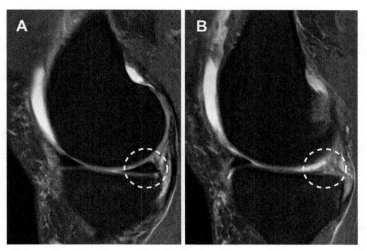

Fig. 3. The "ghost sign" is a characteristic indication for a meniscus root tear, with a radiologically defined presence (*A*) and sudden absence (*B*) of a well-defined meniscus structure, between sagittal plane cuts on an MRI.

outcomes of both lateral and medial posterior root repairs, with age not factoring into differential outcomes.[76]

On comparison of the transtibial pull-out repair technique versus nonoperative treatment of the lateral meniscus posterior root repair, performed in concomitance with ACL reconstruction, Pan and colleagues[75] found that both patient groups obtained significant improvement in Lysholm and IKDC scores, but the repair group reported a reduced occurrence of the development of OA. Given the common occurrence of lateral meniscus posterior avulsions with ACL injuries, a modification of this technique to account for potential tunnel convergence was performed in a case series, in which positive outcomes were similarly reported.[74]

To better generalize treatment protocols for posterior meniscal root tears, LaPrade and colleagues[76] performed the anatomic transtibial pull-out technique on patients ranging from 18 to 65 years of age, who either sustained a medial or lateral posterior root tear. A significant improvement was reported for postoperative outcomes and patient satisfaction, regardless of the age or laterality of meniscal injury. The decision of meniscal root repair had previously been considered an age-related factor,[81] although now it seems other factors should be more heavily considered, including OA grade, high BMI, or postoperative rehabilitation protocol compliance.[76,82]

DETAILED ANATOMIC TRANSTIBIAL PULL-OUT REPAIR SURGICAL TECHNIQUE

A radial root tear of the posterior horn of the medial meniscus (shown in **Fig. 4**) is the most common indication for a root repair, ideally within the first centimeter of the attachment of the meniscus to ensure the correct restoration of biomechanics.[21,83] Also, restoration of joint loading capacity of the meniscus is essential, by ensuring the meniscus is pulled back into the joint as part of the surgical repair, recreating the cushioning effect of the medial meniscus.[21,44,84]

The surgical arthroscopic incisions should be placed adjacent to the edges of the patellar tendon, both medially and laterally,[85] with vertical incisions for potential size expansion when accommodating surgical instruments. Following removal of scar tissue distal and medial to the PCL and along the medial edge of the intercondylar notch; the presence of significant osteophytes in the posteromedial aspect of the notch hindering posterior horn visualization may require a posteromedial arthroscopic notchplasty. For chronic root tears, sufficient mobilization of the meniscus laterally should be performed, to reduce meniscal extrusion. Release by a scissor-biter of the inferior and/or superior aspects of the meniscus can be performed through to the anterior margin of the medial collateral ligament attachment, ensuring pull back of the meniscus into the joint. One can perform a release of the meniscotibial portion of

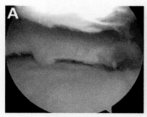 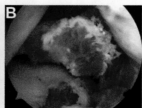 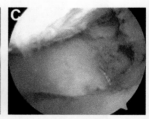

Fig. 4. A radial tear of the medial meniscus is a clear indication of disruption to the meniscal root and can be visualized as a detachment from its posterior tibial insertion (*A, B*). Repair should be performed by positioning tunnels at the anatomic attachment of the posterior root and pulling the root securely to the tibia (*C*).

the joint capsule, under the extruded medial meniscus, which will allow the joint to gap open 1 to 2 mm and significantly improve visualization and placement of surgical instruments.

Medial compartments characterized as "tight" should be managed with use of a spinal needle and trephination of the meniscofemoral portion of the medial collateral ligament at its attachment site,[86–88] increasing access to the medial compartment of the knee.[89] This method also avoids iatrogenic damage of the medial compartment articular cartilage while placing in self-capture instruments.

Preparation of the bony attachment area for the meniscus root repair follows once meniscus mobility is achieved. A curved curette is used to decorticate the tibia, ensuring the position is as far posterior as possible on the medial tibial plateau. Anterior placement of the posterior attachment point will result in meniscus placement that fails to restore normal contact mechanics, while also placing the repair at risk for overload and potential re-tear.[83] If the meniscus root repair is performed in isolation and without concurrent cruciate ligament reconstruction, the tibial incision is made approximately 2 cm medial to the tibial tubercle, directly down to the bone, and is followed with periosteal elevation. The 2-tunnel repair technique allows for a broad distribution of the meniscus tissue down to the tibia, subsequently resulting in a broad healing site and less likelihood of partial healing or reextrusion.[90,91]

The first cannula is placed using an ACL-type drill, in the decorticated posterior aspect of the tibia, leaving the cannula for later passage of a passing suture. A self-capture device is used to pass a suture through healthy tissue of the meniscal posterior horn, 7 mm posterior to the anterior edge of the meniscus. The suture is then subsequently shuttled down the tibial tunnel using the passing suture of the cannula, and using the self-capture sutures previously passed, ultimately pulling the sutures distally through the tibial tunnel. These steps are repeated for the second suture, anteriorly to the previously passed suture. On tensioning of the transtibial sutures, return of the meniscus into anatomic placement should be confirmed, with inadequate positioning suggesting the potential necessity of a further peripheral capsular release to minimize extrusion.

Surgical completion is achieved following securing of the sutures over a metal button on the tibia, with the knee in flexion, which enables early, postoperative range of motion physiotherapy. Sutures secured over a button are seen as the most optimal method, due to the potential of other means to cut through the cortical bone of the tibia after repeat cycles. Buttons are also beneficial in follow-up appointments, by determining if movement of the suture has occurred in postoperative radiographs.

SUMMARY

It is now well-recognized that meniscal root tears are common and that their repair in an anatomic position best restores joint loading and function. Meniscal root repair in properly indicated patients is highly recommended to prevent or stall the progression of OA.

REFERENCES

1. Bullough PG, Munuera L, Murphy J, et al. The strength of the menisci of the knee as it relates to their fine structure. J Bone Joint Surg Br 1970;52(3):564–7.
2. Fithian DC, Kelly MA, Mow VC. Material properties and structure-function relationships in the menisci. Clin Orthop Relat Res 1990;(252):19–31.
3. Radin EL, de Lamotte F, Maquet P. Role of the menisci in the distribution of stress in the knee. Clin Orthop Relat Res 1984;185:290–4.

4. Hein CN, Deperio JG, Ehrensberger MT, et al. Effects of medial meniscal posterior horn avulsion and repair on meniscal displacement. Knee 2011;18(3):189–92.

5. Ihn JC, Kim SJ, Park IH. In vitro study of contact area and pressure distribution in the human knee after partial and total meniscectomy. Int Orthop 1993;17(4): 214–8.

6. Lerer DB, Umans HR, Hu MX, et al. The role of meniscal root pathology and radial meniscal tear in medial meniscal extrusion. Skeletal Radiol 2004;33(10):569–74.

7. Allaire R, Muriuki M, Gilbertson L, et al. Biomechanical consequences of a tear of the posterior root of the medial meniscus. Similar to total meniscectomy. J Bone Joint Surg Am 2008;90(9):1922–31.

8. Marzo JM, Gurske-DePerio J. Effects of medial meniscus posterior horn avulsion and repair on tibiofemoral contact area and peak contact pressure with clinical implications. Am J Sports Med 2009;37(1):124–9.

9. Kenny C. Radial displacement of the medial meniscus and Fairbank's signs. Clin Orthop Relat Res 1997;339:163–73.

10. Kim JG, Lee YS, Bae TS, et al. Tibiofemoral contact mechanics following posterior root of medial meniscus tear, repair, meniscectomy, and allograft transplantation. Knee Surg Sports Traumatol Arthrosc 2013;21(9):2121–5.

11. Koenig JH, Ranawat AS, Umans HR, et al. Meniscal root tears: diagnosis and treatment. Arthroscopy 2009;25(9):1025–32.

12. Kopf S, Colvin AC, Muriuki M, et al. Meniscal root suturing techniques: implications for root fixation. Am J Sports Med 2011;39(10):2141–6.

13. Papalia R, Vasta S, Franceschi F, et al. Meniscal root tears: from basic science to ultimate surgery. Br Med Bull 2013;106:91–115.

14. Shelbourne KD, Roberson TA, Gray T. Long-term evaluation of posterior lateral meniscus root tears left in situ at the time of anterior cruciate ligament reconstruction. Am J Sports Med 2011;39(7):1439–43.

15. Sung JH, Ha JK, Lee DW, et al. Meniscal extrusion and spontaneous osteonecrosis with root tear of medial meniscus: comparison with horizontal tear. Arthroscopy 2013;29(4):726–32.

16. Bhatia S, LaPrade CM, Ellman MB, et al. Meniscal root tears: significance, diagnosis, and treatment. Am J Sports Med 2014;42(12):3016–30.

17. Chung KS, Ha JK, Yeom CH, et al. Comparison of clinical and radiologic results between partial meniscectomy and refixation of medial meniscus posterior root tears: a minimum 5-year follow-up. Arthroscopy 2015;31(10):1941–50.

18. Krych AJ, Johnson NR, Mohan R, et al. Partial meniscectomy provides no benefit for symptomatic degenerative medial meniscus posterior root tears. Knee Surg Sports Traumatol Arthrosc 2018;26(4):1117–22.

19. Krych AJ, Reardon PJ, Johnson NR, et al. Non-operative management of medial meniscus posterior horn root tears is associated with worsening arthritis and poor clinical outcome at 5-year follow-up. Knee Surg Sports Traumatol Arthrosc 2017; 25(2):383–9.

20. LaPrade CM, Jansson KS, Dornan G, et al. Altered tibiofemoral contact mechanics due to lateral meniscus posterior horn root avulsions and radial tears can be restored with in situ pull-out suture repairs. J Bone Joint Surg Am 2014; 96(6):471–9.

21. Padalecki JR, Jansson KS, Smith SD, et al. Biomechanical consequences of a complete radial tear adjacent to the medial meniscus posterior root attachment site: in situ pull-out repair restores derangement of joint mechanics. Am J Sports Med 2014;42(3):699–707.

22. Faucett SC, Geisler BP, Chahla J, et al. Meniscus root repair vs meniscectomy or nonoperative management to prevent knee osteoarthritis after medial meniscus root tears: clinical and economic effectiveness. Am J Sports Med 2019;47(3): 762–9.

23. Kim SB, Ha JK, Lee SW, et al. Medial meniscus root tear refixation: comparison of clinical, radiologic, and arthroscopic findings with medial meniscectomy. Arthroscopy 2011;27(3):346–54.

24. Johnson DL, Swenson TM, Livesay GA, et al. Insertion-site anatomy of the human menisci: gross, arthroscopic, and topographical anatomy as a basis for meniscal transplantation. Arthroscopy 1995;11(4):386–94.

25. Brody JM, Hulstyn MJ, Fleming BC, et al. The meniscal roots: gross anatomic correlation with 3-T MRI findings. AJR Am J Roentgenol 2007;188(5):W446–50.

26. Jacobsen K. Area intercondylaris tibiae: osseous surface structure and its relation to soft tissue structures and applications to radiography. J Anat 1974; 117(Pt 3):605–18.

27. Kohn D, Moreno B. Meniscus insertion anatomy as a basis for meniscus replacement: a morphological cadaveric study. Arthroscopy 1995;11(1):96–103.

28. Ellman MB, LaPrade CM, Smith SD, et al. Structural properties of the meniscal roots. Am J Sports Med 2014;42(8):1881–7.

29. Bhatia S, Korth K, Van Thiel GS, et al. Effect of reamer design on posteriorization of the tibial tunnel during endoscopic transtibial anterior cruciate ligament reconstruction. Am J Sports Med 2013;41(6):1282–9.

30. Berlet GC, Fowler PJ. The anterior horn of the medical meniscus. An anatomic study of its insertion. Am J Sports Med 1998;26(4):540–3.

31. Ziegler CG, Pietrini SD, Westerhaus BD, et al. Arthroscopically pertinent landmarks for tunnel positioning in single-bundle and double-bundle anterior cruciate ligament reconstructions. Am J Sports Med 2011;39(4):743–52.

32. Johannsen AM, Civitarese DM, Padalecki JR, et al. Qualitative and quantitative anatomic analysis of the posterior root attachments of the medial and lateral menisci. Am J Sports Med 2012;40(10):2342–7.

33. Hauch KN, Villegas DF, Haut Donahue TL. Geometry, time-dependent and failure properties of human meniscal attachments. J Biomech 2010;43(3):463–8.

34. Benjamin M, Evans EJ, Rao RD, et al. Quantitative differences in the histology of the attachment zones of the meniscal horns in the knee joint of man. J Anat 1991; 177:127–34.

35. Ahmed AM, Burke DL. In-vitro measurement of static pressure distribution in synovial joints–Part I: Tibial surface of the knee. J Biomech Eng 1983;105(3): 216–25.

36. Fukubayashi T, Kurosawa H. The contact area and pressure distribution pattern of the knee. A study of normal and osteoarthrotic knee joints. Acta Orthop Scand 1980;51(6):871–9.

37. Kettelkamp DB, Jacobs AW. Tibiofemoral contact area–determination and implications. J Bone Joint Surg Am 1972;54(2):349–56.

38. Messner K, Gao J. The menisci of the knee joint. Anatomical and functional characteristics, and a rationale for clinical treatment. J Anat 1998;193(Pt 2):161–78.

39. Walker PS, Erkman MJ. The role of the menisci in force transmission across the knee. Clin Orthop Relat Res 1975;(109):184–92.

40. Fairbank TJ. Knee joint changes after meniscectomy. J Bone Joint Surg Br 1948; 30B(4):664–70.

41. Shrive NG, O'Connor JJ, Goodfellow JW. Load-bearing in the knee joint. Clin Orthop Relat Res 1978;131:279–87.

42. LaPrade CM, James EW, Cram TR, et al. Meniscal root tears: a classification system based on tear morphology. Am J Sports Med 2015;43(2):363–9.
43. Karim AR, Cherian JJ, Jauregui JJ, et al. Osteonecrosis of the knee: review. Ann Transl Med 2015;3(1):6.
44. Geeslin AG, Civitarese D, Turnbull TL, et al. Influence of lateral meniscal posterior root avulsions and the meniscofemoral ligaments on tibiofemoral contact mechanics. Knee Surg Sports Traumatol Arthrosc 2016;24(5):1469–77.
45. Hunter DJ, Zhang YQ, Niu JB, et al. The association of meniscal pathologic changes with cartilage loss in symptomatic knee osteoarthritis. Arthritis Rheum 2006;54(3):795–801.
46. Sharma L, Eckstein F, Song J, et al. Relationship of meniscal damage, meniscal extrusion, malalignment, and joint laxity to subsequent cartilage loss in osteoarthritic knees. Arthritis Rheum 2008;58(6):1716–26.
47. Jorgensen U, Sonne-Holm S, Lauridsen F, et al. Long-term follow-up of meniscectomy in athletes. A prospective longitudinal study. J Bone Joint Surg Br 1987;69(1):80–3.
48. McNicholas MJ, Rowley DI, McGurty D, et al. Total meniscectomy in adolescence. A thirty-year follow-up. J Bone Joint Surg Br 2000;82(2):217–21.
49. Simpson DA, Thomas NP, Aichroth PM. Open and closed meniscectomy. A comparative analysis. J Bone Joint Surg Br 1986;68(2):301–4.
50. Seedhom BB, Dowson D, Wright V. Proceedings: functions of the menisci. A preliminary study. Ann Rheum Dis 1974;33(1):111.
51. Frank JM, Moatshe G, Brady AW, et al. Lateral meniscus posterior root and meniscofemoral ligaments as stabilizing structures in the ACL-deficient knee: a biomechanical study. Orthop J Sports Med 2017;5(6). 2325967117695756.
52. Noyes FR, Bassett RW, Grood ES, et al. Arthroscopy in acute traumatic hemarthrosis of the knee. Incidence of anterior cruciate tears and other injuries. J Bone Joint Surg Am 1980;62(5):687–95, 757.
53. Shybut TB, Vega CE, Haddad J, et al. Effect of lateral meniscal root tear on the stability of the anterior cruciate ligament-deficient knee. Am J Sports Med 2015;43(4):905–11.
54. Kan A, Oshida M, Oshida S, et al. Anatomical significance of a posterior horn of medial meniscus: the relationship between its radial tear and cartilage degradation of joint surface. Sports Med Arthrosc Rehabil Ther Technol 2010;2:1.
55. Nelson FR, Craig J, Francois H, et al. Subchondral insufficiency fractures and spontaneous osteonecrosis of the knee may not be related to osteoporosis. Arch Osteoporos 2014;9:194.
56. Robertson DD, Armfield DR, Towers JD, et al. Meniscal root injury and spontaneous osteonecrosis of the knee: an observation. J Bone Joint Surg Br 2009;91(2):190–5.
57. Yamagami R, Taketomi S, Inui H, et al. The role of medial meniscus posterior root tear and proximal tibial morphology in the development of spontaneous osteonecrosis and osteoarthritis of the knee. Knee 2017;24(2):390–5.
58. Yao L, Stanczak J, Boutin RD. Presumptive subarticular stress reactions of the knee: MRI detection and association with meniscal tear patterns. Skeletal Radiol 2004;33(5):260–4.
59. LaPrade RF, Engebretsen AH, Ly TV, et al. The anatomy of the medial part of the knee. J Bone Joint Surg Am 2007;89(9):2000–10.
60. Hussain ZB, Chahla J, Mandelbaum BR, et al. The role of meniscal tears in spontaneous osteonecrosis of the knee: a systematic review of suspected etiology and a call to revisit nomenclature. Am J Sports Med 2019;47(2):501–7.

61. Lee DW, Ha JK, Kim JG. Medial meniscus posterior root tear: a comprehensive review. Knee Surg Relat Res 2014;26(3):125–34.
62. Seil R, Duck K, Pape D. A clinical sign to detect root avulsions of the posterior horn of the medial meniscus. Knee Surg Sports Traumatol Arthrosc 2011; 19(12):2072–5.
63. Hwang BY, Kim SJ, Lee SW, et al. Risk factors for medial meniscus posterior root tear. Am J Sports Med 2012;40(7):1606–10.
64. De Smet AA, Mukherjee R. Clinical, MRI, and arthroscopic findings associated with failure to diagnose a lateral meniscal tear on knee MRI. AJR Am J Roentgenol 2008;190(1):22–6.
65. Choi SH, Bae S, Ji SK, et al. The MRI findings of meniscal root tear of the medial meniscus: emphasis on coronal, sagittal and axial images. Knee Surg Sports Traumatol Arthrosc 2012;20(10):2098–103.
66. Lee SY, Jee WH, Kim JM. Radial tear of the medial meniscal root: reliability and accuracy of MRI for diagnosis. AJR Am J Roentgenol 2008;191(1):81–5.
67. Costa CR, Morrison WB, Carrino JA. Medial meniscus extrusion on knee MRI: is extent associated with severity of degeneration or type of tear? AJR Am J Roentgenol 2004;183(1):17–23.
68. LaPrade RF, LaPrade CM, James EW. Recent advances in posterior meniscal root repair techniques. J Am Acad Orthop Surg 2015;23(2):71–6.
69. Ozkoc G, Circi E, Gonc U, et al. Radial tears in the root of the posterior horn of the medial meniscus. Knee Surg Sports Traumatol Arthrosc 2008;16(9):849–54.
70. Kim JH, Chung JH, Lee DH, et al. Arthroscopic suture anchor repair versus pull-out suture repair in posterior root tear of the medial meniscus: a prospective comparison study. Arthroscopy 2011;27(12):1644–53.
71. Ahn JH, Lee YS, Yoo JC, et al. Results of arthroscopic all-inside repair for lateral meniscus root tear in patients undergoing concomitant anterior cruciate ligament reconstruction. Arthroscopy 2010;26(1):67–75.
72. Ahn JH, Wang JH, Yoo JC. Arthroscopic all-inside suture repair of medial meniscus lesion in anterior cruciate ligament–deficient knees: results of second-look arthroscopies in 39 cases. Arthroscopy 2004;20(9):936–45.
73. West R, Kim J, Armfield D, et al. Lateral meniscal root tears associated with anterior cruciate ligament injury: classification and management. Arthroscopy 2004; 20:32–3.
74. LaPrade CM, James EW, LaPrade RF. A modified transtibial pull-out repair for posterior root avulsions of the lateral meniscus with concomitant anterior cruciate ligament reconstruction: a report of two cases. JBJS Case Connect 2014; 4(4):e96.
75. Pan F, Hua S, Ma Z. Surgical treatment of combined posterior root tears of the lateral meniscus and ACL tears. Med Sci Monit 2015;21:1345–9.
76. LaPrade RF, Matheny LM, Moulton SG, et al. Posterior meniscal root repairs: outcomes of an anatomic transtibial pull-out technique. Am J Sports Med 2017; 45(4):884–91.
77. Ahn JH, Wang JH, Lim HC, et al. Double transosseous pull out suture technique for transection of posterior horn of medial meniscus. Arch Orthop Trauma Surg 2009;129(3):387–92.
78. Griffith CJ, LaPrade RF, Fritts HM, et al. Posterior root avulsion fracture of the medial meniscus in an adolescent female patient with surgical reattachment. Am J Sports Med 2008;36(4):789–92.

79. Kim YM, Rhee KJ, Lee JK, et al. Arthroscopic pullout repair of a complete radial tear of the tibial attachment site of the medial meniscus posterior horn. Arthroscopy 2006;22(7):795.e1-4.
80. Marzo JM, Kumar BA. Primary repair of medial meniscal avulsions: 2 case studies. Am J Sports Med 2007;35(8):1380–3.
81. Feucht MJ, Kuhle J, Bode G, et al. Arthroscopic transtibial pullout repair for posterior medial meniscus root tears: a systematic review of clinical, radiographic, and second-look arthroscopic results. Arthroscopy 2015;31(9):1808–16.
82. Moon HK, Koh YG, Kim YC, et al. Prognostic factors of arthroscopic pull-out repair for a posterior root tear of the medial meniscus. Am J Sports Med 2012; 40(5):1138–43.
83. LaPrade CM, Foad A, Smith SD, et al. Biomechanical consequences of a nonanatomic posterior medial meniscal root repair. Am J Sports Med 2015;43(4): 912–20.
84. Steineman BD, LaPrade RF, Santangelo KS, et al. Early osteoarthritis after untreated anterior meniscal root tears: an in vivo animal study. Orthop J Sports Med 2017;5(4). 2325967117702452.
85. Pache S, Aman ZS, Kennedy M, et al. Meniscal root tears: current concepts review. Arch Bone Jt Surg 2018;6(4):250–9.
86. Claret G, Montanana J, Rios J, et al. The effect of percutaneous release of the medial collateral ligament in arthroscopic medial meniscectomy on functional outcome. Knee 2016;23(2):251–5.
87. Fakioglu O, Ozsoy MH, Ozdemir HM, et al. Percutaneous medial collateral ligament release in arthroscopic medial meniscectomy in tight knees. Knee Surg Sports Traumatol Arthrosc 2013;21(7):1540–5.
88. Todor A, Caterev S, Nistor DV. Outside-in deep medial collateral ligament release during arthroscopic medial meniscus surgery. Arthrosc Tech 2016;5(4):e781–5.
89. Chung KS, Ha JK, Ra HJ, et al. Does release of the superficial medial collateral ligament result in clinically harmful effects after the fixation of medial meniscus posterior root tears? Arthroscopy 2017;33(1):199–208.
90. Chahla J, Moulton SG, LaPrade CM, et al. Posterior meniscal root repair: the transtibial double tunnel pullout technique. Arthrosc Tech 2016;5(2):e291–6.
91. LaPrade CM, LaPrade MD, Turnbull TL, et al. Biomechanical evaluation of the transtibial pull-out technique for posterior medial meniscal root repairs using 1 and 2 transtibial bone tunnels. Am J Sports Med 2015;43(4):899–904.

Ramp Lesions
An Unrecognized Posteromedial Instability?

Bertrand Sonnery-Cottet, MD[a],*, Raphael Serra Cruz, MD[b,c,d],
Thais Dutra Vieira, MD[a], Rodrigo A. Goes, MD, MSc[b],
Adnan Saithna, MD[e,f]

KEYWORDS

- Ramp lesion • Hidden lesion • Meniscus • Meniscocapsular tear
- Meniscotibial ligament • Posteromedial corner • Meniscal instability • Meniscal tear

KEY POINTS

- Meniscal ramp lesions are a "hot topic" because of increasing recognition that they have important biomechanical consequences and also that they occur much more frequently than was previously understood.
- Historically, ramp lesions have been underdiagnosed because of the low sensitivity of MRI and inadequate visualization through standard arthroscopic anterior viewing portals.
- A systematic exploration of the posteromedial compartment of the knee via a trans-notch approach is needed to confirm or refute the presence of a meniscal ramp lesion.
- If left untreated, meniscal ramp lesions may contribute to residual anteroposterior instability in the anterior cruciate ligament–reconstructed knee and may also result in failure of meniscal repair.
- Recent epidemiologic data and definition of risk factors helps to inform an appropriate index of suspicion, identification, and adequate treatment of ramp lesions.

INTRODUCTION

Meniscal ramp lesions were studied by Hamberg and colleagues[1] in the 1980s but at that time were described only as "injuries of the posterior aspect of the medial

Disclosure Statement: B. Sonnery-Cottet receives royalties from, is a paid consultant for, receives research support from, and has made presentations for Arthrex. A. Saithna is a paid consultant for Arthrex Inc.
[a] Centre Orthopédique Santy, FIFA Medical Centre of Excellence, Groupe Ramsay-Générale de Santé, Hôpital Privé Jean Mermoz, 24 Avenue Paul Santy, Lyon 69008, France; [b] Instituto Nacional de Traumatologia e Ortopedia, 500 Avendia Brasil, Caju, Rio de Janeiro, 20940-070, Brazil; [c] Hospital São Vicente de Paulo, Rio de Janeiro, Rio de Janeiro, Brazil; [d] Instituto Brasil de Tecnologias da Saúde, Rio de Janeiro, Rio de Janeiro, Brazil; [e] Sano Orthopedics, 2000 SE Blue Pkwy, Kansas City, MO 64063, USA; [f] Department of Specialty Medicine (Trauma & Orthopedic Surgery), Kansas City University, Kansas City, MO, USA
* Corresponding author.
E-mail address: sonnerycottet@aol.com

meniscus." Later, Strobel[2] introduced the term *ramp lesion* and characterized the injury as a longitudinal tear, 2.5 cm in length, located at the meniscocapsular junction. In 1991, Morgan[3] described a surgical technique for arthroscopic repair of ramp lesions using a suture hook through a posteromedial portal, and in 2004 Ahn and colleagues[4] reported a series providing clinical outcomes of repair.

Despite this long history of recognition of ramp lesions, the topic has been infrequently studied over the past few decades, until a recent resurgence in interest. This lack of prior importance attributed to the topic is likely a consequence of an underestimation of their incidence due to a high rate of missed diagnoses, insufficient knowledge about their biomechanical consequences, and an intuitive sense that these lesions could heal spontaneously. The recent interest in these injuries heralds an increasing recognition of their importance and an emerging concept of their association with posteromedial knee instability. The contemporary literature describes these injuries as tears at the posterior meniscocapsular junction and/or tears of the posterior meniscotibial ligament.[5–8] The expression "hidden lesion," also has been recently used to describe this injury, and the term refers to the difficulty in identifying ramp lesions from standard anterior arthroscopic portals,[6,9] and also with preoperative MRI, which has low sensititvty.[10–12]

Ramp lesions are hypothesized to occur through a number of possible mechanisms. The most simple is as a result of high forces transmitted through the posteromedial capsule during valgus strain, internal rotation of the tibia, and axial loading at the time of an anterior cruciate ligament (ACL) injury.[9] The contrecoup injury mechanism,[13] a compensatory varus alignment and internal rotation of the femur after the initial pivot-shift mechanism, also offers a potential mechanism because it results in impaction between the medial femoral condyle and the medial aspect of the tibial plateau, thus trapping the meniscus. Similarly, Hughston[14] also suggested these lesions could occur as a result of the meniscus becoming trapped between the femur and tibia, but attributed this to the increased anterior tibial translation that occurs as a result of an ACL injury. Hughston[14] and others[9,13,15] have also suggested a potentially important role for the semimembranosus muscle-tendon complex, which in cadaveric study has been found to have a firm attachment to the medial meniscocapsular area in most specimens (86%).[16] This close anatomic relationship between the semimembranosus tendon and the meniscocapsular region often can be visualized at the time of ramp repair (**Fig. 1**). It is hypothesized that contraction of the semimembranosus, secondary to excessive anterior translation of the tibia during an ACL tear or the subsequent contrecoup mechanism may stress this posteromedial area, resulting in a meniscocapsular tear ± meniscotibial ligament injury and posteromedial instability.[14,16]

The emerging concept of ramp lesions representing a posteromedial instability is based on increasing recognition of the potentially important role of these injuries in knee stability. Ahn and colleagues[17] and Peltier and colleagues[18] have demonstrated an increase in anteroposterior instability in ACL-deficient cadaveric knees on creation of ramp lesions and others have also demonstrated significant increases in both internal[18] and external[18,19] rotation laxity at all knee flexion angles on creation of ramp lesions ± meniscotibial ligament injuries. Peltier and colleagues[18] concluded that these lesions appear to play a significant role in knee stability and also that ramp lesions increase the forces in the ACL. These reports are further supported with the work of numerous other investigators who have demonstrated that isolated ACL reconstruction fails to restore normal joint kinematics and results in residual laxity in the presence of a ramp lesion.[4,18,19] Furthermore, it has been demonstrated that repair

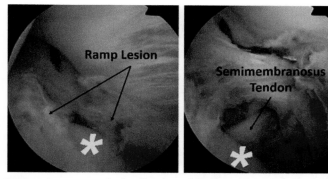

Fig. 1. Arthroscopic trans-notch visualization of the posteromedial compartment of the left knee (* = posteromedial tibial plateau). Retraction of the ramp lesion using an arthroscopy probe placed through the posteromedial portal reveals the close anatomic relationship between the semimembranosus tendon and the meniscocapsular region.

of these lesions abolishes[17,19,20] the pathologic increase in laxity and therefore provides a biomechanical rationale for identifying and repairing these lesions.

Ramp lesions are reported to occur frequently (9.3%–24.0%) in ACL-deficient knees, including in children and adolescents,[10,12,17,20,21] but Seil and colleagues[21] identified an even higher rate of 41% in those with a contact rather than noncontact mechanism of injury. Additional previously reported risk factors for the occurrence of ramp lesions in ACL-deficient knees include male gender, patients younger than 30 years, revision ACL reconstruction, chronic injuries, preoperative side-to-side anteroposterior laxity difference of 6 mm or more, and the presence of concomitant lateral meniscal tears.[22] The presence of any of these factors should raise the index of suspicion for the existence of a ramp lesion.

OBJECTIVE DIAGNOSIS

The accurate detection and treatment of these lesions is essential for restoring knee kinematics and abolishing residual knee laxity. When ramp lesions are overlooked in an ACL reconstruction, anteroposterior and rotational instabilities persist,[14,23,24] increasing the risk of failure of the reconstruction.[25] Because of the high incidence of ramp lesions, surgeons must be highly suspicious of this diagnosis when evaluating a patient with ACL rupture and be aware that there are no specific physical examination tests for ramp lesions.[26]

MRI can be helpful in the detection of a ramp lesion, but it is important to note that it has low to moderate sensitivity and a recognized rate of missed diagnoses.[12] Recently, a broad range of sensitivities of both 1.5T[25,27,28] and 3T[27,28] MRI for the detection of ramp lesions has been reported by DePhillipo and colleagues[27] (48%), Hatayama and colleagues[28] (71.7%), and Arner and colleagues[25] (53.9%–84.6%), with a high specificity (>90%).[25,28] The most specific sign in the MRI evaluation of ramp lesions is the hyperintense signal that can be observed between the meniscus and the capsule[29] **(Fig. 2)**. However, most acute knee MRI evaluations are performed with the knee in full extension, which reduces the meniscocapsular gap, and can lead to false-negative tests.[29] The MRI detected presence of bone bruising in the postero-medial tibial plateau has also been associated with ramp lesions, at a rate

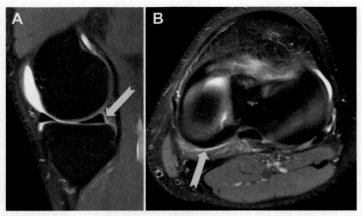

Fig. 2. T2-weighted MRI. (*A*) Sagittal section showing a hyperintense signal in the posterior meniscocapsular junction of the medial meniscus (*arrow*). (*B*) Axial section showing the same lesion (*arrow*). Observe the difficulty in establishing this diagnosis only by conventional imaging.

that varies from 38.5% for Hatayama and colleagues,[28] 66.3% for Kumar and colleagues,[30] and 72.0% for DePhillipo and colleagues.[27]

Arthroscopy is considered gold standard for diagnosis of ramp lesions.[6] However, it is not without pitfalls.[28] Forty percent of ramp lesions are not identified through standard anterior portal visualization and inspection of the posterior compartment via a trans-notch view, and posteromedial probing is required to identify them.[6,7] This is of particular importance, because these missed tears are repairable.[6,31]

CLASSIFICATION

Ramp lesions may be classified into 5 types according to their morphology[7] (**Fig. 3**):

Type 1: Meniscocapsular lesions. These lesions are very peripherally located in the synovial sheath. Mobility at probing is very low.

Type 2: Partial superior lesions. These lesions are stable and can be diagnosed only by a trans-notch approach. Mobility at probing is low.

Type 3: Partial inferior or *hidden lesions.* The lesions are typically subtle or not immediately visible even with trans-notch visualization but can be strongly suggested by significant mobility on probing and also by identification of abnormal tissue quality on needling.[5]

Type 4: A complete tear of the red-red zone. Mobility at probing is very high.

Type 5: A double tear involving the meniscocapsular junction and a second more anterior tear of the posterior horn.

TREATMENT OPTIONS

As these lesions occur, by definition, in a well-vascularized zone, isolated tears that are small (less than 10 mm) and stable may amenable to conservative treatment.[32] If these conditions are not met, suture of the tear is recommended. One of the most popular surgical techniques for treating meniscal ramp lesions is the use of a posteromedial portal suture hook device. This is used to pass a suture through the injured

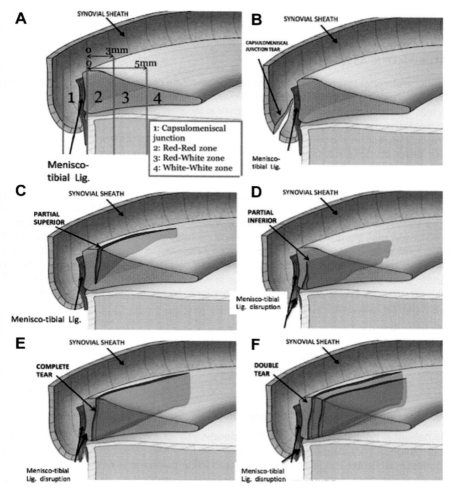

Fig. 3. Ramp lesion classification as proposed by Thaunat and colleagues.[7] (*A*) Illustration demonstrating the posterior meniscus-capsular region and the areas of meniscus vascularization. (*B*) Type 1: Meniscocapsular lesion, located in the synovial sheath. (*C*) Type 2: Upper partial lesion. (*D*) Type 3: Lower lesion ("hidden lesion"). (*E*) Type 4: Complete injury in the red-red area. (*F*) Type 5: Double tear. Lig., ligament. (*From* Thaunat M, Fayard JM, Guimaraes TM, Jan N, Murphy CG, Sonnery-Cottet B. Classification and Surgical Repair of Ramp Lesions of the Medial Meniscus. *Arthroscopy techniques.* Aug 2016;5(4):e871-e875; with permission.)

area, which is then tied with sliding knots (described later in this article). More recently, some investigators have proposed alternative treatments like a classic all-inside suture technique[33] or even abrasion and trephination of stable lesions (without repair), when they measure less than 1.5 cm, at the time an ACL reconstruction.[32] Although these studies provide important information, they do not provide sufficient evidence to guide optimal treatment. In contrast, some surgeons have suggested that acute repair is necessary for ramp lesions because the capsular portion of the torn meniscus has a tendency to retract inferiorly, away from the tibial plateau, making it less likely for the tissue to heal spontaneously, thus requiring a specific posteromedial approach for the repair.[4]

ARTHROSCOPIC ASSESSMENT

An important characteristic of the ramp lesion and one of the reasons why it has been underdiagnosed over the years is the difficulty in observing the tear via classic anterior portals, because the medial femoral condyle is located between the arthroscope and the posterior meniscocapsular junction, where it occurs.[6] This is particularly true in varus knees and in those knees with a tight medial compartment. Some strategies have been proposed to improve visualization of the posteromedial aspect of the knee, including the use of a leg holder for joint distraction along with a large inflow cannula[34]; or pie crusting of the medial collateral ligament.[35] Despite application of these techniques, the view of the peripheral area of the meniscus remains restricted.[6] To better assess this region, a trans-notch approach is recommended because it provides better visualization of the posterior meniscocapsular junction.[6,7] Although a ramp lesion may be suspected by increased mobility of the meniscus, it is essential to perform a direct visualization of the posterior meniscocapsular junction, because some of these tears (types I and II) may seem stable when inspected through anterior portals, even after probing.[7] Observing this scenario, Sonnery-Cottet and colleagues[6] have proposed a systematic arthroscopic exploration of the knee joint,[6,7] using a 30° scope, which includes 4 steps:

Step 1: Standard arthroscopic exploration
Step 2: Exploration of posteromedial compartment and probing the meniscocapsular junction with a needle
Step 3: Creation of a posteromedial portal
Step 4: Meniscal repair procedure

Step 1: Standard Arthroscopic Exploration

The patient is positioned supine on the operating table with a tourniquet applied high on the thigh. A foot support is used to maintain the knee at 90° of flexion during the procedure, while allowing it to be manipulated through full range of motion, as needed (**Fig. 4**). A standard high lateral parapatellar portal is created for visualization with the arthroscope, while a medial parapatellar portal is created for instrumentation.

The presence of a meniscal tear is then evaluated by meticulous probing of the meniscal tissue. The mobility of the meniscus at probing may lead the surgeon to suspect the presence of a posterior tear even if it is not visible by standard anterior viewing, because ramp lesions classified as types III, IV, and V may be highly mobile when pulled.

Step 2: Exploration of Posteromedial Compartment and Probing the Meniscocapsular Junction with a Needle

Trans-notch visualization of the posteromedial compartment is performed. The arthroscope is introduced in the anterolateral portal with the knee positioned at 90° of flexion and then advanced through a triangle limited by the medial femoral condyle, the posterior cruciate ligament, and the tibial spines (**Fig. 5**A). To facilitate the passage through this space, a valgus force is applied (**Fig. 5**B) first in extension and then in flexion. If passage remains difficult, the use of a blunt trocar may be helpful. Tibial internal rotation may improve visualization of the tear by causing posterior tibial plateau subluxation and a posterior translation of the medial segment. With this maneuver,

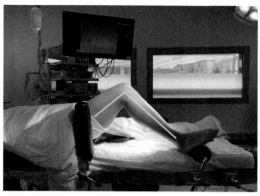

Fig. 4. Positioning of the patient on the operating table, with a support under the ipsilateral foot, sustaining the knee at 90° of flexion during the procedure while allowing it to be manipulated as needed.

two-thirds of the peripheral lesions from the posterior segment up to the middle segment can be seen (**Fig. 5C**).[36] In this position, the 30° optical lens may be adjusted for optimal visualization of the meniscocapsular junction to assess the presence of a ramp lesion without the need for a 70° scope.[7] The posterior horn of the medial meniscus can then be explored with a needle to detect a ramp lesion. With the arthroscope positioned in the trans-notch view, transillumination allows the surgeon to observe the nerves and veins that must be avoided. The knee is positioned at 90° of flexion to minimize the risk of injury to neurovascular structures and a needle is introduced above the hamstring tendons, 1 cm posterior to the medial tibiofemoral joint line, pointing toward the lesion (**Fig. 6**). A hidden lesion (type 3) may be found by dissecting the synovial tissue with the needle over the tear. This type of lesion may be suspected, by holding an appropriate index of suspicion based on the presence of risk factors and also if the surgeon notes high mobility of the meniscus at probing during the standard anterior portal arthroscopic evaluation.

Step 3: Creation of a Posteromedial Portal

After arthroscopically checking the adequate placement of the guiding needle via trans-notch view (**Fig. 7**A), the needle is removed and a No. 11 scalpel is then used

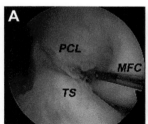
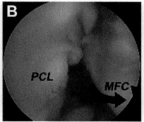
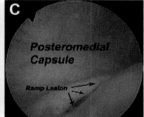

Fig. 5. Arthroscopic view with a 30° scope of a right knee through the anterolateral portal. (*A*) Probe is inserted through the anteromedial portal in the space between the posterior cruciate ligament (PCL) and the medial femoral condyle (MFC). (*B*) Passage of the arthroscope through the space between the PCL and the MFC after a valgus force is applied. (*C*) Image obtained via trans-notch visualization of the posteromedial region of the knee, observing the posteromedial capsule and the meniscal ramp lesion. TS, tibial spine.

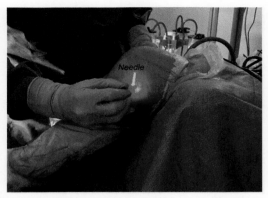

Fig. 6. External image of the knee demonstrating how transillumination with the arthroscope positioned in the trans-notch view helps avoiding neurovascular structures during the creation of the posteromedial portal.

to make a small incision over the posteromedial skin and capsule (**Fig. 7**B), creating the posteromedial portal. There is no need for a cannula.

Step 4: Meniscal Repair Procedure

We describe a technique for repair of ramp lesions by the placement of all-inside sutures with the aid of a curved suture hook device (**Fig. 8**), introduced through the posteromedial portal. A left curved hook device is used for a right knee and vice-versa. After correct identification of the tear and debridement of its edges with a shaver (**Fig. 9**A) or a meniscal rasp, the curved hook device loaded with a No. 0 absorbable monofilament suture (polydioxanone) is introduced through the posteromedial portal (**Fig. 9**B). It is then manipulated to make the sharp tip penetrate the peripheral wall of the medial meniscus from outside to inside (**Fig. 9**C) and then penetrate the inner portion of the tear so that both parts are held together (**Fig. 9**D). The suture is then progressed through the device. A grasper is used to retrieve the free end of the suture via the posteromedial portal (**Fig. 9**E). A sliding knot is tied with the aid of a knot pusher (**Fig. 9**F) and then cut. It is the preference of the authors to place sutures at a distance of 10 mm apart, beginning at the most posterior aspect of the tear to the most anterior one (**Fig 10**). Internal rotation of the foot helps keep the medial femoral

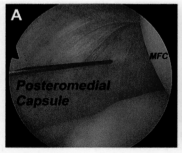
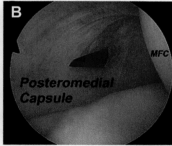

Fig. 7. Arthroscopic image through trans-notch vision showing 2 steps for the creation of the posteromedial portal. (*A*) Insertion of the needle to verify the correct positioning of the portal and (*B*) creation of the posteromedial portal with a no. 11 scalpel. MFC, medial femoral condyle.

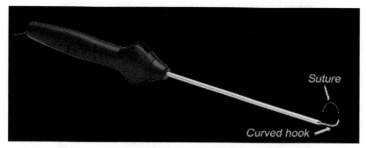

Fig. 8. Image of a curved hook device, with the tip curvature pointing to the left side (ideal for suturing meniscal ramp lesion on a right knee).

condyle away from the posterior segment of the meniscus and facilitates the procedure. After an adequate number of sutures are placed, stabilization of the ramp lesion is tested by probing, with the knee positioned in extension and valgus. If the tear extends anteriorly through the posterior horn and/or body of the meniscus, it should be repaired with the surgeon's preferred technique.

REHABILITATION PROTOCOL

There is no consensus in the literature regarding rehabilitation following ramp repair. Most investigators choose to use their standard ACL rehabilitation protocol.[6,10,31,37] In the case of isolated ramp lesions, a standard meniscal repair rehabilitation protocol should be followed.[31] Most protocols agree that early knee motion is beneficial; however, knee hyperflexion is associated with anterior tibial translation, which can increase the stress on the repair.[12] In our practice, the postoperative management of an ACL

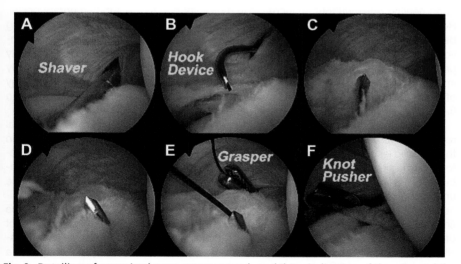

Fig. 9. Detailing of a meniscal ramp suture procedure. (*A*) Revitalization of the edges of the lesion using a shaver. (*B*) Suture device inserted through the posteromedial portal. (*C*) Penetration of the peripheral edge of the lesion. (*D*) Penetration of the suture device through the inner portion of the tear, encompassing both ends of the lesion. (*E*) Progression of the suture, which is then captured out of the knee with the aid of a grasper. (*F*) First stitch being completed using a knot pusher.

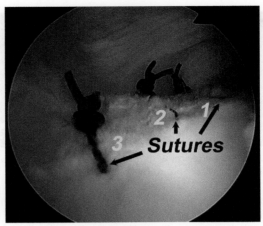

Fig. 10. Final arthroscopic aspect of a meniscal ramp repair, as seen by trans-notch view, in which 3 stitches were required to close the lesion. Numbers represent the sequence of suturing.

reconstruction associated with ramp repair is modified by restriction of the active and passive range of motion to 0 to 90° of flexion during the first 6 weeks. Progression to full weight bearing is allowed by postoperative week 3. Jogging is permitted after week 12 to 16, pivot activity at 6 months, and full activity at 9 months for all patients.[36]

OUTCOMES

Although several investigators have reported clinical outcomes of repair of ramp lesions, the number of publications is fairly limited.[4,10,22,36,38] Jan and colleagues[39] reported that arthroscopic suture hook repair via a posteromedial portal provides good healing rates without an increase in morbidity due to the supplementary portal. Reported failure rates range from 2.6%[4] to 12.0%,[38] with 30% of failures occurring between 2[17] and 4 years after the index procedure.[22,40] Typically the new lesion involves a smaller and more central part of the meniscus, anterior to the previously passed sutures. Often there is the appearance of a "postage-stamp" effect, possibly implicating the suture hook and/or presence of nonabsorbable sutures in the etiology of the new lesion.[39] However, this pattern leads to a smaller secondary resection than had partial meniscectomy been performed initially.[41]

It is a well-recognized phenomenon that there is an increased failure rate of meniscal repairs in ACL-deficient knees due to abnormal knee kinematics and excessive loads on the repaired lesion.[40,42] It is therefore unsurprising to note that the secondary meniscectomy rate is significantly reduced (twofold) in those patients who have undergone a combined ACLR and anterolateral ligament reconstruction (ALLR) when compared with those undergoing isolated ACLR. This is because isolated ACLR fails to restore normal knee kinematics in those knees in which a combined ACL and anterolateral injury exists.[43] These findings support the results of previous study that has demonstrated the protective effect of ALLR on medial meniscal repairs.[22,38] In addition, it is valuable to recognize the possibility that the important biomechanical consequences of these injuries may risk a greater failure rate of ACL grafts in knees with unrepaired ramp lesions.[37]

SUMMARY

Meniscal ramp lesions are common but frequently underrecognized in the ACL-injured knee. It is important to highlight that both preoperative MRI and arthroscopic evaluation via classic anterior portals are associated with high rates of missed diagnoses. For that reason, a systematic exploration of the posteromedial compartment is advocated in all ACL-injured knees. Failure to recognize and repair ramp lesions is associated with persistent anterior and rotational knee laxity, suggesting it makes part of a posteromedial instability, in the setting of an ACL tear. Concomitant suture repair of these lesions, via a posteromedial portal, can restore normal biomechanics and is associated with excellent clinical outcomes.

AUTHORS' OPINION

Interesting fact: All over the world, in orthopedic meetings, the meniscal root lesion is more extensively debated than the ramp lesion. This is despite the fact that ramp lesions are a lot more common (24% in ACLR in our experience). This greater focus on root tears is perhaps because of the well-recognized loss of hoop force distribution and profound biomechanical consequences of root tears. However, it is increasingly recognized that ramp lesions also have important biomechanical consequences including persistent anteroposterior (AP) and rotational laxity and an association with higher ACL graft failure rates. It is the authors' opinion that ramp lesions require further study and greater attention because of their underrecognized role in posteromedial knee instability.

Changing patterns: The authors have observed a decrease in the failure rate for all types of medial meniscus suture repair since 2012, from 25% to 7%, with a mean follow-up of 5 years. This observation is attributed to the systematic exploration of the posteromedial compartment, allowing us to discover and repair these previously underrecognized ramp lesions. It is our opinion that the lower rate of failure of all types of medial meniscus repair is a function of improved knee kinematics, through abolishing the greater AP and rotational laxity associated with ramp lesions and also due to the better quality of repair as a result of improved lesion access and debridement via a posteromedial portal.

Technical Tip: When evaluating the posteromedial compartment, it is important to avoid missed diagnoses of hidden lesions. There are tears in which the superior surface often appears subtlety abnormal but the tear is not apparent unless it is probed with a needle and the intact superficial fibers are separated revealing the ramp lesion.

REFERENCES

1. Hamberg P, Gillquist J, Lysholm J. Suture of new and old peripheral meniscus tears. J Bone Joint Surg Am 1983;65(2):193–7.
2. Strobel MJ. Menisci. Manual of arthroscopic surgery. New York: Springer; 1988. p. 171–8.
3. Morgan CD. The "all-inside" meniscus repair. Arthroscopy 1991;7(1):120–5.
4. Ahn JH, Kim SH, Yoo JC, et al. All-inside suture technique using two posteromedial portals in a medial meniscus posterior horn tear. Arthroscopy 2004;20(1):101–8.
5. Smigielski R, Becker R, Zdanowicz U, et al. Medial meniscus anatomy-from basic science to treatment. Knee Surg Sports Traumatol Arthrosc 2015;23(1):8–14.
6. Sonnery-Cottet B, Conteduca J, Thaunat M, et al. Hidden lesions of the posterior horn of the medial meniscus: a systematic arthroscopic exploration of the concealed portion of the knee. Am J Sports Med 2014;42(4):921–6.
7. Thaunat M, Fayard JM, Guimaraes TM, et al. Classification and surgical repair of ramp lesions of the medial meniscus. Arthrosc Tech 2016;5(4):e871–5.

8. Pedersen RR. The medial and posteromedial ligamentous and capsular structures of the knee: review of anatomy and relevant imaging findings. Semin Musculoskelet Radiol 2016;20(1):12–25.

9. Laprade RF. The Menisci—a comprehensive review of their anatomy, biomechanical function and surgical treatment. Springer-Verlag Berlin Heidelberg; 2017.

10. Liu X, Feng H, Zhang H, et al. Arthroscopic prevalence of ramp lesion in 868 patients with anterior cruciate ligament injury. Am J Sports Med 2011;39(4): 832–7.

11. Seil R, VanGiffen N, Pape D. Thirty years of arthroscopic meniscal suture: what's left to be done? Orthop Traumatol Surg Res 2009;95(8 Suppl 1):S85–96.

12. Bollen SR. Posteromedial meniscocapsular injury associated with rupture of the anterior cruciate ligament: a previously unrecognised association. J Bone Joint Surg Br 2010;92(2):222–3.

13. Yoon KH, Yoo JH, Kim KI. Bone contusion and associated meniscal and medial collateral ligament injury in patients with anterior cruciate ligament rupture. J Bone Joint Surg Am 2011;93(16):1510–8.

14. Hughston JC. Knee ligaments: injury and repair. Saint Louis (MO): Mosby; 1993.

15. Smith JP 3rd, Barrett GR. Medial and lateral meniscal tear patterns in anterior cruciate ligament-deficient knees. A prospective analysis of 575 tears. Am J Sports Med 2001;29(4):415–9.

16. DePhillipo NN, Moatshe G, Chahla J, et al. Quantitative and qualitative assessment of the posterior medial meniscus anatomy: defining meniscal ramp lesions. Am J Sports Med 2019;47(2):372–8.

17. Ahn JH, Bae TS, Kang KS, et al. Longitudinal tear of the medial meniscus posterior horn in the anterior cruciate ligament-deficient knee significantly influences anterior stability. Am J Sports Med 2011;39(10):2187–93.

18. Peltier A, Lording T, Maubisson L, et al. The role of the meniscotibial ligament in posteromedial rotational knee stability. Knee Surg Sports Traumatol Arthrosc 2015;23(10):2967–73.

19. Stephen JM, Halewood C, Kittl C, et al. Posteromedial meniscocapsular lesions increase tibiofemoral joint laxity with anterior cruciate ligament deficiency, and their repair reduces laxity. Am J Sports Med 2016;44(2):400–8.

20. Reider B. Ramped up. Am J Sports Med 2017;45(5):1001–3.

21. Seil R, Mouton C, Coquay J, et al. Ramp lesions associated with ACL injuries are more likely to be present in contact injuries and complete ACL tears. Knee Surg Sports Traumatol Arthrosc 2018;26(4):1080–5.

22. Sonnery-Cottet B, Praz C, Rosenstiel N, et al. Epidemiological evaluation of meniscal ramp lesions in 3214 anterior cruciate ligament-injured knees from the SANTI Study Group Database: a risk factor analysis and study of secondary meniscectomy rates following 769 ramp repairs. Am J Sports Med 2018;46(13): 3189–97.

23. Noyes FR, Chen RC, Barber-Westin SD, et al. Greater than 10-year results of red-white longitudinal meniscal repairs in patients 20 years of age or younger. Am J Sports Med 2011;39(5):1008–17.

24. Mariani PP. Posterior horn instability of the medial meniscus a sign of posterior meniscotibial ligament insufficiency. Knee Surg Sports Traumatol Arthrosc 2011;19(7):1148–53.

25. Arner JW, Herbst E, Burnham JM, et al. MRI can accurately detect meniscal ramp lesions of the knee. Knee Surg Sports Traumatol Arthrosc 2017;25(12):3955–60.

26. Bronstein RD, Schaffer JC. Physical examination of the knee: meniscus, cartilage, and patellofemoral conditions. J Am Acad Orthop Surg 2017;25(5):365–74.

27. DePhillipo NN, Cinque ME, Chahla J, et al. Incidence and detection of meniscal ramp lesions on magnetic resonance imaging in patients with anterior cruciate ligament reconstruction. Am J Sports Med 2017;45(10):2233–7.

28. Hatayama K, Terauchi M, Saito K, et al. Magnetic resonance imaging diagnosis of medial meniscal ramp lesions in patients with anterior cruciate ligament injuries. Arthroscopy 2018;34(5):1631–7.

29. Hash TW 2nd. Magnetic resonance imaging of the knee. Sports Health 2013;5(1): 78–107.

30. Kumar NS, Spencer T, Cote MP, et al. Is edema at the posterior medial tibial plateau indicative of a ramp lesion? an examination of 307 patients with anterior cruciate ligament reconstruction and medial meniscal tears. Orthop J Sports Med 2018;6(6). 2325967118780089.

31. Chahla J, Dean CS, Moatshe G, et al. Meniscal ramp lesions: anatomy, incidence, diagnosis, and treatment. Orthop J Sports Med 2016;4(7). 2325967116657815.

32. Liu X, Feng H, Hong L, et al. A prospective randomized control trial of arthroscopic surgery for stable ramp lesion of the medial meniscus. Zhonghua Wai Ke Za Zhi 2017;55(3):161–5 [in Chinese].

33. Chen Z, Li WP, Yang R, et al. Meniscal ramp lesion repair using the FasT-fix technique: evaluating healing and patient outcomes with second-look arthroscopy. J Knee Surg 2018;31(8):710–5.

34. Carson WG Jr. Arthroscopic techniques to improve access to posterior meniscal lesions. Clin Sports Med 1990;9(3):619–32.

35. Fakioglu O, Ozsoy MH, Ozdemir HM, et al. Percutaneous medial collateral ligament release in arthroscopic medial meniscectomy in tight knees. Knee Surg Sports Traumatol Arthrosc 2013;21(7):1540–5.

36. Thaunat M, Jan N, Fayard JM, et al. Repair of meniscal ramp lesions through a posteromedial portal during anterior cruciate ligament reconstruction: outcome study with a minimum 2-year follow-up. Arthroscopy 2016;32(11):2269–77.

37. Li WP, Chen Z, Song B, et al. The FasT-fix repair technique for ramp lesion of the medial meniscus. Case Rep Orthop 2015;27(1):56–60.

38. Sonnery-Cottet B, Saithna A, Blakeney WG, et al. Anterolateral ligament reconstruction protects the repaired medial meniscus: a comparative study of 383 anterior cruciate ligament reconstructions from the SANTI Study Group with a minimum follow-up of 2 years. Am J Sports Med 2018;46(8):1819–26.

39. Jan N, Sonnery-Cottet B, Fayard JM, et al. Complications in posteromedial arthroscopic suture of the medial meniscus. Orthop Traumatol Surg Res 2016;102(8s): S287–93.

40. Rochecongar G, Plaweski S, Azar M, et al. Management of combined anterior or posterior cruciate ligament and posterolateral corner injuries: a systematic review. Orthop Traumatol Surg Res 2014;100(8 Suppl):S371–8.

41. Pujol N, Beaufils P. Healing results of meniscal tears left in situ during anterior cruciate ligament reconstruction: a review of clinical studies. Knee Surg Sports Traumatol Arthrosc 2009;17(4):396–401.

42. Duchman KR, Westermann RW, Spindler KP, et al. The fate of meniscus tears left in situ at the time of anterior cruciate ligament reconstruction: a 6-year follow-up study from the MOON Cohort. Am J Sports Med 2015;43(11):2688–95.

43. Inderhaug E, Stephen JM, Williams A, et al. Anterolateral tenodesis or anterolateral ligament complex reconstruction: effect of flexion angle at graft fixation when combined with ACL reconstruction. Am J Sports Med 2017;45(13):3089–97.

Meniscus Scaffolds for Partial Meniscus Defects

Francesca de Caro, MD[a], Francesco Perdisa, MD[b], Aad Dhollander, MD, PT, PhD[c],
Rene Verdonk, MD, PhD[d], Peter Verdonk, MD, PhD[e],*

KEYWORDS

• Meniscus • Scaffold • Actifit • CMI • Meniscectomy

KEY POINTS

• Meniscus scaffolds represent a safe and viable treatment for symptomatic partial meniscus defects in the well-aligned, stable knee with limited cartilage degeneration.
• Meniscus scaffolds provide significant improvement of clinical outcome at short and midterm follow-up, with an acceptable failure rate and complication rate.
• In most cases, MRI shows a reduced size of the implant, with hyperintense signal. The clinical relevance remains unclear.
• The chondroprotective effect of meniscus scaffolds remains to be proven.

INTRODUCTION

Meniscectomy is one of the most common procedures in orthopedic surgery, capable of returning the knee to a satisfactory function when a meniscal tear occurs.[1] However, over the years, several concerns have arisen about its detrimental effects on the joint status in the medium to long term. It is now acknowledged that loss of meniscal tissue permanently alters knee biomechanics and homeostasis with secondary degenerative changes to the articular cartilage and higher risk of developing symptomatic osteoarthritis (OA).[2] Hence, meniscus repair and substitution have gained significant interest. Unfortunately, the effectiveness of meniscal repair strictly relies on the tissue quality and defect location with respect to the vascular supply; tears in the vascularized "red" peripheral zone are more likely to heal, whereas the more common lesions in the avascular "white" zone have poor healing potential.[3–7] Unfortunately, meniscectomy is unavoidable in more than 90% of cases.

[a] Department of Orthopaedic Surgery, Humanitas Castelli, via Mazzini, n. 11, Bergamo, Italy; [b] SC Chirurgia Protesica dei Reimpianti di Anca e di Ginocchio, IRCCS Istituto Ortopedico Rizzoli, via di Barbiano, Bologna 40136, Italy; [c] Department of Orthopaedic Surgery, KLINA Hospital, Augustijnslei 100, Brasschaat 2930, Belgium; [d] Department of Orthopaedic Surgery, Universite Libre de Bruxelles, Avenue Franklin Roosevelt 50, Bruxelles 1050, Belgium; [e] Orthoca, Kielsevest 14, Antwerp 2018, Belgium
* Corresponding author. Orthoca, Stevenslei 20, Deurne 2100, Belgium.
E-mail address: pverdonk@yahoo.com

Clin Sports Med 39 (2020) 83–92
https://doi.org/10.1016/j.csm.2019.08.011
0278-5919/20/© 2019 Elsevier Inc. All rights reserved.

In the past decades, alternative meniscus substitution strategies have been developed to replace symptomatic loss of meniscal tissue. Meniscal allograft transplantation and meniscus prostheses have been used to replace a complete or subtotal loss of meniscal substance, whereas scaffolds have been developed for segmental meniscus defects.[8,9] Meniscus allograft transplantation is a well-established procedure with extensive literature highlighting the results for long-term follow-up. However, the role and indication of a meniscus scaffold for the biological treatment of a segmental defect remain more controversial. The general goal is to save or replace the damaged meniscal tissue with the final goal to provide early pain relief, healing of the damaged or absent tissue, and prevention of secondary joint degeneration in the long term. The effectiveness of scaffolds in terms of clinical improvement and chondroprotection still can be improved. This narrative review aims at highlighting the current state of meniscus scaffold surgery and the advancements being made.

General Concept of the Meniscus Scaffold

Meniscus scaffolds are 3-dimensional biocompatible structures capable of supporting meniscuslike fibrocartilaginous tissue regeneration in segmental meniscus defects (**Fig. 1**). Two constructs for meniscal replacement are available on the market: the first is made of bovine collagen derived from purified bovine Achilles tendon with collagen fibers enriched with glycosaminoglycans to aid cellular ingrowth. The scaffold is highly bioresorbable (12–18 months) and highly porous (collagen meniscus implant [CMI]; Stryker, Kalamazoo, MI). The second more recent scaffold consists of a synthetic polyurethane-based material with flexible segments made from polycaprolactone 80% and stiff segments made from urethane 20% (Actifit; Orteq Sports Medicine, London, UK).[10] The scaffold is slowly biodegradable with an estimated degradation time of 4 to 6 years and is highly porous. Both implants come in a specific configuration for medial or lateral meniscus defects.

Indications and Contraindications

Meniscus scaffold implantation represents a novel biological solution for the treatment of patients with symptomatic partial meniscus defects with limited signs of cartilage degeneration. Since the negative impact of meniscectomy in anterior cruciate ligament (ACL)-injured knees on long-term cartilage degeneration has recently been established, prophylactic meniscus reconstruction using a scaffold in the ACL reconstructed knee with partial meniscectomy could be another indication.

The key inclusion criteria are (1) irreparable medial or lateral meniscal tear or partial meniscus loss with intact rim. The meniscus substitute is not intended for the treatment of total or subtotal meniscus defects; ideally, the defect length should be limited

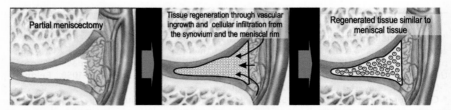

Fig. 1. Basic concept on meniscus scaffolds. The meniscus scaffold should be attached to the vascular rim of the meniscus. Cells derived from that rim and the synovium will grow into the scaffold and regenerate a hybrid tissue of fibrous and fibrochondrocytic mensicuslike tissue.

to 5 to 6 cm; (2) skeletally mature patients; (3) age 16 to 50 years; (4) stable knee joint or knee joint stabilization procedure within 12 weeks of index procedure; and (5) International Cartilage Repair Society (ICRS) classification $\leq$3.

The key exclusion criteria are (1) total meniscus loss or unstable segmental rim defect; (2) multiple areas of partial meniscus loss that could not be treated by a single scaffold; (3) any significant malalignment (varus or valgus); (4) ICRS classification greater than 3; and (5) body mass index $\geq$35. Of importance, the presence of condylar squaring, a structural phenomenon often observed years after meniscectomy, is to be considered a contraindication, as it becomes structurally impossible to introduce a triangular-shaped scaffold into a flattened joint line.

Surgical Technique

The surgical technique is similar for both the devices, involving the arthroscopic resection of the damaged tissue and subsequent implantation of a custom-sized, porous material, which is finally sutured to the meniscal rim and capsule using standard inside-out, outside-in, or all-inside sutures. A partial meniscectomy with surgical debridement back to the vascularized zone of the damaged portion of the meniscus is performed. The meniscus rim should be continuous, this is of particular importance to the popliteal hiatus of the lateral meniscus. In this area, a complete loss of the tissue in front of the popliteus tendon is often referred to as a partial defect but should be considered a total loss and is therefore a contraindication for a meniscus scaffold. After debridement, the resulting void is measured for sizing along the peripheral edge using the meniscal ruler guide and ruler supplied with the scaffold. The scaffold is cut to fit and using a blunt-nosed grasper, placed into the knee joint through the anteromedial or anterolateral portal and sutured to the native meniscus. The suturing techniques used are all-inside, inside-out, or outside-in depending on the area to be sutured and the surgeon's experience and preference.

Histologic Data

Histologic evidence of tissue ingrowth and regrowth remains scarce. The first clinical article describing histology after CMI was published in 2008 by Rodkey and colleagues.[11] Based on the histologic evaluations performed 1 year after implantation, the collagen meniscus implant appears to provide a scaffold for the formation of hybrid fibrous and meniscuslike fibrochondrocytic matrix by the host. In nearly all cases in which remnants of the CMI could be identified, there was evidence of infiltration into the interstices of the CMI with maturing fibrous connective tissue differentiating toward meniscuslike fibrochondrocytic tissue. All of these cases demonstrated some degree of assimilation of the CMI into a newly developing fibrochondrocytic matrix. Visual estimates indicated that approximately 10% to 25% of the CMI remained at 1 year. An incidental, rare finding (observed in <5% of the cases) was inflammation of the synovium in the biopsy specimen of the CMI, but none of these cases was associated with any clinical findings of synovitis at the time of the second-look arthroscopy.

An early publication 1 year after implantation of the polyurethane scaffold showed fully vital material with no signs of inflammatory reaction, necrosis, or cell death, illustrating that the scaffold is biocompatible and supports successful new tissue ingrowth.[12] Moreover, a distinct organization of tissue was observed, with 3 layers based on the presence or absence of vessel structures, cellular morphology, and extracellular matrix (ECM) composition. This particular organization with vascular and avascular tissue with a collagenous matrix resembles that of native human meniscus tissue. When comparing the biopsy findings of the inner free edge of the scaffold-meniscus with the native meniscus tissue, layer 1 resembles the peripheral red, vascularized zone typically rich in meniscus cells of the fusiform (fibroblastlike) cell type and thus rich in type I collagens. Layer 2 resembles the middle red-white zone of the native human meniscus containing a mixture of oval and polygonal fibro-chondroblastlike cells and fibroblastlike cells while being completely avascular. Layer 3 resembles the white or inner third zone with fibrochondroblastlike cells, character-ized by its avascularity; nevertheless, the observed ECM is still immature. This char-acteristic organization suggests that ingrowth is started superficially and that a maturation process occurs in an inbound direction. It should be noted, however, that fully mature meniscuslike tissue was not observed at the 12-month time-point. These clinical histologic results are supportive of data previously reported in animal studies that describe an active fibrovascular ingrowth derived from the synovium following total meniscal replacement with the meniscus implant.[13] Over time, this fibrovascular front slowly retracted, leaving behind tissue that resembled fibrocarti-lage within the scaffold.[13]

A recent comparative study reported that biopsy samples from the CMI group showed more fibrous tissue that was rich in spindle and rounded fibroblastlike cells and blood vessels.[14] The Actifit biopsy samples appeared completely avascular with more cartilaginouslike appearance consisting of chondroblastlike roundish, large, and active cells. Over time, there was a greater percentage of smaller cells that had completely differentiated into chondrocytes, surrounded by a capsule and inserted in gaps, with few cells displaying a typical columnar arrangement. All the biopsy sam-ples showed vital cell and matrix structures with no evidence of necrosis. In 3 of the 11 Actifit patients who underwent second-look arthroscopy, histologic evaluation showed presence of plasma cells, macrophages, and rare lymphocytes, which could be a result of foreign body reaction.

Clinical Outcome

Both implants, either based on collagen or polyurethane, showed promising short-term clinical results and stable satisfactory outcomes up to midterm and long-term evaluation. Clinical follow-up studies report outcomes for CMI ranging from 6 months to 12 years, whereas the longest clinical follow-up study on Actifit reports up to 8 years. Overall, significant improvement has been documented in all studies using a wide range of clinical outcome scores: Lysholm, Visual Analog Scale (VAS) pain, International Knee Documentation Committee (IKDC), Tegner, Knee injury and Osteoarthritis Outcome Score (KOOS), Cincinnati, a patient self-assessment scale and a satisfaction scale, EuroQol (EQ)-5D, Knee Society Score (KSS), University of California Los Angeles, Short Form (SF)-36, and an activity scale. Typically, patients will progressively improve over the first year with an approximate improvement of 30 points on Lysholm (maximum 100) and 3.5 points on the VAS score (maximum 10). These clinical results remain stable over time, although few studies report long-term clinical outcomes. Monllau and colleagues[15] reports 83% good and excellent results at 10-year follow-up for 22 patients treated with the CMI device. The typical 30 points improvement of the Lysholm score was present, improving from 59.9 (range, 30–90) to 89.6 (range, 78–100; $P<.001$) and 87.56 (range, 59–100; $P<.001$) at 1-year and 10-year follow-up, respectively. A significant improvement of all the clinical scores from preoperative status to final follow-up (9.6 years mean follow-up) was reported by Bulgheroni and colleagues[16] in a randomized trial aiming to compare the clinical, objective, and radiographic long-term results of patients with ACL rupture and partial medial meniscus defects treated with ACL reconstruc-tion and partial medial meniscectomy or medial CMI implant. Even if all the clinical scores increased over time, no statistically significant differences were found between these 2 groups. Zaffagnini and colleagues[17] report results in a prospective study evaluating patients treated with medial CMI implantation versus partial medial meniscectomy. The CMI group showed significantly lower VAS for pain, higher objective IKDC, and Tegner scores compared with the meniscectomy group at minimum 10-year follow-up. The SF-36 and Lyshom scores did not show a statistically significant differences between both groups. A recent meta-analysis on 613 Actifit patients reports that both VAS and Tegner scores improved significantly and remained stable up to 72 months. This suggests that stabilization of the pain allows activity level to remain unchanged over time.[10] Schüttler and colleagues[18] report on 18 Actifit patients with a follow-up of 4 years demonstrating significant improvement of VAS from 5 preoperatively to 1 at 4 years of follow-up. In a similar study by Leroy and colleagues[19] with a minimal follow-up of 5 years, 15 patients improved from 5.3 and 50 preoperative VAS and subjective IKDC scores respectively to 2.9 and 79 at a mean follow-up of 6 years (range 5–8 years). Another recent meta-analysis by Houck and colleagues[20] showed similar clinical outcome for both CMI and Actifit patients. The preoperative status of cartilage damage is proven to affect the clinical outcomes, irrespective of the type of scaffold used. It has been proven that cartilage damage should not exceed ICRS grade 2 to obtain predictable results after meniscal implantation.

Scaffold implantation along with concomitant procedures does not influence clinical outcome, and often implicates a slower recovery. Some investigators therefore do not recommend to proceed to combine surgeries, such as ACL reconstruction or high tibial osteotomies.[21] It is still debated whether patients with an acute lesion or those with a chronic lesion (previous surgeries in the treated knee) have better results. These controversial findings can be explained by the rapid clinical improvement offered by a simple meniscectomy, but current evidence tends to support the use of meniscal scaffolds for chronic lesions, with better clinical outcomes at longer follow-up. A small number of complications has been reported with a total rate of 12.6%.[10] These include pain, effusion, infections, suture removals, debridement of nonintegrated scaffold, tear of tissue scaffold, nerve branch included in a suture, and excessive scar tissue formation. Failures are variously defined in each article, going from infection due to the implant, mechanical blocking, or chronic synovitis. Most investigators consider a failure any unplanned second operation on the index knee including but not limited to implant removal, osteotomies, and total joint arthroplasty. The lack of a commonly accepted definition of failure makes a comparison of failed patients among different studies very difficult and a meaningful analysis impossible. Failure rates have been described to increase over time defined by progression of the osteoarthritic disease or pain, with a comparable reported rate of 9.9% at a mean follow-up of 40 months and 6.7% at a mean follow-up of 44 months, for the Actifit and CMI patients, respectively.[10]

Radiological Outcome

Only a few articles reporting the MRI results of meniscal scaffolds have been published, and even fewer investigators have reported the long-term MRI outcomes of these procedures (**Figs. 2** and **3**). The Genovese classification is the most commonly used classification to evaluate the scaffold quality by means of morphology/size and signal intensity, despite low interobserver and intraobserver reliability.[22] Generally, a reduction in size of the scaffold is found, with a persistency of signal hyperintensity. This hyperintense signal tends to diminish over the years showing scaffold maturation, cellular ingrowth, and collagen network creation, but never reaches the same low

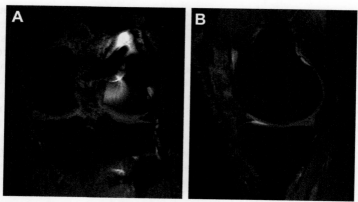

Fig. 2. (*A*) Coronal MRI showing polyurethane scaffold on the medial meniscus. Observe the high signal from the scaffold and the slight extrusion of the medial meniscus. Normal signal intensity of the lateral meniscus. (*B*) Sagittal MRI showing the posterior horn of the medial meniscus repaired with a polyurethane meniscus scaffold.

signal of the normal fibrocartilaginous meniscus. These MRI findings have raised several concerns despite their clinical significance remaining unclear. Patients receiving CMI scaffolds had higher grades for Genovese morphology and signal intensity when compared with Actifit scaffold patients. On MRI, extrusion is more frequently observed in the Actifit-treated patients with no defined correlation with clinical outcomes. These data are reported in a recent meta-analysis by Young-Soo Shin,[23] where despite a worsening cartilage status and meniscal extrusion between baseline and final follow-up was found, patients demonstrated significant functional improvement and pain relief when compared with baseline scores. Moreover, preoperative coronal meniscal extrusion strongly predicts postoperative clinical and morphologic outcomes.[24] Therefore, absence of such extrusion at preoperative MRI should be added as a criterion for patient selection for meniscal scaffold implantation. In patients with post-partial-meniscectomy syndrome and a sufficiently thick meniscal rim, the possibility that a meniscal allograft may be more appropriate than a substitute should

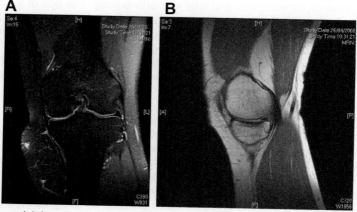

Fig. 3. Coronal (*A*) and sagittal (*B*) MRI showing the midbody and posterior horn of the medial meniscus repaired with a CMI scaffold. Notice the reduced size of the regenerated tissue.

be considered.[19] No significant progression of the degenerative process is found at short-term and midterm follow-up according to the ICRS or the Outerbridge scores. These results are confirmed at longer-term follow-up up to 10 years with radiographic evaluation demonstrating no development or progression of degenerative knee joint disease. Significantly less medial joint space narrowing was found in the CMI group compared with the meniscectomy controls in only one comparative study by Zaffagnini and colleagues.[17] However, study limitations do not allow clear conclusions to be drawn on the chondroprotective effects of the newly formed meniscus.

Postoperative Treatments and Rehabilitation

To ensure protection of the newly formed fragile tissue and to provide optimum conditions for healing, all patients are required to undergo a conservative rehabilitation program similar to that for a meniscal allograft. The rehabilitation protocol lasts 16 to 24 weeks, with the patient non–weight bearing for the first 3 weeks. Partial weight bearing is permitted from week 4 onward, with a gradual increase in loading up to 100% load at 9 weeks postimplantation. The progressive weight bearing is initiated in stages, increasing by 10 kg per week for patients weighing $\leq$60 kg and by 15 kg per week for patients weighing more than 60 kg to $\leq$90 kg. Full weight bearing with an unloader brace is allowed from week 9 onward, and without the use of the unloader brace from week 14 onward. Gradual resumption of sports is generally commenced as of 6 months at the discretion of the responsible orthopedic surgeon; however, contact sports are to recommence only after 9 months.

Discussion

Based on the existing short, midterm, and long-term data, meniscus scaffolds represent a safe and reliable treatment of a symptomatic segmental meniscus defect. Although most patients suffering a partial meniscectomy do not develop early-onset clinical symptoms, a subset of them will present themselves with pain, swelling, and early articular cartilage degeneration.[2,25] Treatment options include conservative therapy and surgery. It is generally accepted that alignment and stability of the knee joint should be assessed and corrected before meniscus substitution. Moreover, in the case of malalignment or instability in association with segmental meniscus loss, an isolated corrective osteotomy or knee ligament reconstruction is highly likely to provide lasting clinical benefit to the patient.[26] The benefit of additional meniscus substitution using scaffolds in such cases remains questionable.[21] However, in the well-aligned and stable knee with limited articular cartilage degeneration suffering from segmental loss of medial or lateral meniscus, a meniscus scaffold provides significant clinical improvement. In general, midterm MRI data show the meniscus regenerated tissue has a smaller volume and high signal intensity, illustrating immature meniscus-like tissue. Extrusion of the meniscus is also a common finding.[24,27,28] The clinical relevance of these MRI findings remains unclear. The chondroprotective effect remains to be proven in a randomized clinical trial. Similar to meniscus allograft research, basic knowledge on speed of onset and natural progression of articular cartilage degeneration after segmental loss of meniscus tissue in the symptomatic population is lacking. The further understanding of why a certain subgroup of patients develops early-onset symptoms or degeneration is currently a hot topic within the research community. Another area of research is the observed extrusion of meniscus that also occurs after meniscectomy and meniscus transplantation and is most likely induced by the loss of hoop fibers. Histologically, biopsies taken after implantation have never shown full restoration of essential structural elements of the human meniscus, such as hoop fibers, or of the structural organization of native meniscus tissue.[6,12–14] The histologic finding of less organized immature meniscuslike tissue consisting of a hybrid fibrous and fibrochondrocytic tissue also correlates with the higher signal intensity as observed on the MRI. Although meniscus scaffolds provide a safe and biodegradable matrix for cellular ingrowth, further improvement of the scaffold technology could be achieved by incorporating growth factors, cells or other active biologicals to accelerate healing.[29–32] Fast recovery, a reduced length of rehab and a swift return to (sports) activities are considered attractive to both the patient and the health care system, whereas the current clinical improvement takes 1 year.

SUMMARY

The meniscus is a crucial player in knee homeostasis and its preservation is now considered necessary to obtain satisfactory clinical results, above all in the long-term follow-up to avoid the future onset of arthritis. Even when a repair is impossible or failed, different innovative options using biological or synthetic scaffolds are now available to regenerate meniscuslike tissue, with the aim to allow a satisfactory clinical improvement to patients. However, the role of any of these procedures in terms of chondroprotection is questionable, and the overall outcomes in the long term still can be improved.

REFERENCES

1. Lyman S, Hidaka C, Valdez AS, et al. Risk factors for meniscectomy after meniscal repair. Am J Sports Med 2013;41(12):2772–8.
2. Heijink A, Gomoll AH, Madry H, et al. Biomechanical considerations in the pathogenesis of osteoarthritis of the knee. Knee Surg Sports Traumatol Arthrosc 2012; 20(3):423–35.
3. Longo UG, Campi S, Romeo G, et al. Biological strategies to enhance healing of the avascular area of the meniscus. Stem Cells Int 2012;2012:528359.
4. DeHaven KE, Sebastianelli WJ. Open meniscus repair. Indications, technique, and results. Clin Sports Med 1990;9:577–87.
5. Beaufils P. Meniscal lesions. Rev Prat 1998;48(16):1773–9.
6. Goodwillie AD, Myers K, Sgaglione NA. Current strategies and approaches to meniscal repair. J Knee Surg 2014;27(6):423–34.
7. Zaffagnini S, Grassi A, Marcheggiani Muccioli GM, et al. MRI evaluation of a collagen meniscus implant: a systematic review. Knee Surg Sports Traumatol Arthrosc 2015;23(11):3228–37.
8. Verdonk R, Van Daele P, Claus B, et al. Viable meniscus transplantation. Orthopade 2014;23(2):153–9.
9. Zur G, Linder-Ganz E, Elsner JJ, et al. Chondroprotective effects of a polycarbonate-urethane meniscal implant: histopathological results in a sheep model. Knee Surg Sports Traumatol Arthrosc 2011;19(2):255–63.
10. Filardo G, Andriolo L, Kon E, et al. Meniscal scaffolds: results and indications. A systematic literature review. Int Orthop 2015;39(1):35–46.
11. Rodkey WG, DeHaven KE, Montgomery WH, et al. Comparison of the collagen meniscus implant with partial meniscectomy. A prospective randomized trial. J Bone Joint Surg Am 2008;90(7):1413–26.
12. Verdonk R, Verdonk P, Huysse W, et al. Tissue ingrowth after implantation of a novel, biodegradable polyurethane scaffold for treatment of partial meniscal lesions. Am J Sports Med 2011;39(4):774–82.

13. Tienen TG, Heijkants RG, de Groot JH, et al. Replacement of the knee meniscus by a porous polymer implant: a study in dogs. Am J Sports Med 2006;34(1): 64–71.

14. Bulgheroni E, Grassi A, Campagnolo M, et al. Comparative study of collagen versus synthetic-based meniscal scaffolds in treating meniscal deficiency in young active population. Cartilage 2016;7(1):29–38.

15. Monllau JC, Gelber PE, Abat F, et al. Outcome after partial medial meniscus substitution with the collagen meniscal implant at a minimum of 10 years' follow-up. Arthroscopy 2011;27(7):933–43.

16. Bulgheroni E, Grassi A, Bulgheroni P, et al. Long-term outcomes of medial CMI implant versus partial medial meniscectomy in patients with concomitant ACL reconstruction. Knee Surg Sports Traumatol Arthrosc 2015;23:3221–7.

17. Zaffagnini S, Marcheggiani Muccioli GM, Lopomo N, et al. Prospective long-term outcomes of the medial collagen meniscus implant versus partial medial meniscectomy. A minimum 10-year follow-up study. Am J Sports Med 2011;39(5). https://doi.org/10.1177/0363546510391179.

18. Schüttler KF, Haberhauer F, Gesslein M, et al. Midterm follow-up after implantation of a polyurethane meniscal scaffold for segmental medial meniscus loss: maintenance of good clinical and MRI outcome. Knee Surg Sports Traumatol Arthrosc 2016;24(5):1478–84.

19. Leroy A, Beaufils P, Faivre B, et al. Actifit(®) polyurethane meniscal scaffold: MRI and functional outcomes after a minimum follow-up of 5 years. Orthop Traumatol Surg Res 2017;103(4):609–14.

20. Houck DA, Kraeutler MJ, Belk JC, et al. Similar clinical outcomes following collagen or polyurethane meniscal scaffold implantation: a systematic review. Knee Surg Sports Traumatol Arthrosc 2018;26:2259–69.

21. Gelber PE, Isart A, Erquicia JI, et al. Partial meniscus substitution with a polyurethane scaffold does not improve outcome after an open-wedge high tibial osteotomy. Knee Surg Sports Traumatol Arthrosc 2015;23:334–9.

22. Hirschmann A, Schiapparelli FF, Schenk L, et al. The Genovese grading scale is not reliable for MR assessment of collagen meniscus implants. Knee 2017;(24):9–15.

23. Young-Soo S, Hoon-Nyun L, Hyun-Bo S, et al. Polyurethane meniscal scaffolds lead to better clinical outcomes but worse articular cartilage status and greater absolute meniscal extrusion. Knee Surg Sports Traumatol Arthrosc 2018;26: 2227–38.

24. Faivre B, Bouyarmane H, Lonjon G, et al. Actifit® scaffold implantation: influence of preoperative meniscal extrusion on morphological and clinical outcomes. Orthop Traumatol Surg Res 2015;101(6):703–8.

25. Paxton ES, Stock MV, Brophy RH. Meniscal repair versus partial meniscectomy: a systematic review comparing reoperation rates and clinical outcomes. Arthroscopy 2011;27(9):1275–88.

26. Arnold MP, Hirschmann MT, Verdonk PC. See the whole picture: knee preserving therapy needs more than surface repair. Knee Surg Sports Traumatol Arthrosc 2012;20(2):195–6.

27. De Coninck T, Huysse W, Willemot L, et al. Two-year follow-up study on clinical and radiological outcomes of polyurethane meniscal scaffolds. Am J Sports Med 2013 Jan;41(1):64–72.

28. Gelber PE, Petrica AM, Isart A, et al. The magnetic resonance aspect of a polyurethane meniscal scaffold is worse in advanced cartilage defects without

deterioration of clinical outcomes after a minimum two-year follow-up. Knee 2015;(21):389–94.

29. Moran CJ, Busilacchi A, Lee CA, et al. Biological augmentation and tissue engineering approaches in meniscus surgery. Arthroscopy 2015;31(5):944–55.

30. Griffin JW, Hadeed MM, Werner BC, et al. Platelet-rich plasma in meniscal repair: does augmentation improve surgical outcomes? Clin Orthop Relat Res 2015;473: 1665–72.

31. Pak J, Lee JH, Lee SH. Regenerative repair of damaged meniscus with autologous adipose tissue-derived stem cells. Biomed Res Int 2014;2014:436029.

32. Koch M, Achatz FP, Lang S, et al. Tissue engineering of large full-size meniscus defects by apolyurethane scaffold: accelerated regeneration by mesenchymal stromal cells. Stem Cells Int 2018;2018:8207071.

Meniscal Allograft Transplants

Taylor M. Southworth, BS[a], Neal B. Naveen, BS[a], Tracy M. Tauro, BS, BA[a], Jorge Chahla, MD, PhD[a], Brian J. Cole, MD, MBA[b,c],*

KEYWORDS

- Meniscal allograft transplantation • Meniscus • Knee • Sports medicine

KEY POINTS

- In young patients with persistent pain after total meniscectomy, meniscal allograft transplantation may be indicated to alleviate symptoms and delay the onset of osteoarthritis.
- Ideal candidates are those who have failed conservative management and meniscectomy, with minimal to no osteoarthritis, a low to normal body mass index, and are younger.
- There are several different techniques used in meniscal allograft transplantation, which are broadly categorized into using bony fixation (using bone plugs or a bridge-in-slot technique) and soft tissue fixation.
- Outcomes in patients with meniscal allograft transplantation are promising, with long-term favorable graft survival rates in patients undergoing isolated procedures and with concomitant anterior cruciate ligament reconstruction or a cartilage preservation procedure.

INTRODUCTION

The menisci act as shock absorbers, by decreasing tibiofemoral contact area and contact pressure, thus enhancing the stability of the knee joint[1-4]. Removal of the meniscus via partial or total meniscectomy can, therefore, result in altered biomechanics of the knee in a manner that depends on the amount of meniscus removed.[2,5-9] Meniscal deficiency, such as in patients who have previously

Disclosure Statement: Dr B.J. Cole would like make the following disclosures: Aesculap/B. Braun: Research support; Arthrex, Inc: IP royalties; Paid consultant; Research support; Athletico: Other financial or material support; JRF Ortho: Other financial or material support; National Institutes of Health (NIAMS & NICHD): Research support; Ossio: Stock or stock options; Regentis: Paid consultant, Research support, Stock or stock options; Smith & Nephew: Other financial or material support. All other authors have nothing to disclose.
[a] Department of Orthopaedics, Midwest Orthopaedics at Rush, 1611 West Harrison Street, Chicago, IL 60612, USA; [b] Department of Orthopedics, Rush University, 1611 West Harrison Street, Chicago, IL 60612, USA; [c] Department of Surgery, Rush OPH, Midwest Orthopaedics at Rush, 1611 West Harrison Street, Chicago, IL 60612, USA
* Corresponding author. 1611 West Harrison Street, Chicago, IL 60612.
E-mail address: bcole@rushortho.com

undergone a meniscectomy, can lead to the onset and progression of knee osteoarthritis (OA).[10,11] Additionally, for some patients with meniscal pathology, the symptoms of pain, swelling, instability, and functional limitation do not subside after initial meniscectomy.[12] In these patients with persistent pain in a meniscal deficient knee, meniscal allograft transplantation (MAT) may be indicated to restore the force distribution across the knee and reduce symptoms (**Box 1**).[12–15] Because MAT is considered a salvage procedure, it is still relatively rare with an estimated 3295 performed from 2007 to 2011 and an incidence of 0.24 procedures per year per 100,000 patients.[16,17] Although MAT is less common than other meniscal procedures,[18] it gives patients with debilitating pain and functional limitations a viable treatment option that may improve symptoms and function, and it may contribute to a more biomechanically stable knee.[19–30]

PATIENT EVALUATION AND PREOPERATIVE PLANNING

Careful patient selection is crucial for successful outcomes after MAT. To determine if a patient is an appropriate candidate for this procedure, a thorough history and physical examination is essential. Ideal candidates are relatively young patients (too young for knee arthroplasty), have undergone a partial or total meniscectomy, and continue to have joint line pain specific to the meniscectomized compartment with Kellgren-Lawrence grade 2 OA or less.[31] There has not been a firm consensus on the upper age limit of MAT, but a review of the current literature indicates that most physicians do not perform MAT in patients more than 45 to 55 years old because patients with meniscal deficiency over this age often have significant arthritis.[12,27,32–36]

Box 1
Indications and contraindications for meniscal allograft transplant

Indications for meniscal allograft transplant

- Less than 55 years old

- Meniscus deficient

- Unicompartmental pain at the joint line

- Functional limitation

- Pain is the predominant symptom

- No significant OA (Kellgren-Lawrence grades 1–2)

Contraindications for meniscal allograft transplant

- Diffuse arthritic changes

- Inflammatory arthritis

- Synovial disease

- Skeletal immaturity

- Joint infection, previous or active

- Marked obesity

- Asymptomatic patients

Note: Malalignment, ligamentous insufficiency, and chondral defects are not absolute contraindications to MAT. These pathologies do; however, need to be addressed concomitantly or via a staged procedure to receive optimal patient outcomes.

Physeal status should be assessed carefully in younger patients to avoid causing a physeal arrest and alignment deformities. Obesity should be considered as a relative contraindication to perform MAT; some authors contraindicate this procedure in patients with a body mass index of more than 30 because it increases the load within the knee compartments, resulting in an increased risk of allograft failure.[37]

Imaging

It is important to review radiographs, including anteroposterior weight bearing views, lateral non-weight bearing views, Rosenberg views (posteroanterior 45° flexion weight bearing views), and merchant views (axial views of the patellofemoral joint) (**Fig. 1**), because the ideal candidate for MAT does not have radiographic evidence of diffuse OA. Candidates for MAT should present with radiographs showing minimal joint space narrowing, no osteophytes, and no significant bony flattening in the involved compartment. These views should be obtained with a sizing marker to determine the graft size needed for MAT.[12] Mechanical axis views should also be reviewed to evaluate the patient's alignment and potential need for a realignment procedure concurrently or before the transplant. An MRI should be obtained to evaluate the meniscus, specifically the amount of meniscus remaining (**Fig. 2**). The MRI will also assess for any subchondral edema, cartilage damage, or ligamentous insufficiency, because focal chondral defects or ligamentous pathology may need to be addressed concomitantly.

Diagnostic Arthroscopy

Before MAT, the senior author (BJC) recommends the patient undergo a diagnostic arthroscopy to further evaluate and confirm the status of the meniscus (**Fig. 3**), cartilage damage, and concomitant pathologies. The diagnostic arthroscopy helps to elucidate other possible causes of knee pain to ensure the patient is an appropriate MAT candidate. This diagnostic arthroscopy is ideally completed within 6 months of

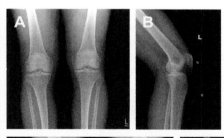
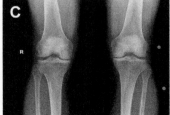
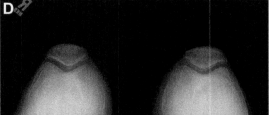

Fig. 1. Radiographical imaging needed before MAT to evaluate evidence of OA as well as for sizing of the meniscal graft. (*A*) Anteroposterior views of bilateral knees. (*B*) Non-weight bearing lateral view of operative knee with sizing marker. (*C*) Rosenberg view of bilateral knees (posteroanterior 45° flexion weight bearing view) with a sizing marker. (*D*) Merchant view of bilateral knees.

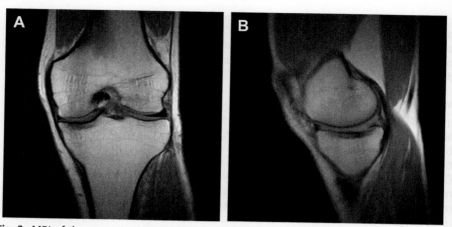

Fig. 2. MRI of the operative knee. (*A*) Coronal view of the left knee showing medial meniscal deficiency. (*B*) Sagittal view of the left knee with evidence of medial meniscal deficiency.

MAT in the absence of outside index information that would otherwise verify the intra-articular pathology.

Graft Selection and Sizing

Preoperative radiographs with sizing markers are essential for ordering a size-matched meniscal allograft. Meniscal allografts are matched to the patient's laterality, specific compartment, and size. Size matching is important because an improperly sized meniscus can lead to increased contact pressures in unwanted areas.[38] Sizing is as described by Pollard and colleagues,[39] on anteroposterior films in which 2 vertical lines are drawn perpendicular to the joint line and are used to measure meniscal width. In a medial meniscus, the first line is tangential to the medial tibial metaphyseal margin and the second is through the peak of the medial tibial eminence. For a lateral meniscus, the first line is tangential to the lateral tibial margin and the second is through the peak of the lateral tibial eminence. The distance between these 2 lines is said to be the meniscal width. Of note, it is important to measure from the margin

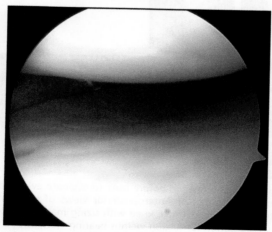

Fig. 3. Diagnostic arthroscopy revealing right knee medial meniscus deficiency.

of the tibial metaphysis rather than the joint space. Meniscal length is measured on lateral radiographs in a similar manner. The first line is drawn at the anterior tibial surface above the tuberosity and the second is a parallel line tangent to the posterior margin of the tibial plateau. The medial meniscus length is 0.8 times this distance, and the lateral meniscal length is 0.7 times the distance.

In the senior author's practice, fresh-frozen allografts are preferred. Fresh-frozen meniscal allografts are able to be stored for 5 years at −80°C in a physiologic solution with an antibiotic.[40] Although freezing the meniscus has been shown to result in decreased cell viability, this has not been reported to have negative effects on patient outcomes or graft survivorship.[41,42] Other graft options include cryopreserved and fresh grafts. Because fresh grafts do not offer the same ability to plan in advance, fresh-frozen allografts ease the burden on both the physician and patient. Meniscal allografts have shown excellent integration and repopulation with host trabeculae when a bony bed is used[43] with minor risk of immunologic reaction.

SURGICAL TECHNIQUE

The senior author's preferred technique, bone bridge in slot, and positioning have been described previously.[23,44–46]

Patient Positioning

After induction with general anesthesia, the patient is positioned supine on the operating table with the foot of the bed dropped and the hips in line with the end of the bed. The contralateral leg is positioned in a well-leg holder in flexion, abduction, and external rotation. The operative knee is positioned in a thigh holder with a tourniquet in place and allowed to hang off the end of the bed. Standard preoperative antibiotics are administered before any incisions. An examination under anesthesia is performed to assess ligamentous stability. The patient limb is then prepped and draped sterilely.

Arthroscopy

The senior author performs the same technique for both medial and lateral MATs. After creation of the anterolateral and anteromedial portals, arthroscopy is performed to evaluate once more for focal chondral defects or ligamentous insufficiency. After the evaluation of concomitant pathologies via arthroscopy, the remaining meniscus in the index compartment is debrided taking care to not violate the capsule. This should be done until there is a 1- to 2-mm peripheral rim remaining with punctate bleeding. The anterior and posterior horn remnants can serve as a footprint for allograft insertion. The residual meniscal rim is left in place to prevent radial displacement of the allograft and function as a firm bed for meniscal fixation.[47,48] A limited notchplasty can be performed at this time to enhance visualization and ease of graft passage. The anterior cruciate ligament fibers at the tibial insertion should be released, as minimally as possible, to allow for visualization of the medial tibial spine.

A posteromedial or posterolateral approach is made starting one-third of the way above the level of the joint line and extending two-thirds of the way below the level of the joint line, which will later be used to pass the sutures (as described elsewhere).[23,44,46] Next, a 3-cm transpatellar tendon incision is made, into which a 4.5-mm burr is inserted to create a provisional slot, in line with the insertion of the anterior and posterior horns. After a depth gauge is inserted into the slot to verify appropriate depth (usually 10 mm), a guide pin is placed directly underneath and seated in the posterior cortex to establish the bottom of the slot. Fluoroscopic guidance may be used to ensure proper placement of the guide pin and to not violate the posterior cortex. An

8-mm cannulated reamer is placed over the guidewire, and a box cutter osteotome is used to widen the slot to 8 mm wide and 10 mm deep. A rasp is then used to even out all the edges in the slot and to maximize congruency with the bone bridge.

Graft Preparation

The meniscal allograft is prepared on the back table during arthroscopy. The meniscal allograft is delivered by the tissue bank as a hemiplateau with attached meniscus, with all nonmensical tissue removed. The graft is debrided so only true attachment sites remain and is then prepared to dimensions appropriate for the arthroscopic tibial slot preparation (**Fig. 4**). Of note, the bone bridge is undersized by 1 mm as a preventive measure for ease of graft passage and minimization of potential bridge fracture. As a standard, the bone bridge is cut to a width of 7 mm and a height of 10 mm. Excess bone beyond the posterior horn attachment is removed to ensure proper alignment of the bone bridge posterior wall and posterior edge of the slot. To help with graft insertion, excess bone beyond the anterior horn is preserved. The junction of the posterior horn and middle third of the meniscus are secured using a no. 0 polydioxanone with a vertical mattress traction suture (**Fig. 5**). In the event that the anterior horn is larger, the bone bridge width on the anterior horn insertion should be appropriately increased, with the remaining bone bridge cut to 7 mm.

Graft Insertion

First, the arthroscope is placed in the corresponding compartment portal (ie, anteromedial for medial MAT), and a repair cannula is placed in the contralateral portal, aiming toward the intended position of the junction of the middle and posterior portions of the graft.

A flexible suture-passing wire is then inserted through the meniscal repair cannula, and out the posterolateral/posteromedial portal. The ends from the traction stitch of the graft are threaded through the loop of the suture passing wire, which is retrieved

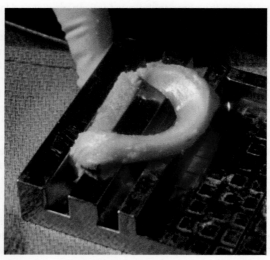

Fig. 4. Medial meniscal allograft after debridement so only true attachments remain. The graft is placed into a sizer to appropriately match the size of the tibial slot prepared in the knee.

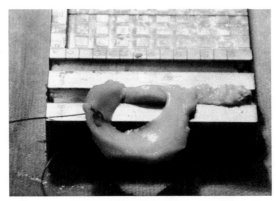

Fig. 5. A vertical mattress traction suture is placed in the graft approximately two-thirds of the way from the posterior horn.

from the transpatellar incision. The wire and sutures are then pulled through the posterolateral/posteromedial incision, and the meniscus is carefully inserted through the anterior incision, while simultaneously pulling on the polydioxanone traction suture and applying the appropriate stress (varus for a lateral MAT and valgus stress for a medial MAT) to insert the bridge into its position (**Fig. 6**). Proper reduction of the meniscus and visualization of the bone block in the bridge is then done arthroscopically. After a few cycles of flexion and extension to ensure appropriate graft placement relative to the condyles, a 4.75 or 5.75 mm Swivelock anchor (Arthrex, Naples, FL) is placed to fix the bone bridge (**Fig. 7**). Eight to 10 vertical mattress sutures are then placed using an inside-out technique, taking care to not tie them until any concomitant procedures are complete (**Fig. 8**). The anterior horn of the meniscus is repaired with an outside-in technique. After concomitant procedures are complete, the inside-out sutures are tied while the knee is in full extension.

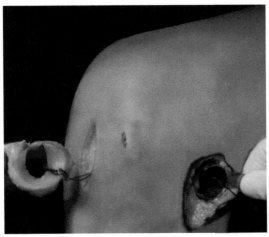

Fig. 6. The meniscus allograft is inserted through the anterior incision while the polydioxanone traction suture is pulled through the medial or lateral arthrotomy for medial and lateral meniscal allograft transplants, respectively.

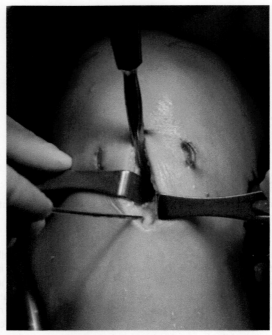

Fig. 7. Visualization of the appropriate placement of the 4.75 or 5.75 mm anchor to fix the meniscal allograft into the tibial bone slot.

Concomitant Procedures

Concomitant procedures, when indicated, can and should be performed at the time of MAT or via staged procedure. These may include high tibial or distal femoral osteotomies for varus or valgus malalignment, respectively, ligamentous procedures for ligament insufficiency or rupture, and cartilage procedures, such as microfracture, autologous chondrocyte implantation, osteochondral allograft, or osteochondral autograft, for focal chondral defects. Any chondral defects should be addressed after the MAT, because the frequent varus/valgus manipulations associated with the MAT procedure can cause improper seating of the osteochondral graft. The concomitant procedure may alter the postoperative rehabilitation protocol slightly, all of which should be discussed with the patient preoperatively.

Closure

The posterolateral/posteromedial lesions are closed in a layered fashion, and portal holes are closed with 3-0 nylon interrupted sutures. After closure, local anesthesia is injected to maximize postoperative pain relief.

Rehabilitation

The postoperative rehabilitation protocol recommended by the senior author (BJC) is as follows. The patient is made heel touch weight bearing with crutches for the first 6 weeks and can progress to full weight bearing 6 to 8 weeks postoperatively. The patient is restricted from weight bearing with flexion greater than 90° for the first 8 weeks. The brace is locked in full extension for sleeping and all activities for the first 2 weeks,

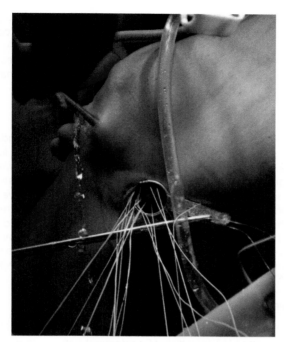

Fig. 8. Vertical mattress sutures are placed via an inside-out technique to secure the meniscus in place and are left untied until all concomitant procedures are completed.

after which time the brace is locked at 0° to 90° and can be removed at night. Before 6 weeks, all exercises should be done with the brace. After this timepoint, activities can be done without the brace as tolerated. The brace can be discontinued 8 weeks postoperatively. The patient should avoid any tibial rotation for 8 weeks to protect the meniscus. Range of motion should be limited to 0° to 90° when non-weight bearing for the first 2 weeks and then can progress as tolerated over weeks 2 to 8. The patient should have full range of motion by weeks 8 to 12. After 8 weeks, hamstring work, lunges, proprioception exercises, and stationary bike can begin and progress as tolerated through 20 weeks. Around 6 months, the patient is able to advance to sport-specific drills, running, and jumping after physician clearance.

OUTCOMES

There are many variables that make MAT outcomes difficult to assess and generalize. These include conjoined analysis of medial and lateral MATs, different graft types (fresh, cryopreserved, and fresh frozen), a variety of concomitant procedures, differing techniques and surgeon experience, and the low levels of evidence of current studies.[49] Thus, with many of the studies reporting on patients undergoing concomitant realignment, cartilage or ligamentous procedures, it can be difficult to ascertain the contribution of an MAT on the patient's clinical outcome. When looking at short and long-term MAT outcomes with and without concomitant procedures, studies typically evaluate patient-reported outcome measures, return to activity, subsequent procedures, complications, graft survival, and failures, often defined as the need for revision MAT or the progression to arthroplasty. Additionally, recently an emphasis has been put on determining the minimal clinically important difference (MCID) and patient acceptable symptomatic state (PASS) in patient-reported outcome measures. Other important outcomes after MAT include the progression of OA as well as graft extrusion and the clinical implications of these. Overall reported results have been encouraging mainly for the treatment of the symptoms and functional improvement. A summary of many of these studies is included in **Table 1**.

IMAGING

Saltzman and colleagues[50] studied 60 MRI scans of patients who underwent isolated MAT to evaluate subchondral bone marrow lesions. Patients were followed up at a mean of 4.9 ± 2.3 years. A significant correlation was noted between the Welsch and colleagues grading system, based on lesion size, and Knee Injury and Osteoarthritis Outcome Score (KOOS), Western Ontario and McMaster Universities Osteoarthritis Index (WOMAC), and Marx patient reported outcomes. A correlation was also noted between the Costa-Paz and colleagues grading system, based on appearance and location, and postoperative satisfaction. There were no significant differences in graft survivorship between those with more severe subchondral bone marrow lesions. These findings can help to further refine the patient population who will have the most success after MAT.

CONCOMITANT PROCEDURES

McCormick and colleagues[19] reported on the largest case series, with 172 consecutive patients undergoing MAT (of whom 59 underwent concomitant procedures), with a 2-year survival rate of greater than 95%, with a similar survivorship found in other studies as well. Seventy-three percent of patients who underwent subsequent surgery did so within the first 2 years postoperatively. In patients who did not undergo subsequent procedures, there was a 98% graft survival rate, compared with 88% survival rate in those who underwent concomitant procedures. The failure rate, which was defined as the rate of revision or conversion to total knee arthroplasty, was low at 4.7%.

Cole and colleagues[20] analyzed isolated and concomitant MAT in 22 patients with a mean follow-up of 8.5 ± 1.3 years. All patients reported significant improvements postoperatively on all scoring scales with a mean postoperative satisfaction of 8.8 out of 10. Patients also reported a significant increase in the overall condition of their knee. Some patient outcome scores continued to improve 2-year after the index procedure and some showed a small decrease over time; however, most scores were maintained. Three patients were identified as failures at 24 months, 54 months, and 68 months for undergoing either revision MAT (24, 54 months) or unicompartmental arthroplasty (68 months). Of note, the authors found that MAT performed with appropriately indicated concomitant procedures showed statistically significant greater improvements in Lysholm, KOOS Pain, and KOOS Quality of Life as compared with the improvements seen with isolated MAT.

Frank and colleagues[51] evaluated 100 patients undergoing osteochondral allograft transplantation (OCA) with or without MAT. Both groups showed statistically significant improvements in Lysholm, International Knee Document Committee (IKDC), KOOS, WOMAC, and Short Form (SF)-12 physical scores as compared with preoperative scores. There were no significant differences in reoperation rates, time to reoperation, failure rates, or improvement in patient-reported clinical outcome scores between the groups. The graft survival rate was noted to be 86% at 5 years in those who underwent OCA and MAT. Similarly, Saltzman and colleagues[24] studied 91

Table 1
Studies examining clinical outcomes after meniscal allograft transplant

Author	No. of Patients	Laterality	Graft Preservation Technique	Mean Age (y)	Mean F/u (y)	Mean BMI (kg/m^2)	Time to Surgery (y)	Workers Comp	Concomitant Procedures	Clinical/ Radiographic Outcomes	Failures, Complications	Overall Survival Rate/ Reoperation Rate	Conclusion
Lee et al,[56] 2019	130 (4 studies)	NR	NR	25.1 ± 6.2	NR	NR	NR	NR	NR.	Return to sport ranged from 7.6 to 16.5 mo.	NR.	3/4 studies reported reoperation rates of 12%, 25%, and 30% of athletes.	67%–85.7% of athletes returned to sport within an average of 7.6–16.5 mo after MAT, which was longer and lower rate than those undergoing partial meniscectomies. There were no significant differences between patients with different degrees of chondral damage or in laterality.

(continued on next page)

Table 1 (continued)

Author	No. of Patients	Laterality	Graft Preservation Technique	Mean Age (y)	Mean F/u (y)	Mean BMI (kg/m²)	Time to Surgery (y)	Workers Comp	Concomitant Procedures	Clinical/ Radiographic Outcomes	Failures, Complications	Overall Survival Rate/ Reoperation Rate	Conclusion
Liu et al,[65] 2019	98	57 medial, 41 lateral	Fresh frozen	29.4 ± 9.0	≥1 y	26.8 ± 5.2	NR	NR	82 (84%): (n = 10) ACLR, (n = 4) chondroplasty, (n = 12) MFx, (n = 3) OAT, (n = 50) OCA, (n = 6) ACI, (n = 4) HTO, (n = 3) DFO.	Of the 34 patients who completed satisfaction surveys, MCID and PASS were established for Lysholm, IKDC, and KOOS; 28 patients were satisfied with their surgery and 6 were not satisfied.	NR.	NR.	Patients who had lower scores preoperatively were more likely to achieve the thresholds for MCID and PASS established by this study. Workers' compensation patients and patients with higher BMIs were less likely to achieve these values for certain outcome measures.

| Lee et al,[63] 2018 | 53 patients who underwent lateral MAT with the keyhole technique assigned to either (n = 25) standard rehabilitation or delayed rehabilitation (n = 28; ie, 3 wk immobilization followed by use of unloading braces for 9 wk) | All lateral | Fresh frozen | 30.6 | 2.1 | NR | NR | NR | None. | The number of patients and absolute/relative percent extrusion was greater in the group assigned to standard rehabilitation. Significant correlations between coronal graft extrusion and postoperative joint space width was found. | None. | NR. | Patients who underwent the delayed rehabilitation program had statistically less extrusion on coronal MRI at 24 mo as well as less progression of OA compared with those in the standard program, although no differences in clinical outcomes between the groups were observed. |

(continued on next page)

Table 1
(continued)

Author	No. of Patients	Laterality	Graft Preservation Technique	Mean Age (y)	Mean F/u (y)	Mean BMI (kg/m²)	Time to Surgery (y)	Workers Comp	Concomitant Procedures	Clinical/Radiographic Outcomes	Failures, Complications	Overall Survival Rate/Reoperation Rate	Conclusion
Masferrer-Pino et al,[62] 2018	LMAT: 15 with bony fixation, 14 with suture fixation through bone tunnel after capsulodesis	All lateral	Fresh frozen	38.2	2.1	NR	NR	NR	Not discussed.	After excluding the first 4 cases, which showed the worst cases of extrusion from the analysis as a learning curve for the new technique, there was a significantly lower percentage of extrusion seen in the capsulodesis group at 36–48 mo of F/u.	NR.	NR.	Although the capsulodesis technique in LMAT presented a lesser degree of meniscal extrusion than the bone bridge fixation if the first 4 cases were excluded, clinical outcome did not differ significantly between the 2 groups.
Saltzman et al,[50] 2018	60 patients undergoing isolated MAT	27 medial, 13 lateral	NR	26.1 ± 9.3	58.8 ± 27.6	25.5 ± 5.2	NR	25%	None.	Significant improvements in IKDC, KOOS Pain, and SF-12 physical were noted postoperatively ≥2 y.	4 (15%): (n = 2) total meniscectomies, (n = 1) TKA, (n = 1) revision MAT at postoperative 30.84 ± 16.80 mo.	95% graft survival at 24 mo and 87% graft survival at 60 mo. 11 Revisions: (n = 4) partial meniscectomy, (n = 2) total meniscectomy, (n = 1) revision MAT, (n = 1) plica excision, (n = 1) OCA, (n = 1) de novo NT, (n = 1) synovectomy	Increasing BML size correlates with worse postoperative pain scores and lower activity ratings but no significant differences in graft survivorship was found based on gradings.

Study	Total	Graft site	Graft	Age	F/U (mo)	BMI		%	Procedures	PROs	Complications	Survivorship/Failures	Conclusions
Frank et al,[51] 2018	100: 50 with OCA + MAT, 50 MAT	29 medial, 29 lateral	Fresh frozen	31.7 ± 9.8	4.9 ± 2.7	25.0 ± 4.8	NR	14%	50: (n = 45) OCA + MAT, (n = 3) OCA + MAT + DFO, (n = 2) OCA + HTO + DFO.	Both groups showed statistically significant improvements in Lysholm, IKDC, KOOS, WOMAC and SF-12 physical scores as compared with preoperative scores.	2 (4%): local cellulitis (n = 1), postoperative arthrofibrosis requiring adhesiolysis; 17 reoperations.	86% at 3.34 y; 7 failures.	At final F/u, patients in both groups experienced statistically significant improvements in Lysholm, IKCD, KOOS, WOMAC, and SF-12 physical subscale outcomes, with no significant differences in PROs between the groups. There were no significant differences between complication rates or reoperations between the 2 groups.
Saltzman et al,[24] 2018	91: 22 with no defect (Outerbridge 0/I), 69 with full thickness defect (Outerbridge IV)	NR	Fresh frozen	28.6	4.5 ± 2.6	25.7	NR	NR	10 in no defect group: (n = 2) realignment procedures, (n = 8) ACLR. 69 cartilage procedures in full thickness group: (n = 48) OCA, (n = 13) ACI, (n = 9) MFx, (n = 3) OAT, (n = 1) de novo NT, (n = 7) realignment, (n = 8) ACLR.	No significant differences in postoperative or final F/u delta patient reported outcomes, number of subsequent surgeries, or failures between the no defect (grade 0/I) and full thickness defect (grade IV) groups.	1 complication in the full-thickness defect group, with 0 in no defect group. Three failures: 1 (5%) in no defect group, 2 (3.3%) in full thickness defect group.	10: 2 (10%) in no defect group, 8 (12.9%) in full thickness group. 86% survivorship in both full-thickness and no defect group.	Chondral damage that is treated with cartilage restoration at the time of MAT may not affect the clinical outcomes of MAT.

(continued on next page)

Table 1
(continued)

Author	No. of Patients	Laterality	Graft Preservation Technique	Mean Age (y)	Mean F/u (y)	Mean BMI (kg/m²)	Time to Surgery (y)	Workers Comp	Concomitant Procedures	Clinical/Radiographic Outcomes	Failures, Complications	Overall Survival Rate/Reoperation Rate	Conclusion
Kim et al,[61] 2018	46	All lateral	Fresh frozen	31.6 ± 10.8	51.1 ± 7.1	NR	NR	NR	4: (n = 2) ACLR, (n = 2) MFx.	Relative extrusion in the coronal plane did not differ significantly at 6 wk, 1 y, and 3–5 y postoperatively in either the coronal or sagittal plane	NR	NR	Extrusion following LMAT did not significantly progress in either plane during F/u at 3–5 y.
Riboh et al,[22] 2016	32	5 Medial, 27 Lateral	Fresh-frozen	15.4 ± 1.0, (range 13–16)	7.2 ± 3.2	22.1 ± 3.6	NR	NR	13 (41%): (n = 10) ACI, (n = 2) ACLR, (n = 1) ACI biopsy, (n = 1) OAT, (n = 3) OCA, (n = 1) HTO.	Significant improvements were seen in Lysholm, IKDC, WOMAC pain, function and stiffness, SF-12 physical, and all KOOS subscores except KOOS Symptoms. IKDC significantly declined from 2 y to final F/u.	No revisions or failures.	6% meniscal reoperation rate: (n = 2) debridements for torn MAT, overall reoperation rate 22% (n = 8).	Improvements in functional outcomes for adolescent patients was seen after MAT with a low meniscal reoperation rate.

Study	Patients	Medial/Lateral	Graft	Age			Follow-up		Concomitant	Outcomes	Failures	Survival/Reoperations	Conclusions
Saltzman et al,[54] 2016	40 patients undergoing combined MAT with ACLR	33 medial, 7 lateral	Cryopreserved	30.3 ± 9.6	5.7 ± 3.2	27.7 ± 4.2	9.1 ± 6.6	17.5%	19: (n = 9) HWR, (n = 9)OCA.	Significant improvement in all PROs analyzed except for Tegner score, which significantly decreased, WOMAC stiffness, and SF-12 scores. 9/18 athletes returned to sport.	8: (n = 2) graft failures at 7.3 y, (n = 6) arthroplasty 8.3 y. Two minor complications involving surgical drainage.	98% graft survival rate at 1.7 y, 84% at 5 y and 45% at 10 y; 14 reoperations: most commonly (n = 8) debridement, (n = 4) partial meniscectomy, 2 HW.	Concomitant ACLR/MAT can provide significant improvement in clinical outcomes and knee stability for patients.
Zaffagnini et al,[55] 2016	89	45 medial, 44 lateral	Fresh frozen	38.5 ± 11.2	4.2 ± 1.9	23.8 ± 6.1	1.2 ± 0.9 from index meniscectomy	None	41 (45%): (n = 12) HTO, (n = 1) HTO + ACLR, (n = 1) HTO + OCA, (n = 2) DFO, (n = 9) ACLR, (n = 2) revision ACLR, (n = 2) mosaicplasty, (n = 3) OCA, (n = 9) MFx.	At latest F/u, patients who returned to sport had significantly better Tegner scores and KOOS subscores (ADL, QoL, KOOS total) as well as higher knee function, and global satisfaction than those who did not return to sport.	1 failure: UKA.	11 (12%): (n = 3) partial meniscectomy, (n = 3) arthroscopic debridement, (n = 1) peroneal nerve release, (n = 1) UKA, (n = 3) HWR, (n = 1) patellar tendon repair.	49% were able to return to preinjury level of play and 74% were able to return to sport after 8.6 ± 4.1 mo, and those who returned to sport had superior subjective outcomes to those who did not return to sport.

(continued on next page)

Table 1
(continued)

Author	No. of Patients	Laterality	Graft Preservation Technique	Mean Age (y)	Mean F/u (y)	Mean BMI (kg/m²)	Time to Surgery (y)	Workers Comp	Concomitant Procedures	Clinical/ Radiographic Outcomes	Failures, Complications	Overall Survival Rate/ Reoperation Rate	Conclusion
Roumazeille et al,[33] 2015	22	2 medial, 20 lateral	Fresh frozen	37 ± 7.5	4.4 ± 1.6	NR	NR	NR	5 ACLR.	10/14 grafts were fully or partially healed (Henning's criteria). At final F/u, the extrusion had increasing to 3.6 ± 1.9 mm, a relative percentage of extrusion of 46% ± 29.9%, and all KOOS subscales and IKDC scores had improved significantly.	1 hematoma.	2 second-look arthroscopies.	MAT without bone plugs achieved good clinical outcomes and graft healing. No correlation was found between percent extrusion and graft healing, and despite meniscus extrusion in most patients on MRI, pain and knee function scores were significantly improved compared with baseline.

| McCormick et al,[19] 2014 | 172 | NR | Fresh frozen | 34.4 ± 10.3 | 4.9 | 25 ± 3.4 | 1.75 (range 0.2–8.9 y), 73% within 2 y | 10% | 119 (60%): MAT + cartilage procedure (n = 37), MAT + Cartilage procedure + osteotomy (n = 14), MAT + ACLR (n = 11), MAT + osteotomy (n = 8). | NR. | 64 (32%): debridement/ scar excision/ MUA (n = 38), treatment of progressive disease (n = 17), graft repair or debridement <50%, second look arthroscopy (n = 3), revision MAT/ arthroplasty (n = 8). | 88% in revision MAT or TKA, 98% in patients with no subsequent procedures. A 32% reoperation rate for MAT, with a mean 95% allograft survival at 5 y. 73% of patients who underwent secondary surgery did so at mean of 21 mo. | There was a 32% reoperation rate for MAT, and those requiring secondary surgery within 2 y of the MAT had an OR of 8.4 for a subsequent revision MAT or TKA. |

(continued on next page)

Table 1 (*continued*)

Author	No. of Patients	Laterality	Graft Preservation Technique	Mean Age (y)	Mean F/u (y)	Mean BMI (kg/m²)	Time to index Surgery (y)	Workers Comp	Concomitant Procedures	Clinical/ Radiographic Outcomes	Failures, Complications	Overall Survival Rate/ Reoperation Rate	Conclusion
Yanke et al,[64] 2014	8 revision MAT	2 medial, 6 lateral	Fresh frozen	31.6 ± 10.2	3.8 ± 1.3	NR	Time to index procedure was 3.45 ± 2.52 y	NR	4: (n = 1) ACLR, (n = 1) DFO, (n = 2) OCA.	Patients demonstrated significant improvements in IKDC, KOOS pain scores, and subjective symptom rating scale. No significant differences were seen in Outerbridge grading between initial and revision. Seven of 8 patients reported they would undergo the procedure again.	2 TKA.	75% at final F/u.	Revision MAT achieved high patient satisfaction and improvement in IKDC and KOOS, showing that outcomes after revision MAT would be improved compared with preoperative conditions, with no correlation between preoperative radiographic evidence and outcomes after revision MAT.

Marcacci et al,[32] 2014	12 male professional soccer players	6 medial, 6 lateral	Fresh frozen	24.5 ± 3.6	23.2 ± 1.1	3.1 ± 2.6 y from meni-sectomy to MAT	7: (n = 3) MFx, (n = 1) OCA, (n = 2) ACLR, (n = 1) ACI biopsy.	NR	92% of players returned to soccer at a mean 10.5 ± 2.6 mo postoperatively. Tegner, Lysholm, IKDC, WOMAC, and VAS pain were significantly improved 12 mo after surgery and were stable at 36 mo.	1 failure: patient was treated for infection but stopped playing soccer.	NR.	Return to sport in soccer players after MAT was 75% at 36 mo F/u, with a mean time to return to previous athletic level of 16.5 mo.

(continued on next page)

Table 1
(continued)

Author	No. of Patients	Laterality	Graft Preservation Technique	Mean Age (y)	Mean F/u (y)	Mean BMI (kg/m²)	Time to Surgery (y)	Workers Comp	Concomitant Procedures	Clinical/ Radiographic Outcomes	Failures, Complications	Overall Survival Rate/ Reoperation Rate	Conclusion
Harris et al,[53] 2014	35 patients undergoing cartilage procedure with (n = 15) and without concomitant MAT	NR	Fresh frozen	29.6 ± 10.5	3.7 ± 1.7	23.9 ± 4.1	2.51 ± 3.52	NR	15: (n = 1) LMAT + MFx, (n = 8) LMAT + ACI, (n = 1) LMAT + OAT, (n = 4) LMAT + OCA (n = 1) LMAT + DFO + OCA.	At F/u, patients undergoing isolated articular cartilage surgery had a significantly higher KOOS QoL subscore than did those undergoing articular cartilage surgery and lateral MAT, with no other significant postoperative differences in any outcome score between the 2 groups.	1 patient with superficial wound infection.	No conversions to TKA or MAT revisions; 14% overall reoperation rate: (n = 1) lateral release, (n = 1) partial lateral meniscectomy, (n = 5) chondroplasty, (n = 1) revision OCA.	When indicated, meniscal deficiency, malalignment, and chondral defects can be addressed concomitantly without compromising clinical outcomes.

Chalmers et al,[25] 2013	13 high school or college athletes	3 medial, 10 lateral	Fresh frozen	19.3	3.3	NR	23.9 ± 23.5 from index meniscectomy	None	7: (n = 3) ACLR, (n = 2) OCA, (n = 1) OCA + DFO, (n = 1) MFx.	Significant improvements in IKDC, Lysholm, KOOS pain, symptoms, activity of daily living, and sport subscores at final F/u.	1 failure: LMAT.	3 (23%): (n = 1) revision MAT, (n = 1) partial meniscectomy, (n = 1) meniscal repair.	77% returned to their previous level of activity and 70% returned to their desired level of play, with a mean time to return to previous athletic level of 16.5 mo with significant improvement in clinical and functional outcomes.
Cole et al,[20] 2012	22	13 medial, 9 lateral	Fresh frozen	32.5 ± 12.3	8.5 ± 1.3	8 patients with BMI <25, 14 with BMI >25	None from index meniscectomy	NR	14 (64%): ACI (n = 5), ACL revision (n = 3), Mfx (n = 2), OCA (n = 2), OAT (n = 2), HWR (n = 3), PCL thermal shrinkage (n = 1).	Mean postoperative satisfaction was 8.8/10; 77% RTS at mean of 17 mo. At 7 y postoperatively, the Overall Knee Condition, IKDC, Lysholm, and all 5 KOOS subgroup scores improved significantly (P < .05) compared with baseline.	3 patients were identified as failures at 24 mo, 54 mo and 68 mo for undergoing either revision MAT (24, 54 mo) or unicompartmental arthroplasty (68 mo).	88% survivorship.	MAT performed with appropriately indicated concomitant procedures showed statistically significant greater improvements in Lysholm, KOOS Pain, and KOOS QoL as compared with the improvements seen with isolated MAT.

(continued on next page)

Table 1
(continued)

Author	No. of Patients	Laterality	Graft Preservation Technique	Mean Age (y)	Mean F/u (y)	Mean BMI (kg/m²)	Time to Surgery (y)	Workers Comp	Concomitant Procedures	Clinical/Radiographic Outcomes	Failures, Complications	Overall Survival Rate/Reoperation Rate	Conclusion
Rue et al,[52] 2008	31: 16 with ACI and 15 with OCA	20 medial, 11 lateral	Majority cryopreserved, those after 2004 fresh frozen	29.9	3.1	NR	NR	4 (13%)	3 in OCA group: 1 HTO, 2 HWR.	Significant improvements in Lysholm, IKDC, KOOS, Noyes Symptom scores in both groups. Absolute outcome scores for ACI were significantly better than those for OCA in IKDC and KOOS (all subscores).	2 failures: revision MAT (3 y), complete meniscectomy (2.4 y).	94% survival at a mean of 3.1 y.	Outcomes of combined cartilage and MAT procedures are comparable to reports of these procedures performed in isolation.

Abbreviations: ACI, autologous chondrocyte implantation; ACLR, anterior cruciate ligament reconstruction; ADL, activities of daily living; BMI, body mass index; BML, bone marrow lesion; de novo NT, de novo natural tissue; DFO, distal femoral osteotomy; F/u, follow-up; HTO, high tibial osteotomy; HW, hardware; HWR, hardware removal; IKDC, International Knee Document Committee; KOOS, Knee Injury and Osteoarthritis Outcome Score; LMAT, lateral meniscal allograft transplantation; MFx, microfracture; MMAT, medial meniscal allograft transplant; MUA, manipulation under anesthesia; NR, not reported; OAT, osteochondral autograft; OCA, osteochondral allograft; OR, odds ratio; PROs, patient-reported outcomes; QoL, quality of life; SF-12, Short Form-12; TKA, total knee arthroplasty; UKA, unicompartmental knee arthroplasty; VAS, visual analog scale; WOMAC, Western Ontario and McMaster Universities Osteoarthritis Index.

patients undergoing either isolated MAT or MAT plus cartilage procedure (OCA, autologous chondrocyte implantation, microfracture, osteochondral autograft, de novo juvenile particulate cartilage implantation) for a mean follow-up of 4.48 ± 2.63 years and 3.84 ± 2.47 years, respectively. The study found no significant differences in postoperative patient-reported outcomes, number of subsequent surgeries, or failures between the 2 groups. Furthermore, Rue and colleagues[52] analyzed 29 patients undergoing MAT with either autologous chondrocyte implantation or OCA with a mean follow-up of 3.1 years and found that there were significant improvements in all patient reported outcomes except the SF-12. Two patients were considered failures. Harris and colleagues[53] analyzed 18 patients undergoing MAT, osteotomy, and a cartilage procedure with a mean follow-up of 6.5 ± 3.2 years and found that there were significant improvements in KOOS pain, KOOS activities of daily living, KOOS sports and recreation, KOOS quality of life, IKDC, and Lysholm. Additionally, although there was a 55.5% reoperation rate, most commonly for lysis of adhesions, only 1 patient converted to knee arthroplasty and only 1 patient underwent revision cartilage and meniscal transplant surgery. These results suggest that, when indicated, meniscal deficiency, malalignment, and chondral defects can be addressed concomitantly without compromising clinical outcomes.

Studies have also evaluated the performance of MAT concomitantly with anterior cruciate ligament reconstruction. Saltzman and colleagues[54] evaluated 40 patients undergoing anterior cruciate ligament reconstruction and MAT with a mean follow-up of 5.7 ± 3.2 years. The study noted a significant improvement in all patient-reported outcomes analyzed except for Tegner score, which significantly decreased, WOMAC stiffness, and SF-12 scores. The authors found a 98% graft survival rate at 1.7 years, 84% at 5 years, and 45% at 10 years, suggesting that, when indicated, anterior cruciate ligament reconstruction can be performed concomitantly with MAT without negatively affecting patient outcomes.

MENISCAL ALLOGRAFT TRANSPLANTATION IN HIGH-LEVEL ATHLETES AND ADOLESCENTS

Outcomes in young patients following MAT have also been another main area of investigation for several authors. It was previously thought that open physes were a contraindication for MAT. Riboh and colleagues[22] investigated 32 patients ages 13 to 16 with a mean follow-up of 7.2 ± 3.2 years. Significant improvements were seen in Lysholm, IKDC, WOMAC pain, function and stiffness, SF-12 physical, as well as all KOOS subscores, except KOOS symptoms. Of note, at final follow-up, the only outcome score that had significantly declined from 2-year follow-up was IKDC. In terms of meniscal reoperation, however, the rate was only 6%, and both patients underwent debridement for a torn meniscal allograft. There were no revision MAT procedures required and no documented failures.

Marcacci and colleagues[32] studied 12 male professional soccer players who underwent MAT. The authors reported 92% returned to soccer at a mean 10.5 ± 2.6 months postoperatively. At the 1-year follow-up, 67% were playing at their preinjury level. At the 3-year follow-up, 75% were still playing professional soccer and 17% were playing semiprofessionally. In a retrospective case series, Chalmers and colleagues[25] evaluated MAT in 13 high school-level and higher athletes regarding return to their preinjury level of play with a mean follow-up of 3.3 years. Postoperatively, 77% returned to their previous level of activity and 70% returned to their desired level of play. The mean time to return to previous athletic level was 16.5 months. Zaffagnini and colleagues[55] studied 89 active patients who underwent MAT without bone plugs with a mean follow-up of 4.2 ± 1.9 years and found that 49% were able to return to preinjury level of play and 74% were able to return to sport after 8.6 ± 4.1 months. In systematic reviews, Lee and colleagues[56] found that 67% to 85.7% of athletes returned to sport anywhere from 7.6 to 16.5 months after surgery.

Graft Extrusion

Another important factor when considering patient outcomes is the extrusion of the meniscal allograft or the displacement of the meniscus with respect to the central margin of the tibial plateau.[57] Although the long-term clinical effect of meniscal allograft extrusion still needs to be evaluated, several studies have begun using MRI to measure extrusion during follow-up because extrusion has been shown to be a sign of arthritis.[58,59] Additionally, extrusion of the graft puts the graft in a nonanatomic position and leads to biomechanical disadvantages.[60] Because the prevention and delay of OA are among the main goals for MAT, minimizing extrusion and determining the clinical implications is an important and timely task, although it remains a controversial topic because studies have not found clinical outcome scores to correlate with meniscal allograft extrusion thus far.

Roumazeille and colleagues[33] studied MAT without bone plugs and found that meniscal extrusion, defined as the distance from the periphery of the graft to medial border of the tibia in the coronal plane, was present in 75% of patients evaluated via MRI at 6 months postoperatively. Interestingly, no correlation was found between percent extrusion and graft healing. These patients continued to report significant improvements in pain and knee function scores. Similarly, Kim and colleagues[61] found that, in 30 patients who underwent MAT, there was no significant change or progression in the extrusion measured on MRI at 3 or 12 months postoperatively. Furthermore, the amount of extrusion was not found to correlate with postoperative outcomes.

To evaluate surgical techniques that might reduce extrusion, Masferrer-Pino and colleagues[62] compared the standard bridge in slot technique to a capsulodesis, in which a capsular fixation suture was passed through each of the transtibial tunnels to add a fixation point of the capsule to the tibial plateau. Although the initial statistical analysis of 29 patients revealed no significant difference in extrusion at follow-up (36–48 months), when the authors removed the first 4 cases of capsulodesis from the analysis as a learning curve for the new technique as the worst cases of extrusion in this group were seen in the first 4 patients, there was a significantly lower percentage of extrusion seen in the capsulodesis group. These extrusion results, however, did not transfer to clinical outcomes because there were no significant differences in outcome scores between the groups.

In a cohort study evaluating 53 patients who underwent lateral MAT with the keyhole technique, Lee and colleagues[63] used a delayed rehabilitation program that involved immobilization of the knee in full extension with varus force applied via a long leg cast for 3 week postoperatively, followed by continuous passive range of motion exercise 0° to 90° for 3 additional weeks and 0° to 120° for the next 6 weeks. After the cast was removed, patients wore a lateral unloading brace for 9 weeks. The control group underwent a standard rehabilitation program of immobilization in extension for 5 to 7 days followed by continuous passive range of motion starting at 7 days. The patients wore a hinged brace locked in full extension during partial weight bearing for 3 weeks with movement restrictions of 0° to 90° starting at 3 weeks and 0° to 120° at 6 weeks. The authors found that patients who underwent the delayed rehabilitation program had statistically less extrusion on coronal MRI at 24 months as well as less progression of OA. Although no differences in clinical outcomes between the groups were observed, more investigation needs to be done to assess the clinical impact of meniscal extrusion.

REVISION MENISCAL ALLOGRAFT TRANSPLANTATION

In the small percentage of patients who underwent revision MAT, Yanke and colleagues[64] prospectively analyzed 8 patients with a mean follow-up after revision MAT of 3.83 ± 1.3 years. The average time to revision MAT from index procedure was 3.45 ± 2.52 years. These patients demonstrated significant improvements in IKDC, KOOS pain scores, and subjective symptom rating scale. Comparison of Outerbridge grading at the time of initial MAT and revision MAT showed no significant differences. Overall, these patients showed significant improvements and 7 of the 8 patients stated they would undergo the procedure again, including the patient who progressed to arthroplasty, suggesting that the pain relief and gain of function associated with the procedure, albeit for a short time for this patient, is significantly improved compared with preoperative pain and function levels.

MINIMAL CLINICALLY IMPORTANT DIFFERENCE AND PATIENT ACCEPTABLE SYMPTOMATIC STATE

More recently, an emphasis has been placed on establishing thresholds to establish MCID for patients undergoing MAT. Liu and colleagues[65] evaluated 98 patients to analyze the short-term outcomes and determine the MCID and PASS with respect to patient reported outcomes. The MCID and PASS were determined for Lysholm score (MCID, 12.3; PASS, 66.5), IKDC (9.9; 36.0), KOOS Pain (9.9; 43.0), KOOS Symptoms (9.7; 73.0), KOOS Activities of Daily Living (9.5; 74.5), KOOS Sport (13.3; 22.5), and KOOS Quality of Life (14.6; 53.0). The study found that workers' compensation patients and patients with higher body mass indexes were less likely to achieve these values for certain outcome measures. Additionally, patients who had lower scores preoperatively were more likely to achieve these thresholds in most outcome measures. Physicians should use these correlations to help counsel patients preoperatively about MAT outcomes as well as to fine-tune patient selection for MAT.

SUMMARY

Because meniscectomy can lead to the onset and progression of OA by altering the biomechanics and contact pressures of the knee, it is essential to develop treatment options to address this effect. In patients less than 55 years old with a deficient meniscus, persistent pain after meniscectomy, and correctable concomitant pathology, MAT provides a viable option for pain and symptom relief and possibly the delay in the onset of OA. Short- and long-term outcomes are promising for MAT, although more investigation is needed into the clinical effects of meniscal extrusion and techniques to minimize extrusion.

REFERENCES

1. Andersson-Molina H, Karlsson H, Rockborn P. Arthroscopic partial and total meniscectomy: a long-term follow-up study with matched controls. Arthroscopy 2002;18(2):183–9.
2. Baratz M, Fu F, Mengato R. Meniscal tears: the effect of meniscectomy and of repair on intraarticular contact areas and stress in the human knee. A preliminary report. Am J Sports Med 1986;14(4):270–5.

3. Cox J, Nye C, Schaefer W, et al. The degenerative effects of partial and total resection of the medial meniscus in dogs' knees. Clin Orthop Relat Res 1975; 109:178–83.

4. Walker PS, Erkman MJ. The role of the menisci in force transmission across the knee. Clin Orthop Relat Res 1975;(109):184–92. Available at: http://www.ncbi. nlm.nih.gov/pubmed/1173360.

5. Brown M, Farrell J, Kluczynski M, et al. Biomechanical effects of a horizontal medial meniscus tear and subsequent leaflet resection. Am J Sports Med 2016;44:850–4.

6. Koh J, Yi S, Ren Y, et al. Tibiofemoral contact mechanics with horizontal cleavage tear and resection of the medial meniscus in the human knee. J Bone Joint Surg Am 2016;98:1829–36.

7. Goyal K, Pan T, Tran D, et al. Vertical tears of the lateral meniscus: effects on in vitro tibiofemoral joint mechanics. Orthop J Sports Med 2014;2. 2325967114541237.

8. Ode G, Van Thiel G, McArthur S, et al. Effects of serial sectioning and repair of radial tears in the lateral meniscus. Am J Sports Med 2012;40:1863–70.

9. Bedi A, Kelly N, Baad M, et al. Dynamic contact mechanics of radial tears of the lateral meniscus: implications for treatment. Arthroscopy 2012;28:372–81.

10. Johnson R, Kettelkamp D, Clark W, et al. Factors effecting late results after meniscectomy. J Bone Joint Surg Am 1974;56:719–29.

11. Fairbank J, Pynsent P, van Poortvliet J, et al. Mechanical factors in the incidence of knee pain in adolescents and young adults. J Bone Joint Surg Br 1984;66(5): 685–93.

12. Alford W, Cole BJ. The indications and technique for meniscal transplant. Orthop Clin North Am 2005;36(4):469–84.

13. McCulloch PC, Dolce D, Jones HL, et al. Comparison of kinematics and tibiofemoral contact pressures for native and transplanted lateral menisci. Orthop J Sports Med 2016;4(12):1–9.

14. Spang JT, Dang ABC, Mazzocca A, et al. The effect of medial meniscectomy and meniscal allograft transplantation on knee and anterior cruciate ligament biomechanics. Arthroscopy 2010;26(2):192–201.

15. Seedhom BB, Hargreaves DJ. Transmission of the load in the knee joint with special reference to the role of the menisci: part II: experimental results, discussion and conclusions. Eng Med 1979;8(4):220–8.

16. Myers P, Tudor F. Meniscal allograft transplantation: how should we be doing it? A systematic review. Arthroscopy 2015;31(5):911–25.

17. Cvetanovich GL, Yanke AB, McCormick F, et al. Trends in meniscal allograft transplantation in the United States, 2007 to 2011. Arthroscopy 2015;31(6):1123–7.

18. Abrams GD, Frank RM, Gupta AK, et al. Trends in meniscus repair and meniscectomy in the United States, 2005-2011. Am J Sports Med 2013;41(10):2333–9.

19. Mccormick F, Harris JD, Abrams GD, et al. Survival and reoperation rates after meniscal allograft transplantation analysis of failures for 172 consecutive transplants at a minimum 2-year follow-up. Am J Sports Med 2014. https://doi.org/ 10.1177/0363546513520115.

20. Cole BJ, Saltzman B, Bajaj S, et al. Prospective long-term evaluation of meniscal allograft transplantation procedure: a minimum of 7-year follow-up. J Knee Surg 2012;25(02):165–76.

21. Hommen JP, Applegate GR, Del Pizzo W. Meniscus allograft transplantation: ten-year results of cryopreserved allografts. Arthroscopy 2007;23(4):388–93.

22. Riboh JC, Tilton AK, Cvetanovich GL, et al. Meniscal allograft transplantation in the adolescent population. Arthroscopy 2016;32(6):1133–40.e1.

23. Mascarenhas R, Yanke AB, Frank RM, et al. Meniscal allograft transplantation: preoperative assessment, surgical considerations, and clinical outcomes. J Knee Surg 2014;27(6):443–58.

24. Saltzman BM, Meyer MA, Leroux TS, et al. The influence of full-thickness chondral defects on outcomes following meniscal allograft transplantation: a comparative study. Arthroscopy 2018;34(2):519–29.

25. Chalmers PN, Karas V, Sherman SL, et al. Return to high-level sport after meniscal allograft transplantation. Arthroscopy 2013;29(3):539–44.

26. Abrams GD, Hussey KE, Harris JD, et al. Clinical results of combined meniscus and femoral osteochondral allograft transplantation: minimum 2-year follow-up. Arthroscopy 2014;30(8):964–70.e1.

27. Noyes FR, Barber-westin SD, Rankin M. Meniscal transplantation in symptomatic patients less than fifty years old. J Bone Joint Surg Am 2005;87-A:1392–404.

28. Cotter EJ, Frank RM, Waterman BR, et al. Meniscal allograft transplantation with concomitant osteochondral allograft transplantation. Arthrosc Tech 2017;6(5): e1573–80.

29. Cole BJ, Dennis MG, Lee SJ, et al. Prospective evaluation of allograft meniscus transplantation: a minimum 2-year follow-up. Am J Sports Med 2006;34(6): 919–27.

30. Smith NA, Parsons N, Wright D, et al. A pilot randomized trial of meniscal allograft transplantation versus personalized physiotherapy for patients with a symptomatic meniscal deficient knee compartment. Bone Joint J 2018;100B(1):56–63.

31. Kellgren J, Lawrence J. Radiological assessment of osteoarthritis. Ann Rheum Dis 1957;16:494–502.

32. Marcacci M, Marcheggiani Muccioli GM, Grassi A, et al. Arthroscopic meniscus allograft transplantation in male professional soccer players: a 36-month follow-up study. Am J Sports Med 2014;42(2):382–8.

33. Roumazeille T, Klouche S, Rousselin B, et al. Arthroscopic meniscal allograft transplantation with two tibia tunnels without bone plugs: evaluation of healing on MR arthrography and functional outcomes. Knee Surg Sports Traumatol Arthrosc 2015;23(1):264–9.

34. Kon E, Filardo G, Berruto M, et al. Articular cartilage treatment in high-level male soccer players: a prospective comparative study of arthroscopic second-generation autologous chondrocyte implantation versus microfracture. Am J Sports Med 2011;39(12):2549–57.

35. Marcacci M, Zaffagnini S, Marcheggiani Muccioli GM, et al. Meniscal allograft transplantation without bone plugs: a 3-year minimum follow-up study. Am J Sports Med 2012;40(2):395–403.

36. Ha JK, Sung JH, Shim JC, et al. Medial meniscus allograft transplantation using a modified bone plug technique: clinical, radiologic, and arthroscopic results. Arthroscopy 2011;27(7):944–50.

37. Abat F, Gelber PE, Erquicia JI, et al. Suture-only fixation technique leads to a higher degree of extrusion than bony fixation in meniscal allograft transplantation. Am J Sports Med 2012;40(7):1591–6.

38. Dienst M, Greis P, Ellis B, et al. Effect of lateral meniscal allograft sizing on contact mechanics of the lateral tibial plateau: an experimental study in human cadaveric knee joints. Am J Sports Med 2014;35(1):34–42.

39. Pollard ME, Kang Q, Berg EE. Radiographic sizing for meniscal transplantation. Arthroscopy 1995;11(6):684–7.

40. Schubert T, Cornu O, Delloye C. Organization: types of grafts, conservation, regulation. In: Beaufils P, Verdonk R, editors. The meniscus. 1st edition. London: Springer; 2010. p. 315–21.

41. Elattar M, Dhollander A, Verdonk R, et al. Twenty- six years of meniscal allograft transplantation: is it still experimental? A meta-analysis of 44 trials. Knee Surg Sports Traumatol Arthrosc 2011;19(2):147–57.

42. Smith NA, Parkinson B, Hutchinson CE, et al. Is meniscal allograft transplantation chondroprotective? A systematic review of radiological outcomes. Knee Surg Sports Traumatol Arthrosc 2016;24(9):2923–35.

43. Cole B, Carter T, Rodeo S. Allograft meniscal transplantation: background, techniques, and results. Instr Course Lect 2003;52:383–96.

44. Lee AS, Kang RW, Kroin E, et al. Allograft meniscus transplantation. Sports Med Arthrosc Rev 2012;20(2):106–14.

45. Freedman KB, Cole BJ, Farr J. Arthroscopic meniscus transplantation: Bridge in slot technique. In: Miller MD, Cole BJ, editors. Textbook of Arthroscopy. Philadelphia: Elsevier; 2004. p. 547–54.

46. Rao AJ, Erickson BJ, Cvetanovich GL, et al. The meniscus-deficient knee: biomechanics, evaluation, and treatment options. Orthop J Sports Med 2015; 3(10):1–14.

47. Verdonk PCM, Verstraete KL, Almqvist KF, et al. Meniscal allograft transplantation: long-term clinical results with radiological and magnetic resonance imaging correlations. Knee Surg Sports Traumatol Arthrosc 2006;14(8):694–706.

48. Verdonk P, Depaepe Y, Desmyter S, et al. Normal and transplanted lateral knee menisci: evaluation of extrusion using magnetic resonance imaging and ultrasound. Knee Surg Sports Traumatol Arthrosc 2004;12(5):411–9.

49. Frank RM, Cole BJ. Meniscus transplantation. Curr Rev Musculoskelet Med 2015; 8(4):443–50.

50. Saltzman BM, Cotter EJ, Stephens JP, et al. Preoperative tibial subchondral bone marrow lesion patterns and associations with outcomes after isolated meniscus allograft transplantation. Am J Sports Med 2018;46(5):1175–84.

51. Frank RM, Lee S, Cotter EJ, et al. Outcomes of osteochondral allograft transplantation with and without concomitant meniscus allograft transplantation: a comparative matched group analysis. Am J Sports Med 2018;46(3):573–80.

52. Rue JPH, Yanke AB, Busam ML, et al. Prospective evaluation of concurrent meniscus transplantation and articular cartilage repair: minimum 2-year follow-up. Am J Sports Med 2008;36(9):1770–8.

53. Harris JD, Hussey K, Saltzman BM, et al. Cartilage repair with or without meniscal transplantation and osteotomy for lateral compartment chondral defects of the knee: case series with minimum 2-year follow-up. Orthop J Sports Med 2014; 2(10):1–7.

54. Saltzman BM, Meyer MA, Weber AE, et al. Prospective clinical and radiographic outcomes after concomitant anterior cruciate ligament reconstruction and meniscal allograft transplantation at a mean 5-year follow-up. Am J Sports Med 2017; 45(3):550–62.

55. Zaffagnini S, Grassi A, Muccioli GMM, et al. Is sport activity possible after arthroscopic meniscal allograft transplantation? Am J Sports Med 2016;44(3):625–32.

56. Lee YS, Lee O-S, Lee SH. Return to sports after athletes undergo meniscal surgery. Clin J Sport Med 2017;29(1):1.

57. Lerer D, Umans H, Hu M, et al. The role of meniscal root pathology and radial meniscal tear in medial meniscal extrusion. Skeletal Radiol 2004;33(10):569–74.

58. Gale D, Chaisson CE, Totterman SM, et al. Meniscal subluxation: association with osteoarthritis and joint space narrowing. Osteoarthritis Cartilage 1999;7:526–32.
59. Berthiaume M, Raynauld J, Martel-Pelletier J, et al. Meniscal tear and extrusion are strongly associated with progression of symptomatic knee osteoarthritis as assessed by quantitative magnetic resonance imaging. Ann Rheum Dis 2005; 64:556–63.
60. Lee D-H, Lee C-R, Jeon J-H, et al. Graft extrusion in both the coronal and sagittal planes is greater after medial compared with lateral meniscus allograft transplantation but is unrelated to early clinical outcomes. Am J Sports Med 2015;43: 213–9.
61. Kim J, Lee S, Ha DH, et al. The effects of graft shrinkage and extrusion on early clinical outcomes after meniscal allograft transplantation. J Orthop Surg Res 2018;13(1):181.
62. Masferrer-Pino A, Monllau JC, Ibáñez M, et al. Capsulodesis versus bone trough technique in lateral meniscal allograft transplantation: graft extrusion and functional results. Arthroscopy 2018;34(6):1879–88.
63. Lee DW, Lee JH, Kim DH, et al. Delayed rehabilitation after lateral meniscal allograft transplantation can reduce graft extrusion compared with standard rehabilitation. Am J Sports Med 2018;46(10):2432–40.
64. Yanke AB, Chalmers PN, Frank RM, et al. Clinical outcome of revision meniscal allograft transplantation: minimum 2-year follow-up. Arthroscopy 2014;30(12): 1602–8.
65. Liu JN, Gowd AK, Redondo ML, et al. Establishing clinically significant outcomes after meniscal allograft transplantation. Orthop J Sports Med 2019;7(1):1–9.

Meniscus Repair and Regeneration

A Systematic Review from a Basic and Translational Science Perspective

John Twomey-Kozak, BS, Chathuraka T. Jayasuriya, PhD*

KEYWORDS

- Meniscus • Stem cell • Tissue engineering • Scaffolds • Regenerative medicine

KEY POINTS

- Meniscus injury is one of the most common athletic injuries.
- Current reparative techniques fail to produce long-term improvements, and thus, alternative regenerative medicine applications are being investigated in the meniscus field.
- Acellular and cellular therapies as well as their delivery methods are being investigated for repair and regeneration of meniscus tissue.
- Various progenitor/stem cell types are being investigated as optimal cell sources to help stimulate native tissue regeneration of the meniscus.

INTRODUCTION

The meniscal injury is a major cause of functional impairment in the knee joint. This fibrocartilaginous tissue was once considered to be an unnecessary, vestigial appendage that could be sacrificed with minimal consideration.[1,2] This total meniscectomy technique, although common in the past, has largely been abandoned because long-term results after major meniscectomy reported disappointing and adverse effects, such as the degradation of underlying articular cartilage and subsequent development of early osteoarthritis.[1,3–5] As clinical medicine and basic science have evolved, the meniscus is now properly recognized as a necessary structure in the knee joint that is vital for biomechanical and anatomic purposes.[6] Namely, the menisci are key for knee stability, distributing axial load, shock absorption between the articular cartilage of the tibia and femur, and nutrient distribution for protection of the underlying articular cartilage.[1,6,7]

Department of Orthopaedics, Brown University/Rhode Island Hospital, Box G-A1, Providence, RI 02912, USA
* Corresponding author. Rhode Island Hospital & Warren Alpert Medical School of Brown University, West Coro Building, 1 Hoppin Street, Office 4.313, Providence, RI 02903.
E-mail address: chathuraka_jayasuriya@brown.edu

Clin Sports Med 39 (2020) 125–163
https://doi.org/10.1016/j.csm.2019.08.003   sportsmed.theclinics.com
0278-5919/20/© 2019 Elsevier Inc. All rights reserved.

Biochemical Composition

The meniscus is composed of a dense extracellular matrix (ECM) that consists of 72% water, 22% collagen, and 0.8% glycosaminoglycans (GAGs).[8,9] The remaining dry weight is made up of proteins, glycoproteins, and interspersed cells within the meniscus. These cells are referred to as *fibrochondrocytes*, because they have a marked resemblance to both fibroblasts and chondrocytes and synthesize the ECM and meniscal tissue.[9–11] Type I collagen is expressed abundantly throughout the meniscus, whereas type II collagen is detected in the inner region. The interactions of these collagens, GAGs, and proteins likely account for the compressive load resistance, lubrication, and semielastic deformation properties of the meniscus.[9,12]

Biomechanics and Gross Anatomy

The knee joint capsule houses the menisci, which are smooth, lubricated, crescent-shaped discs composed of fibrocartilaginous tissue with a medial and lateral component. These menisci sit on the natural contours of the tibial plateau between the femoral condyle and tibia of the knee. Joint motion and the biomechanical stressors associated with physical activity are important factors in determining the orientation of the collagen fibers that provide meniscal structure. There are 2 types of structural fibers that make up the meniscus: type I and type II collagen. These fibers are typically oriented based on the layers of the meniscus from surface to core: *superficial* (random orientation), *lamellar* (more organized radially at anterior and posterior horns), and *deep* (oriented circumferentially with some radial fibers) and allow the meniscus to expand under compressive forces to increase contact area of the joint.[6,13]

A capillary network that originates in the synovium provides a direct blood supply to the meniscus, but only in certain "zones" of the meniscus. These zones are named based on the extent of vascularization of each respective region. The peripheral, outer third of the meniscus is known as the "red-red" zone, which has an excellent prognosis for repair because the blood supply is directly provided here.[14,15] The intermediate "red-white" zone receives a limited blood supply and usually has a fair prognosis, as long as it is at the border of the vascular zone. The inner "white-white" zone of the meniscus, however, is completely avascular and presents a poor prognosis for recovery, regeneration, and healing.[15] The lack of blood supply in this region confers difficulties for lesion/injury repair and regeneration of injured meniscus tissue. Current clinical reparative capacity seems to be restricted mainly to the peripheral, "red-red" vascular region of the meniscus, where there is a sufficient blood supply to promote healing. Biological tissue engineering and cell-based therapies constitute preclinical meniscus repair/regeneration strategies that offer much promise for the future.[8,16]

Injury Prevalence and Call for Repair

With a combination of axial loading and rotational forces that generate a shear force, the meniscus is subject to both acute and degenerative injury, making it arguably the most commonly injured tissue in the knee.[17] The epidemiologic data for the incidence and prevalence of meniscus injuries and clinical repair are limited, but seem to be rising every year. Logerstedt and colleagues,[18] Hede and colleagues,[19] and Jones and colleagues[20] reported that the incidence rate of meniscus injury was 0.33 and 0.61 per 1000 person-years, with a prevalence of 12% to 14%. In the United States, of the estimated 850,000 to 1,000,000 cases per year in 2010, 10% to 20% of orthopedic surgeries involved surgical repair of the meniscus.[21,22]

Clinicians and scientists alike agree that meniscal injury is considered an essential predictor of the subsequent development of degenerative joint disease and specifically strongly correlated with the development of early osteoarthritis.[23–25] Therefore, considering the high incidence rate and increased risk of osteoarthritis development, it is critical to develop an ideal method for the prevention, repair, and treatment of injured meniscus tissue. Recent efforts have been directed toward regeneration of native meniscus tissue rather than meniscal resection. Although surgical techniques for mending damaged meniscus tissue have been extensively explored in the clinical setting, these repair attempts continue to fail for various reasons (ie, lack of longevity, tissue avascularity). Thus, it seems ideal to reframe this problem through an alternative perspective from the lens of basic science and regenerative medicine. This avenue, rather than meniscectomy or resection, has become an intriguing idea for addressing meniscal injuries in preclinical models. This review comprehensively details the current methodologies that are being explored in the basic sciences to stimulate better meniscus injury repair. Furthermore, it describes how these preclinical strategies may stand to improve current paradigms of how meniscal injuries are clinically treated through a unique and alternative perspective to traditional clinical methodology.

CURRENT CLINICAL PARADIGM

When clinicians come across an irreparable tear in the meniscus or with patients who have undergone a total or subtotal meniscectomy, meniscal allograft transplantation (MAT) may be considered a preferred modality for knee joint restoration.[26] However, the indications for MAT remain controversial, because meniscal transplantation has been demonstrated to produce unsatisfactory results in the knee, including issues with graft size mismatching, donor incompatibility and sterilization, transplant remodeling and stability, and long-term chondroprotection.[27–29]

With an increasing incidence rate of meniscal injury, the urgent need for an innovative and efficacious repair strategy has become evident. Because of the aforementioned limitations, MAT cannot serve as a "fix-all" model. Because of this, the development of acellular biological scaffolds emerged as an interesting alternative to MAT. The primary goal of using these scaffolds is to use a minimally immunogenic 3-dimensional (3D) tissue-replacement that stimulates migration, proliferation, and integration of endogenous/native cells into the scaffold for the purpose of restoring meniscus function with a secondary goal of chondroprotection with respect to joint-loading function.[30]

Collagen Meniscus Implant

Currently in the United States, there is only 1 Food and Drug Administration–approved cell-free scaffold for meniscus replacement: the collagen meniscus implant (CMI). This scaffold was the first regenerative technique specifically invented and used for meniscus replacement in the clinical setting.[31–33] The CMI is composed primarily of type I collagen fibers and GAGs isolated from bovine Achilles tendon that are sterilized via gamma-irradiation.[34] This scaffold is perforated and porous to allow for ideal cell infiltration for better tissue integration purposes; clinical studies have indeed reported this native cell integration into the CMI.[35] In theory, this scaffold appears to be a better replacement than MAT; because it is less destructive to the joint, its shape can be custom fit, and it is composed of biological tissue, thus virtually eliminating the risk of an immunologic response from donor mismatch.[36] However, there has been debated controversy in terms of efficacy of the CMI. In 1999, Rodkey and colleagues[37] reported that 8 patients who underwent arthroscopic replacement with the CMI at short-term follow-up demonstrated tissue regeneration, no degenerative progression, and chondroprotection of the joint surface. These results were confirmed by radiographs, and the histologic grading was confirmed new fibrocartilage formation. Furthermore, a medium-term follow-up study was done by Bulgheroni and colleagues[38] in 2010, with 34 patients who underwent CMI implantation. These patients were evaluated 2 to 5 years later and showed good to excellent results with chondroprotection, no further degradation of the joint surface, and some newly synthesized tissue that appeared healthy.[38] However, the CMI had rescinded in size and was presenting some clinical challenges. Long-term follow-up studies have demonstrated similar adverse results, because the implant significantly shrank in size after 5 to 6 years, possibly because of degradation, and led to decreased biomechanical function.[39] The dangers of a potential size mismatch in the joint after implantation of the CMI would change the mechanical environment of the knee and decrease the chondroprotection of the underlying cartilage, resulting in further joint damage and likely further the progression of osteoarthritis.[40,41]

Platelet-Rich Plasma/Fibrin

Within the field of orthopedics, the use of platelet-rich plasma (PRP) as a clinical therapeutic technique has seen a rapid increase in popularity. In the United States alone, it is estimated that 86,000 athletes are treated with PRP annually.[42] PRP is an autologous blood product containing numerous growth factors and cytokines that is being implemented as a clinical intervention for musculoskeletal defects, including meniscus injuries.[43] The increased concentration of platelets and growth factors is purported to aid in the native wound-healing process through the stimulation of meniscus cell proliferation and migration, angiogenesis, and matrix synthesis.[42,43] Despite its growing popularity both in medicine and in the mainstream media, the efficacy and usage of this biological treatment remain controversial.

Pujol and colleagues[44] attempted to augment repair and promote meniscal healing through the use of PRP treatment of horizontal meniscal tears. At a minimum of 24 months postoperatively, they reported a slight improvement in functional outcome and MRI-documented healing during midterm follow-up in young patients.[44] Furthermore, Blanke and colleagues[45] treated 10 patients with grade II meniscal lesions with percutaneous injections of PRP in 7-day intervals. Four of 10 patients showed a decrease of the meniscal lesion and relief of pain in a follow-up MRI and pain score after 6 months. In addition to slight pain relief and improved functional outcomes, certain groups have demonstrated the growth factor and immunologic response associated with PRP treatment. Wasterlain and colleagues[42] found that serum growth factors were significantly elevated after PRP injection, which may contribute to a better repair response. It is thought that PRP may augment healing by increasing the levels of growth factors and cytokines localized to the injury site.[46-48]

Although these groups have demonstrated positive results, there are also many others that report either (1) no significant improvements using PRP treatment or (2) adverse outcomes associated with PRP treatment. For example, 1 study conducted at the University of Virginia performed 35 isolated arthroscopic meniscal repairs with and without PRP augmentation and reported no clinical advantage of using PRP over non-PRP after a minimum follow-up of 2 years.[48] Furthermore, Zellner and colleagues[49,50] reported that implantation of a composite matrix loaded with PRP failed to improve meniscal healing in the avascular zone. The PRP-loaded matrix treatment outcome was characterized by poor tear filling without meniscal regeneration after a 3-month period. Available in vitro data reporting on the efficacy of PRP treatment of meniscal tears appear to be mixed as well, with groups finding contrasting results.[47,48,51–53] It should be noted that recent studies have found some success by using various mesenchymal stem cell (MSC) sources supplemented with PRP for meniscus repair[49]; however, this field is still being investigated and needs more published data.

Although some studies have demonstrated the benefits of PRP as a therapeutic for meniscal regeneration and healing, the clinical efficacy and results seem to be mixed and unclear. More clinical studies with larger sample sizes and medium- to long-term follow-ups with measurable outcomes, such as histologic analysis and functional grading of meniscus repair, are needed to determine the true efficacy of PRP.

ACELLULAR MENISCUS REGENERATION AND REPAIR TECHNIQUES IN BASIC/ TRANSLATIONAL SCIENCE
Decellularized Scaffold and Growth Factors

As an alternative method for a biomimetic cell-free scaffold, some have suggested using the process of decellularization of intact, native meniscus tissue in order to preserve the native structure and fiber-level organization. This decellularized scaffold technique is a significant advantage compared with other scaffolds because these retain the naturally occurring collagen networks present in the healthy meniscus. Furthermore, this type of scaffold would have a much lower risk of an adverse immunogenic reaction. However, 1 major challenge associated with using decellularized tissue is the low infiltration of cells into these scaffolds, because of their dense ECM structure as well as improper fitting and mismatch sizing issues in the joint.

In response to this, some groups have suggested using biomimetic, biosynthetic scaffolds coupled with chemotactic agents, such as growth factors, to stimulate native cell migration and infiltration to enhance integration into the scaffold. These growth factors that are used usually play a significant role in limb development. Local delivery or supplementation of growth factors may create a beneficial microenvironment to promote endogenic repair and integration for engineered tissue scaffolds.[54] Growth factors act on target cells to stimulate cellular growth, proliferation, healing, and cellular differentiation. This effect is achieved usually through a receptor-mediated mechanism, whereby a growth factor will bind to its respective receptor and trigger a secondary system of signals or messengers to activate nuclear genes that control different cellular processes.[54,55]

Certain growth factors have been demonstrated to play a key role in the metabolic activity of meniscal fibrochondrocytes (MFCs): regulating development, homeostasis, cell rejuvenation, and regeneration. With this idea in mind, there have been a myriad of different growth factor delivery methods to treat native fibrochondrocytes in both in vivo and in vitro experimental studies with the ultimate goal of optimizing meniscus tissue engineering and repair.[56–58] Specifically, this review focuses on the supplementation of growth factors to MFCs (the native cell of the meniscus) or direct addition of growth factors to meniscal tissue. The most commonly used growth factors for treating meniscal tissue or MFCs seem to be basic fibroblast growth factor (bFGF), transforming growth factor beta-1 and -3 (TGFB1, TGFB3), and insulin-like growth factor-1 (IGF-1), with others being used less frequently (**Table 1**).

Basic fibroblast growth factor
bFGF is a bioactive protein that acts as both a growth factor and a signaling protein that possesses broad mitogenic and cell survival activities, which play a primary role in angiogenesis, mitogenesis of fibroblasts, tyrosine activation, and inhibition of bone morphogenetic proteins (BMPs). When culturing MFCs in monolayer, Hiraide and colleagues[59] and Kasemkijwattana and colleagues[60] found that addition of

Table 1
Effect of different growth factor supplementation on meniscal fibrochondrocytes

Citation Source	Growth Factor Used	Cell Source	Results/Effects	In Vitro/In Vivo
Ionescu et al,[54] 2012	bFGF	None (tissue scaffold)	Short-term delivery-enhanced integration strength of native tissue with scaffold	In vitro explant–scaffold (bovine)
Hiraide et al,[59] 2005	bFGF	MFCs	Enhanced cell proliferation	In vitro–monolayer
Kasemkijwattana et al,[60] 2000	bFGF	MFCs	Enhanced cell proliferation	In vitro–monolayer
Stewart et al,[61] 2007	bFGF	MFCs	Enhanced cell proliferation	In vitro–PGA scaffold culture
Ionescu et al,[54] 2012	bFGF + TGFB3	None (scaffold)	Improved scaffold/tissue integration and enhanced meniscus repair	In vitro–electrospun PCL scaffold
Ionescu et al,[54] 2012	TGFB3	None (tissue scaffold)	Sustained delivery-enhanced integration strength of native tissue with scaffold and increased proteoglycan content	In vitro explant–scaffold (bovine)
Bochyńska et al,[62] 2017	TGFB3	None (scaffold)	Regeneration of articular cartilage underlying meniscus by homing of endogenous cells	In vivo–PCL-HA scaffold (rabbit)
Tarafder et al,[63] 2018	CTGF + TGFB3	None (tissue scaffold)	Remodeling of fibrous matrix into fibrocartilaginous matrix by TGFB3 mechanism, induced recruitment of synovial mesenchymal cells/progenitor cells and meniscal tissue integration through CTGF application	In vitro–loaded fibrin glue scaffold (bovine)
Tanaka et al,[64] 1999	TGFB1	MFCs	Increased collagen and GAG synthesis	In vitro–monolayer
Pangborn & Athanasiou,[65] 2005	TGFB1	MFCs	Increased collagen and GAG synthesis	In vitro–PGA scaffold
Imler et al,[66] 2004	TGFB1	MFCs	Increased collagen and GAG synthesis	In vitro–meniscus explant culture
Marsano et al,[67] 2007	TGFB1	MFCs	Enhanced cell proliferation	In vitro–monolayer

Study	Growth factor	Cell type	Effect	Model
De Mulder et al,[68] 2013	TGFB1	MFCs	Enhanced cell proliferation	In vitro–PU scaffold
Forriol et al,[69] 2014	BMP-7	None	Filled meniscal defect with cellular fibrous tissue	In vivo–intraarticular injection (sheep)
Bhargava et al,[70] 1999	BMP-7 (OP-1)	MFCs	Enhanced cell migration/proliferation	In vitro
Tumia & Johnstone,[71] 2004	IGF-1	MFCs	Enhanced cell proliferation, synthesis of proteoglycans and ECM while inhibiting destruction of matrix	In vitro–monolayer culture
Puetzer et al,[72] 2013	IGF-1	MFCs	Increased levels of collagen and GAG synthesis	In vitro–scaffold culture
Bhargava et al,[70] 1999	IGF-1	MFCs	Enhanced cell migration/homing of cells	In vitro–explant culture
Acosta et al,[73] 2008	IGF-1 + TGFB1	None (tissue scaffold)	Enhanced repair of avascular (white-white) zone of meniscus	In vitro–explant culture
Petersen et al,[74] 2007	VEGF	None (suture coating)	Failure to enhance repair or cell migration	In vivo–VEGF-coated sutures (sheep)
Hidaka et al,[75] 2002	HGF	MFCs	Increased angiogenesis to promote healing response	In vivo–PGA scaffold (mice)
Nishida et al,[76] 2004	CTGF	None (scaffold)	Enhanced articular cartilage regeneration	In vivo–hydrogel collagen scaffold (rat)
Tumia & Johnstone,[77] 2009	PDGF-AB	MFCs	Increased cell proliferation rate and matrix synthesis/formation	In vitro–monolayer culture
Marsano et al,[67] 2007	FGF-2	MFCs/tissue	Enhanced cell proliferation	In vitro–monolayer culture
Pangborn & Athanasiou,[65] 2005	FGF-2	MFCs/tissue	Enhanced collagen synthesis	In vitro–scaffold culture

Abbreviation: PGA, polyglycolic acid.

bFGF resulted in enhanced cell proliferation. Further in vitro studies have demonstrated that bFGF addition resulted in enhanced native tissue integration into various scaffold models and improved meniscus repair.[54,61]

Transforming growth factor-beta

The multifunctional cytokine superfamily, that is, TGFB, is involved in a receptor kinase mechanism that initiates a signaling cascade, which activates many downstream substrates and proteins. The role of TGFB isoforms TGFB1 and TGFB3 in the regulation of differentiation, chemotaxis, cell proliferation, and the immune response has been studied extensively in orthopedic research. In vitro supplementation of TGFB1 and TGFB3 to MFCs in monolayer, synthetic scaffolds, and explant tissue culture models have generally yielded positive results. These positive results include increased GAG and proteoglycan synthesis by native cells, enhanced native cell proliferation, regeneration of articular cartilage, and targeted homing of endogenous cells.[54,62–68]

Insulin Growth Factor-1

IGF-1 is a member of the insulin-related peptide family that plays an important role in childhood growth with continued anabolic effects in adults. IGF-1 is a primary mediator of the effects of growth hormone, which stimulates systemic body growth and is of key interest in the orthopedic research field for musculoskeletal purposes. Addition of IGF-1 to MFCs in monolayer, scaffold culture, and explant culture in vitro resulted in enhanced cell proliferation, increased GAG and proteoglycan production, and better homing of cells.[70–73]

CELL-BASED MENISCAL REGENERATION AND AUGMENTATION TECHNIQUES IN BASIC/TRANSLATIONAL SCIENCE

The cell-based therapeutic potential of human multipotent MSC has long been investigated in the field of meniscal tissue healing and regenerative medicine. This tissue engineering strategy is closer to translation than some might think, and there are even some clinical trials currently underway (ClinicalTrials.gov Identifier: NCT02033525). Currently, groups are investigating several promising cell types and isolation methods to identify ideal MSC sources for meniscus repair. This exploration has produced encouraging but mixed results that are likely due to varying experimental conditions used in each individual investigation. This wide variation has made it difficult to directly compare efficacious outcomes in the field of tissue engineering and regeneration. With an aim to alleviate these difficulties, in 2006, the International Society for Cellular Therapy (ISCT) published a minimal criterion to define human MSCs.[78] First, the MSCs must adhere to tissue culture plastic when maintained in standard culture conditions. Second, the phenotypic profile and epitope expression of MSCs must be at the very minimum: CD105+, CD73+, CD90+ while being CD45−, CD34−, CD14−, CD11b−, CD79a−, or CD19−.[78] Third, MSCs must demonstrate trilineage potential, meaning that they can be differentiated into osteoblasts, adipocytes, and chondroblasts in vitro.[78] In addition, it is thought that these stem cells must be self-renewing and have a high proliferation capacity in the sense that they can perpetually divide/replicate while maintaining an undifferentiated state.[79]

Therefore, this review focuses exclusively on what the authors, in accordance with the ISCT minimal criterion, consider the MSC sources most widely used and most promising in the basic and translational science research setting for cell-based meniscus regeneration: bone marrow-derived mesenchymal stem cells (BM-MSCs), adipose-derived stem cells (ADSCs), synovium-derived stem cells (SDSCs), native MFCs, and progenitor cells, articular cartilage-derived progenitor cells (CPCs).

In the following paragraphs, the authors report on preclinical, in vivo studies with data on meniscal tear augmentation using various cell-based therapies. These data are the focus of **Table 2**, which provides the cell type and quantity used, the animal model that was used, the length of time of the study, the measurements of successful treatment outcomes (histology, MRI, macroscopic, formation of neomeniscal tissue, presence of fibrochondrocytes, and so forth), and finally, the limitations for each cell type.

CELL TYPES AND THEIR PRECLINICAL RESULTS
Bone Marrow Mesenchymal Stem Cells

Cell-based meniscal regeneration strategies using various MSC sources have been well documented in the literature. There is still no true consensus as to which cell source is best for meniscus repair. However, BM-MSCs are often considered the "gold standard" in the field of cell-based regenerative medicine because they are used so frequently and have been thoroughly investigated since they were first discovered by Friedenstein and colleagues in 1968.[30,120,121] These cells are capable of multipotency and exhibit a phenotypic marker profile that is characteristic of MSCs: CD44[+], CD45[−], CD54[−], CD90[+], CD105[+], CD166[+], CD271[+].[78,122]

In 1999, Pittenger and colleagues[123] proposed a method of isolating BM-MSCs autologously from marrow aspirants during minimally invasive surgery that is still used today. Although these cells are relatively easy to collect, they only make up 0.0017% to 0.0201% of bone marrow cells.[124] It has been widely reported that BM-MSCs tend to demonstrate a robust chondrogenic response with elevated COL2A1 and matrix synthesis levels that seem beneficial for meniscus repair. However, these cells also have a harmful tendency to exhibit a hypertrophic phenotype.[125–127] This hypertrophic state has been illustrated specifically in meniscus coculture studies.[128] The propensity of BM-MSCs for hypertrophic differentiation could be detrimental for tissue regeneration and engineering purposes. Currently, the need to address this limitation of the current cell sources used for meniscus repair seems to center on (1) finding a novel and ideal cell source that is more resistant to cellular hypertrophy or (2) modulating BM-MSCs in such a way to dampen hypertrophy. An ideal cell source would be capable of maintaining multipotency while resisting hypertrophy and terminal differentiation in cell-based meniscal tissue engineering applications.

Preclinical applications of bone marrow mesenchymal stem cells results

BM-MSCs are the most thoroughly investigated and most frequently used cell source for meniscal repair in the field of regenerative medicine. These cells have been used in many preclinical meniscal repair studies. They have been used for the repair of meniscal tears[101,103,109–111] and various types of meniscal defects[49] as well as meniscus transections.[100,105] These studies use anywhere from 0.1×10^6 to 30×10^6 BM-MSCs for cell-based treatment depending on the animal model and size of the meniscus injury and range from 3 weeks to 24 months. Furthermore, because BM-MSCs have been widely used for this type of repair, there are many published findings that demonstrate both the advantages and the limitations for using BM-MSCs in many small and larger-animal models (see **Table 2**).

Ferris and colleagues[99] demonstrated in a horse model that intraarticular injection of 15 to 20×10^6 BM-MSCs postoperatively for meniscal lesions resulted in 75% return to some level of work compared with control groups after 24 months. Although this large-animal model is beneficial because it is a good emulator of a human meniscus model, the outcome measurement of "returning to some level of work" is very limited. Furthermore, it is difficult to assess the efficacy of BM-MSC–mediated repair without

Table 2
Various mesenchymal stem cell sources used for meniscus repair/regeneration and their preclinical application

Cell Source	Number of Cells Used	Animal Model	Meniscus Injury Model	Experimental Treatment	Control	Outcome/Results	Reference
SPIO-labeled ADSCs	2×10^6	Rabbit	½ anterior meniscectomy of medial meniscus	SPIO-labeled ADSCs	Saline OR unlabeled ADSCs	12 wk: Targeted ADSC delivery promoted meniscal regeneration + protective effects from OA damage	Qi et al,[80] 2015
Allogeneic rabbit ADSCs	0.1×10^6	Rabbit	Longitudinal lesion in avascular zone	Suture + ADSCs suspended in Matrigel	Suture + Matrigel only	12 wk: Improved healing rate in avascular zone for acute lesions that received suture + ADSCs	Ruiz-Ibán et al,[81] 2011
Autologous sheep ADSCs	20×10^6	Sheep	Medial meniscectomy (and ACL resection)	Autologous chondrogenically induced ADSCs	Culture medium	6 wk: Regenerated de novo cartilage underlying meniscus	Ude et al,[82] 2014
Autologous Human ADSCs	16×10^6	Human	Grade II meniscal tear	Autologous hADSCs + PRP and hyaluronic acid injections	PRP + Hyaluronic acid injections	3 mo: Reduced pain and minimal regeneration of meniscus tissue	Pak et al,[83] 2014
Autologous equine ADSCs	—	Equine	Medial meniscus defect	Autologous ADSCs	Autologous BM-MSCs	12 mo: Some defects appeared to fill in with fibrocartilaginous tissue, others did not heal or fill in	González-Fernández et al,[84] 2016
Human ADSCs	—	Bovine (explant in vitro)	Radial tear on cylindrical explant punch biopsy from inner avascular region of meniscus	Photo-crosslinked hydrogel loaded with ADSCs + TGFB3	TGFB3 only	4 wk and 8 wk: Increased matrix-sulfated proteoglycan deposition and some healing of meniscus	Sasaki et al,[85] 2018

Allogeneic rabbit ADSCs	—	Rabbit	PVA/Ch scaffold seeded with ADSCs	Complete meniscectomy of medial meniscus	Scaffold seeded with articular chondrocytes OR cell-free scaffold	7 mo: Minor meniscus regeneration for articular chondrocyte group (ADSCs had no significant contribution in healing process and lower Col II, Aggrecan, and Col 1)	Moradi et al,[86] 2017
Allogeneic rabbit ADSCs	5×10^4 cells/spheroid (400–500 spheroids)	Rabbit	High-density ADSC spheroid construct (3D culture)	Partial meniscectomy of the medial meniscus	No cells	2, 4, 8, and 12 wk: Mixed results; some rabbits showed beneficial healing effect in the avascular zone of the meniscus	Toratani et al,[87] 2017
Autologous SDSCs	0.25×10^6	Primate	Autologous SDSC aggregate	Partial meniscectomy of medial meniscus + insertional ligament of medial meniscus transection	Intraarticular SDSC injection	8 and 16 wk: Apparent meniscus regeneration in aggregate and control group; SDSC aggregate group had better articular cartilage histology scores *No statistical analysis	Kondo et al,[88] 2017
Allogeneic SDSCs	20×10^6	Micro minipig	Injection of SDSC suspension + suture	Longitudinal tear lesion in medial menisci	Suture only	12 wk: Meniscal healing in SDSC group reported to be significantly better than control group with collagen fibrils present in SDSC group only	Nakagawa et al,[89] 2015
Allogeneic SDSCs	50×10^6	Pig	Intraarticular injection of SDSCs at 0.2 and 4 wk	Partial meniscectomy of medial menisci	Intraarticular injection of PBS	2, 4, 8, 12, and 16 wk: Resected meniscus regeneration enhanced in SDSC group based on histology and MRI + better articular cartilage protection	Hatsushika et al,[90] 2014

(continued on next page)

Table 2
(continued)

Cell Source	Number of Cells Used	Animal Model	Meniscus Injury Model	Experimental Treatment	Control	Outcome/Results	Reference
Syngeneic and allogeneic SDSC	5×10^6	Rat	Partial meniscectomy of medial meniscus	Intraarticular injection of syngeneic SDCs, minor immune mismatch model cell transplantation, major immune mismatch model cell transplantation (for histocompatibility)	Intraarticular injection of PBS	4 wk: Regenerated area of meniscus was larger in minor mismatch and syngeneic SDSC groups than major mismatch group with more cells present (indicated by immunofluorescence)	Okuno et al,[91] 2014
Autologous SDSCs	10×10^6	Rabbit	Partial meniscectomy of medial meniscus	Intraarticular injection of autologous SDSCs in PBS	No cells	1, 3, 4, and 6 mo: Meniscus size was larger in SDSC-treated group initially, but at months 4 and 6 there was no difference; SDSCs adhered to local area of defect; and articular cartilage appeared thicker in SDSC group than control (better histologic scoring)	Hatsushika et al,[92] 2013
SDSCs	0.25×10^6	Rat	Partial meniscectomy	SDSC aggregate	Intraarticular injection of 5×10^6 cell suspension in PBS AND 0.25×10^5 cell suspension in PBS	12 wk: Larger meniscal area and better histologic scores for aggregate groups	Katagiri et al,[93] 2013

Allogeneic SDSCs	0.2×10^6 cells cultured for 3 wk to make 3D construct	Pig	4-mm cylindrical defect in medial meniscus	Cultured SDSC 3D cell/matrix tissue construct (scaffold-free)	No treatment	6 mo: SDSC 3D construct group filled meniscal defect and showed improved tissue integration compared with control	Moriguchi et al,[94] 2013
Allogeneic SDSCs	2×10^6	Rabbit	1.5-mm cylindrical defect in avascular zone of medial meniscus	Allogeneic SDSCs suspended in PBS	PBS only	4, 12, and 24 wk: Mixed results: Quantity of regenerated tissue significant ONLY at 4 and 12 wk. Quality of repair scores significant at 12 and 24 wk. Cells expressed type I and type II collagen at 24 wk	Horie et al,[95] 2012
Allogeneic SDSCs	5×10^6	Rat	Partial meniscectomy of medial meniscus	Intraarticular injection of Luc/LacZ + SDSCs AND BM-MSCs	PBS only	12 wk: Some meniscal regeneration in SDSC group that were LacZ+; SDSCs reportedly differentiated into meniscal cells and promoted regeneration of tissue	Horie et al,[96] 2009
Allogeneic/exogenous SDSCs	—	Rat	Cylindrical defect created in meniscus	Intraarticular injection of GFP-positive SDSCs	PBS only	1 d, 2, 4, 8, and 12 wk: SDSC group expressed type II collagen, attached to the defect site and seemed to have improved histologic scores at week 12, BUT there was NO statistically significant difference between groups	Mizuno et al,[97] 2008

(continued on next page)

Table 2
(continued)

Cell Source	Number of Cells Used	Animal Model	Meniscus Injury Model	Experimental Treatment	Control	Outcome/Results	Reference
Allogeneic SDSCs	—	Rabbits	Full-thickness longitudinal incision on medial meniscus	Fibrin gel loaded with SDSCs + CTGF and TBGFB3	Fibrin alone OR Fibrin + CTGF	6 wk: Fibrocartilaginous tissue integration demonstrated by hematoxylin and eosin and Saf-O fast green stain; tensile testing revealed enhanced biomechanical properties	Tarafder et al,[63] 2018
Autologous BM-MSCs	6×10^6	Sheep	Unilateral medial meniscectomy	Autologous BM-MSCs from iliac crest in HA construct	BMC in HA construct	12 wk: BMC in HA construct allowed for better tissue regeneration than BM-MSCs and this group seemed to inhibit OA progression with a reduction in cartilage and meniscus inflammation. BUT subchondral bone thickness was decreased in both BM-MSC and MSC groups	Desando et al,[98] 2016
Autologous BM-MSCs	$15–20 \times 10^6$	Horse	Meniscal tear	Intraarticular injection of autologous, expanded BM-MSCs into the joint	Surgery only, NO treatment	24 mo: 75% of horses returned to some level of work posttreatment of meniscal injury with BM-MSCs	Ferris et al,[99] 2014

Cells	Cell Number	Animal	Injury	Treatment	Control	Results	Reference
Autologous BM-MSCs	0.1×10^6	Rabbit	4-mm longitudinal tear in avascular zone of medial meniscus	Implantation of autologous BM-MSCs cultured and embedded in hyaluronan/collagen matrix	Suture only, cell-free matrix construct, or PRP	6 and 12 wk: BM-MSC matrix constructs initiated fibrocartilage-like repair tissue and demonstrated better integration and biomechanical properties than any control group	Zellner et al,[50] 2013
Human BM-MSCs and rat BM-MSCs	2×10^6	Rats	Partial meniscectomy	Intraarticular injection of human BM-MSCs or rat BM-MSCs	PBS only	2, 4, and 8 wk: Human BM-MSCs rapidly decreased in number over time, but enhanced meniscal regeneration similar to rat BM-MSCs. Human BM-MSCs increased local expression of Col II and Indian hedgehog (Ihh), with a subset that activated local expression of PTHLH and BMP2	Horie et al,[100] 2012
Human BM-MSCs	2×10^6	Rabbit	Complete radial tear of medial meniscus at the anterior tibial attachment site	Pull-out surgical repair + human BM-MSCs embedded in a matrix gel scaffold	Pull-out surgical repair (NO cells)	2, 4, and 8 wk: n = 20/25 rabbits survived postoperation. Of these, there was no significant difference in regenerative healing or fibrocartilage-like tissue formation between BM-MSC treatment and no cell control group	Hong et al,[101] 2011

(continued on next page)

Table 2
(continued)

Cell Source	Number of Cells Used	Animal Model	Meniscus Injury Model	Experimental Treatment	Control	Outcome/Results	Reference
Autologous BM-MSCs	1.5×10^6	Rabbit	2-mm meniscal tissue punch defect in avascular zone	Hyaluronan-collagen composite matrices loaded with autologous BM-MSCs	PRP loaded in matrices OR autologous bone marrow loaded in matrices OR cell-free matrices	12 wk: Neither bone marrow nor PRP loaded in matrices produced improvements in healing compared with cell-free implants; BM-MSCs loaded in collagen matrix resulted in fibrocartilage-like tissue repair that only partially integrated with the native meniscus	Zellner et al,[49] 2010
Autologous BM-MSCs	$1-2 \times 10^6$	Pig	Radial tear in the avascular zone of the meniscus	Autologous BM-MSCs + sutures and fibrin glue	No treatment OR sutures and fibrin glue alone	8 wk: No complete healing in the no treatment group or with sutures and fibrin glue alone; complete healing was seen in 3 animals and incomplete healing was seen in 5 of the animals in the BM-MSC treated group	Dutton et al,[102] 2010
Autologous BM-MSCs	30×10^6 cells/mL	Goat	Full-thickness meniscal defect in white-white area of meniscus	BM-MSCs transfected with hIGF-1 + calcium alginate gel	Nontransfected BM-MSCs OR calcium alginate gel alone OR no treatment	4, 8, and 16 wk: Defects were filled with fibrocartilage-like tissue composed of cells embedded in matrix spaces of meniscal fibers with enhanced proteoglycan levels in hIGF-1 overexpressed BM-MSCs	Zhang et al,[103] 2009

Autologous BM-MSCs	2.5 × 10^6, then 14 d in culture	Rabbit	Partial meniscectomy of middle 1/3 of meniscus	Autologous BM-MSCs (cultured for 14 d in chondrogenic conditions) loaded into a hyaluronan/gelatin scaffold	Cell-free scaffold OR no treatment	12 wk: Untreated defects showed no healing; cell-free scaffolds showed some repair of fibrocartilaginous tissue; BM-MSC-loaded scaffold had significantly enhanced fibrocartilage repair compared with either control	Angele et al,[104] 2008
BM-MSCs	0.5 × 10^6/mL	Rabbit	Partial meniscectomy of medial meniscus	Type I collagen sponge loaded with autologous BM-MSCs	Cell-free collagen sponge OR periosteal autograft OR no treatment	24 wk: Periosteal autograft differentiated into a bonelike composite that is harmful for meniscus repair; collagen sponge alone supported a fibrous repair response; collagen sponge loaded with BM-MSCs produced fibrocartilaginous tissue similar to native tissue, but the biomechanical function of the meniscus was NOT restored	Walsh et al,[105] 1999
BM-MSCs	~1 × 10^6 cells (from bone marrow aspirant)	Rabbit	1.5-mm full-thickness defect in avascular zone of meniscus	BM-MSCs suspended in fibrin glue	Fibrin glue alone OR no treatment	1, 3, 6, and 12 wk: Defects were smaller in the fibrin glue alone group and the fibrin glue + BM-MSC group; healing response was faster in the fibrin glue + BM-MSC group	Ishimura et al,[106] 1997

(continued on next page)

Table 2
(continued)

Cell Source	Number of Cells Used	Animal Model	Meniscus Injury Model	Experimental Treatment	Control	Outcome/Results	Reference
Allogeneic BM-MSCs	0.3×10^6	Rabbit and rat	Explant culture	Allogeneic rabbit BM-MSCs or rabbit MDSC housed in Matrigel	—	3 wk: BM-MSCs had a high propensity for cartilage hypertrophy and bone formation. MDSCs exhibited greater chondrogenic potential than BM-MSCs	Ding & Huang,[107] 2015
Allogenic horse BM-MSCs	0.2×10^6	Nude mice	Equine meniscal sections	Allogeneic horse BM-MSCs + fibrin glue subcutaneously implanted into rat	PBS OR fibrin glue alone	BM-MSC group showed increased vascularization with increased total bonding of repair and native tissue	Ferris et al,[108] 2012
Autologous BM-MSCs	$11–12 \times 10^6$	Sheep	Meniscal tear of medial meniscus	Intraarticular injection of BM-MSC suspension	Intraarticular injection of suspension medium (NO cells)	6–12 mo: BM-MSC injection group showed no adverse immunologic effects, and meniscus regeneration was demonstrated through histology and macroscopic parameters, BUT these instances were limited and case dependent	Caminal et al,[109] 2014

Cell type	Dose	Animal	Injury model	Treatment	Control	Outcome	Reference
Autologous BM-MSCs	10 × 10^6	Sheep	Complete meniscectomy of the medial meniscus + ACL excision	Intraarticular injection of chondrogenically induced BM-MSCs OR intraarticular injection of basal-culture medium BM-MSCs	Intraarticular injection of basal medium (NO cells)	6 wk: Control group had severe OA and meniscus damage; no significant ICRS scoring was detected between the 2 BM-MSC groups; chondrogenically induced BM-MSC group displayed better meniscus regeneration than basal BM-MSCs and significantly better than the control group	Al Faqeh et al,[110] 2012
Allogeneic BM-MSCs	1 × 10^6 vs 10 × 10^6	Rats	Meniscal tear + ACL tear + articular cartilage defect	Intraarticular injection of allogeneic GFP-positive BM-MSCs	Sham operation OR saline	4 wk: GFP-positive BM-MSCs mobilized to the injury site and contributed to tissue regeneration compared with control groups	Agung et al,[111] 2006
Autologous BM-MSCs	10 × 10^6	Goat	Osteoarthritis (OA) induction through complete meniscectomy of the medial meniscus	Intraarticular injection of autologous BM-MSCs expressing eGFP (retrovirus) suspended in sodium hyaluronan	Sodium hyaluronan alone (NO cells)	26 wk: BM-MSC treatment group displayed meniscus regeneration, with eGFP fluorescent cells located in the newly formed tissue; degeneration of cartilage and the OA phenotype was reduced in the BM-MSC group compared with the control group	Murphy et al,[112] 2003

(continued on next page)

Table 2 (*continued*)

Cell Source	Number of Cells Used	Animal Model	Meniscus Injury Model	Experimental Treatment	Control	Outcome/Results	Reference
Human BM-MSCs	30×10 cells/mL	Rat	Radial cut of the medial meniscus (2 mm × 2 mm excision)	Human BM-MSCs encapsulated in decellularized ECM hydrogel	PBS	8 wk: Significant tissue regeneration in BM-MSC group with higher GAG, type I and type II collagen than control group; some tissue regeneration in control animals	Yuan et al,[113] 2017
Autologous BM-MSCs	—	Rabbit	Total meniscectomy	BM-MSC seeded PCL scaffold meniscus replacement	Cell-free scaffold, sham operation, and total meniscectomy alone	12 and 24 wk: BM-MSC seeded PCL scaffold group had a better gross meniscus appearance with higher expression of type I, II, and III collagen and proteoglycan production found in native fibrochondrocytes + less cartilage degradation than any control group + better tensile and compressive properties in cell-seeded implant	Zhang et al,[114] 2017
Allogeneic BM-MSCs	~4.8×10^6	Rat	Partial meniscectomy (1/2 resection) of the medial meniscus	Allogeneic BM-MSCs cultured in a cell "sheet" from monolayer culture	No treatment	4 and 8 wk: Histologic evaluation revealed regenerated tissue "similar" to native tissue with some collagen bridging as a measure of tissue integration with some alleviation of degenerative cartilage damage compared with the control group	Qi et al,[115] 2016

Allogeneic BM-MSCs	—	Rat	Meniscal defect	Allogeneic rat-derived BM-MSCs were seeded into a scaffold and cultured for 4 wk and then implanted	Cell-free scaffold OR meniscectomy	4 and 8 wk: Expression of extracellular matrices was observed in transplanted tissue 4 wk postsurgery. Articular cartilage was better protected/less damaged in MSC scaffold group than either control group	Yamasaki et al,[116] 2008
Allogeneic human BM-MSCs	—	Rat	Meniscal defect	Allogeneic human GFP-positive BM-MSCs cultured in monolayer and then embedded in fibrin glue and transplanted to injury defect	No treatment OR fibrin glue only (NO cells)	8 wk: GFP-positive BM-MSCs survived and proliferated in the meniscal defects while producing ECM	Izuta et al,[117] 2005
Autologous BM-MSCs	—	Rabbit	Partial meniscectomy of white-red zone	Autologous BM-MSCs loaded in a polyurethane scaffold (Actifit) and sutured into the defect	Polyurethane scaffold alone (Actifit) (NO cells)	6 and 12 wk: Both cell-free and BM-MSC loaded scaffolds led to well-integrated and stable meniscus-like repair tissue with dense vascularization; accelerated healing was achieved by the BM-MSC loaded scaffold	Koch et al,[118] 2018
CPCs	0.1×10^6	Rat (ex vivo)	Radial tear in inner anterior horn	C-PC line 3 + SDF-1 pretreatment OR primary C-PCs + SDF-1 pretreatment	BM-MSCs OR no cell treatment	3, 5, 10, 17, and 20 d: Chondroprogenitors (CPCs) promoted meniscal fibrochondrocyte proliferation and native tissue integration of torn meniscal tissue through progressive; SDF-1/CXCR4 axis is required to successfully fill meniscus tissue tears	Jayasuriya et al,[119] 2018

Abbreviations: eGFP, enhanced green fluorescent protein; GFP, green fluorescent protein.

histologic data, mechanical testing, or MRI analysis. In another larger-animal model, Desando and colleagues[98] performed a unilateral medial meniscectomy in sheep and treated the injury with a Hyaff-11 (HA) construct seeded with either autologous BM-MSCs (6×10^6 cells) or bone marrow concentrate (BMC). After 12 weeks postoperatively, minor joint healing and anti-inflammatory effects were noticed for both groups; however, the BMC group actually allowed for the best meniscus regeneration.[98] Zellner and colleagues[50] conducted a study whereby they created a defect in the avascular zone of a rabbit meniscus and treated the injury with an HA/collagen matrix scaffold that housed 0.1×10^6 autologous BM-MSCs or a cell-free HA/collagen matrix scaffold alone. After 12 weeks, the BM-MSC matrix constructs initiated some fibrocartilage-like tissue repair and exhibited better integration and biomechanical properties than the control group.[50] In 2 more recent studies, Zhang and colleagues[114] and Koch and colleagues[118] performed meniscectomies in rabbits and used 2 different types of scaffolds seeded with BM-MSCs for tissue regeneration and repair. Zhang and colleagues[114] used a polycaprolactone (PCL) scaffold either cell free or seeded with BM-MSCs and showed that after 24 weeks, the BM-MSC–seeded scaffold group had a better gross meniscus appearance with higher expression of type I, II, and III collagen and proteoglycan production found in native fibrochondrocytes with less cartilage degradation than any control group as well as better tensile and compressive properties. In comparison, Koch and colleagues[118] used a cell-free polyurethane Actifit scaffold as a control, or the Actifit implant seeded with BM-MSCs; each implant was sutured in place during the operation. After 12 weeks, the results showed that both the cell-free and the BM-MSC–loaded scaffolds led to well-integrated and stable meniscus-like repair tissue and dense vascularization.[118] The only difference between the groups was that the BM-MSC groups seemed to accelerate the healing response. Yuan and colleagues[113] created a radial cut in a rat meniscus and treated it intraarticularly with human BM-MSCs housed in an injectable, decellularized ECM hydrogel. After 8 weeks postinjection, the meniscus ECM hydrogel was retained and contributed to tissue regeneration and protection from osteoarthritis development as evidenced by macroscopic and microscopic images. Perhaps their most significant findings, however, were that the injured tissue that received the ECM hydrogel + BM-MSC treatment did not demonstrate histologic evidence of mineralization and was moderately negative for type X collagen staining.[113] This study is especially interesting because hypertrophy, senescence, and evidence of adverse terminal differentiation to bone in BM-MSCs have been reported extensively both in vitro and in vivo.[113,127,129] These reports place emphasis on increased type X collagen expression, which has been detected in senescent and degenerative osteoarthritic menisci.[130,131] The limitations with this study, however, include a short length of follow-up time that may not allow for possible hypertrophic development or terminal differentiation to occur, both challenges that naturally arise with using BM-MSCs for meniscus repair. Furthermore, the investigators list the small sample size of rats and a lack of a larger-animal model, such as a rabbit, pig, or sheep, as major limitations that should be addressed in future work.[113]

There have been many studies done to date using different and innovative delivery methods of BM-MSCs for meniscal repair, different quantities of cells, different time periods, and different culturing conditions aiming to treat different types of meniscus injury and regenerate damaged tissue in various animal models. However, the challenge of hypertrophy and mineralization always tends to arise when discussing the use of BM-MSCs as a cell source for meniscus repair. As mentioned before, high expression of hypertrophy and ossification markers generally correlates with calcification and a poor healing response in vivo[132–134] and represents a major challenge with using BM-MSCs for tissue engineering given their high expression of COL10A1 and other hypertrophic markers.[119] Currently, the need to address this limitation in meniscal tissue engineering and regeneration is evident and may focus on finding conditions that can better prevent hypertrophy in BM-MSCs themselves, or through the discovery of a new cell source that is more resistant to hypertrophy altogether.

Adipose-Derived Stem Cells

ADSCs from the infrapatellar fat pad of the knee are considered to be a promising alternative cell source for cartilage and meniscus repair strategies. Zuk and colleagues[135] first introduced ADSCs in 2002, when the group isolated this multipotent, undifferentiated, self-renewing progenitor cell population from digested adipose tissue.[136] This heterogeneous population of cells was derived from the embryonic mesenchyme that contained an easily isolated stroma.[135] Zuk and colleagues isolated these cells and coined the term "processed lipoaspirate (PLA) cells," demonstrating that they can be readily accessed from human adipose tissue. Furthermore, Zuk and colleagues[135] demonstrated that PLA cells expressed a phenotypic profile (CD marker antigens) and genotypic profile (messenger RNA [mRNA] levels and protein analysis) that resembled that of well-defined MSCs.[136] This CD marker profile was $CD90^+$, $CD105^+$, $CD73^+$, $CD44^+$, and $CD166^+$. However, these ADSCs were negative for the hematopoietic markers CD45 and CD34.[137] Histologic analysis using established staining methods have demonstrated the trilineage potential and multipotency of this cell source.[135]

Although these cells are isolated from fatty tissue, they do possess the capability to undergo chondrogenic differentiation to produce proteoglycans and type II collagen. However, studies have demonstrated the limited chondrogenic potential of ADSCs in comparison to BM-MSCs.[125,138] Hamid and colleagues[139] sought to induce chondrogenesis and characterize their capacity. This group found that after 1 week in culture, the expression of chondrogenic genes (collagen type II, ACAN, COMP, ELASTIN, and collagen type XI) was reduced significantly.[139] This dampened chondrogenic capacity may limit their consideration for meniscal and cartilaginous tissue repair. Furthermore, Hamid and colleagues[139] showed that there was a high expression of hypertrophy marker, type X collagen, after 3 weeks of chondrogenic induction. Their results suggest that repeated induction of ADSCs may confer a hypertrophic state that is characterized by increased bone matrix synthesis and a suppressed chondrogenic program. Elevated levels of hypertrophy with concomitant decreased chondrogenic potential would be detrimental in the repair of the fibrocartilaginous meniscus tissue. With the exception of a few studies, it appears to be well demonstrated that BM-MSCs have an enhanced potential for chondrogenesis as compared with ADSCs by measures of GAGs production, type II collagen gene expression and deposition, and pellet size.[125,140,141]

Preclinical applications of adipose-derived stem cells results

ADSCs extracted from the fat pad represent a bioavailable cell type that has been used for various types of tissue repair and regeneration strategies. It has only been within the last decade that ADSCs have been used specifically for meniscal tissue injury and regeneration. Most of the in vivo data currently available focus on meniscus injury in smaller animal models like rabbit,[80,81,87] with a few groups using larger models like equine and bovine (see **Table 2**). These studies range from 12 weeks to a maximum of 12 months in follow-up length after surgical injury and use a range of 0.1×10^6 to 20×10^6 ADSCs for therapeutic cell treatment. Ruiz-Ibán and colleagues[81] used sutures to close a meniscal lesion in the vascular zone of a rabbit and treated the site with ADSCs suspended in a hydrogel. Although they demonstrated neomeniscal tissue formation and reported that the ADSC-treated meniscus group had slight cellularity increase compared with normal tissue, their study is limited because there was no power analysis performed because of the small number of animals that were used per group, and because the length of the study was only 12 weeks, longer-term studies are called for. In another study, Qi and colleagues[80] labeled ADSCs with superparamagnetic iron oxide (SPIO) and used magnets to target specific homing to the injured tissue site after meniscectomy in rabbits. They reported that after 12 weeks there was minimal neomeniscal tissue present that integrated with the host meniscus (confirmed through histologic data), but this tissue was abnormally shaped. Furthermore, the targeting efficiency of the SPIO-labeled ADSCs was admittedly not high, because these cells migrated to other nontargeted tissue.[80] In a short- to medium-term study (7 months), Moradi and colleagues[86] performed a complete meniscectomy in a rabbit and completely replaced the meniscus with a polyvinyl alcohol/chitosan (PVA/Ch) scaffold seeded with ADSCs. They found no significant contribution in the healing process for the scaffold-seeded ADSC group and even found a decreased chondrogenic response with lower Col II, ACAN, and Col I mRNA expression levels present. Lower levels of chondrogenic potential is a typical characteristic of ADSCs, and one that may be a hindrance for meniscal repair. To date, González-Ferndández and colleagues[84] have been the only group to use a large-animal equine model for ADSC-mediated meniscal repair and regeneration. In their study, they created a defect in the medial meniscus of an adult horse and filled it with autologous ADSCs. After 12 months postoperatively, their results were mixed with some defects appearing to be filled with fibrocartilaginous-like tissue, whereas others remained completely unfilled.[84] Because the application of ADSCs for meniscus repair and regeneration has been a recent phenomenon, current studies that are present in the literature lack significant larger-animal data and longer-term follow-up data. Additional studies should, therefore, include longer time points as well as biomechanical and biochemical analysis of the regenerated meniscal tissue to investigate the true efficacy of using ADSCs for meniscal repair and regeneration.

Synovium-Derived Stem Cells

SDSCs are a relatively newly used and promising cell source that is garnering a great deal of attention in the field of meniscus repair. SDSCs are colony-forming cells that can be derived from the synovium of the knee during a simple arthroscopic procedure.[23,142] However, contrary to popular belief, the synovium only contains a small population of multipotent cells that can form colonies.[23,143] Nevertheless, these cells exhibit multipotent capability as well as surface epitope CD markers in accordance with the ISCT-established MSC marker criteria.[144,145] Namely, these ADSCs express CD90, CD166, CD44, CD105, and CD147.[146]

This cell population has been shown to increase in number following injuries to the meniscus.[144,147] An increased presence of SDSCs post-injury suggests that this population may be an important cell source for meniscal repair. In multiple characterization studies comparing SDSCs to BM-MSCs, it has been demonstrated that SDSCs have greater chondrogenic capacity and adipogenic capacity than BM-MSCs.[148-150] Sakaguchi and colleagues[148] also compared the osteogenic capacities of these cell types and found comparably high mineralization levels in BM-MSCs and SDSCs using Alizarin red–positive staining. Furthermore, reverse transcriptase polymerase chain reaction (RT-PCR) results indicated high mRNA expression levels of osteogenic markers RUNX2 and BGLAP in cells derived from the knee synovium (SDSCs).[146,148] Another study done by Pei and colleagues[151] demonstrated that addition of TGF-B3 for chondrogenic induction in vitro resulted in an upregulation of

COL10A1 and ALPL in porcine SDSC pellets compared with TBGF-B1. Although these studies illustrate the aforementioned favorable multipotency of SDSCs, it also points out a potential problem with using these cells to repair the fibrocartilaginous tissue of the meniscus: a high osteogenic capacity may be detrimental for repair in the long term. Stem cell–induced mineralization and calcification of the meniscus could theoretically lead to ineffective repair because these cells become hypertrophic and may potentially serve as a preamble to further joint disease, such as osteoarthritis, in the long term. Therefore, it is ideal that cells used in meniscal repair and tissue regeneration exhibit high chondrogenic capacity, while simultaneously exhibiting low osteogenic and hypertrophy markers. As it stands now, long-term studies are required to fully explore the efficacy of SDSCs in meniscus tissue repair.

Preclinical applications of synovium-derived stem cells results

Similar to ADSCs, SDSCs are a new and promising cell source for meniscal repair. Although this source can be obtained from the synovium during a simple arthroscopic surgery, SDSCs have limited bioavailability because there is only a small population of these colony-forming cells present. Recently, the use of SDSCs for meniscus tissue engineering and repair strategies have been advocated for and investigated heavily.[1,152,153] The literature indicates that groups investigating this cell type for therapeutic repair have been conducting both small- and larger-animal model studies (see **Table 2**). These studies range from 4 weeks to 6-month duration postoperation and use anywhere from 0.20×10^6 to 50×10^6 SDSCs for cell treatment quantity. Hatsushika and colleagues[92] investigated whether intraarticular injection of 10×10^6 SDSCs could enhance meniscal regeneration in a rabbit meniscal defect model. The SDSC and control groups were compared macroscopically and histologically at various time points (1, 3, 4, and 6 months) and showed mixed results. Although the histologic score of the meniscus and chondroprotection was better in the SDSC group, the overall size and macroscopic view of the meniscus between groups were insignificant. As an alternative cell-delivery model to intraarticular injection, Katagiri and colleagues[93] prepared SDSC aggregates in an effort to develop a more practical clinical solution for future human use. They engineered aggregates consisting of 0.25×10^6 SDSCs, placed them on a meniscal defect created in a rat, and found regenerated meniscal tissue that had histologic scores similar to normal menisci after 12 weeks.[93] In addition to small-animal studies, the use of SDSCs for meniscus repair in large animals has been investigated with moderate success.[89,90,94] To comparatively investigate the efficacy of 2 different cell types for repairing a massive meniscal defect, Horie and colleagues[96] injected either 5×10^6 dual luciferase Luc/LacZ+ SDSCs or 5×10^6 BM-MSCs into massive meniscectomized knees of wild-type rats. After 12 weeks, the regenerated meniscal tissue in the SDSC group produced more type II collagen, proliferated at a higher rate than control or BM-MSC group, and appeared macroscopically superior to the control group, but looked identical to the BM-MSC group. However, there were no noticeable differences of regenerated meniscus in morphology or histologic scoring between the SDSC and BM-MSC groups.

   Although these studies have demonstrated that SDSCs and BM-MSCs are comparable in terms of their repair capacity in both small- and larger-animal models, none of them have measured Collagen X or any other markers of cellular hypertrophy or osteoarthritic markers like matrix metallopeptidase either pretreatment or posttreatment. Moreover, because SDSCs are a fairly new cell source that is being used for meniscus repair, more studies in general are needed to better support the findings thus far. Furthermore, the longest time period allowed for in the aforementioned studies was

6 months, which may not be enough time to evaluate proper repair capacity or possible longer-term effects of SDSCs for meniscus repair.

Native Meniscal Fibrochondrocytes + Meniscus-Derived Stem Cells

One of the most recent developments in cell-based meniscus repair/regeneration is meniscus-derived stem cells (MDSCs) or MFCs. The cellular component of the meniscus consists of a population of fibrochondrocytes living within the ECM.[154] Webber and colleagues[155] first coined the term "fibrochondrocytes" to describe these unique cells that they isolated from the menisci of New Zealand white rabbits in their 1985 study. Moon and colleagues[156] and Upton and colleagues[157] suggested that location-specific MFCs respond to changing mechanical environments because the periphery of the meniscus contains cells that better resemble fibroblasts, whereas the inner rim of the meniscus behaves more like chondrocytes. Biomechanically, the periphery of the meniscus is primarily responsible for shock absorption and tensile forces, whereas the inner meniscus acts as a direct point of contact for the femoral condyle and is subject to compressive forces.[156–158] These MFCs display properties of both fibroblasts and chondrocytes, regulating the crucial process of ECM synthesis and deposition in response to the mechanical stimuli present in the joint.[154,158,159] Depending on their position in the meniscus (inner zone vs periphery), MFCs/MDSCs exhibit different morphologies and biochemical properties. For example, MFCs/MDSCs from the inner avascular region have a rounded morphology that resembles articular chondrocytes and are spaced out within ECM.[133,134,160] Conversely, MFCs/MDSCs isolated from the outer fibrous region are spindle shaped and form gap junctions with many other neighboring cells.[133,134,160]

These MDSCs are reported to be highly adherent to tissue culture plastic, like all MSCs. Furthermore, these individual cells that migrate out of the tissue and adhere to the plastic tend to exhibit high colony-forming efficiency, exhibit trilineage potential, and express common MSC markers, including CD44, CD90, and Nanog.[23]

A significant challenge associated with using autologous MDSCs/MFCs for meniscus regeneration and repair is their extremely sparse population in the meniscus.[160–163] Perhaps an even larger problem, however, is the counterintuitive and invasive surgical technique that is required to isolate and extract this cell type. A piece of meniscus tissue would need to be excised from an intact meniscus, diced into small pieces, digested with a protease such as collagenase or pronase, expanded in monolayer culture, and then collected for application. This process is lengthy and fairly common, but more importantly, one that involves injuring a healthy meniscus. This process may mechanically compromise the tissue, thus decreasing the tibiofemoral contact area and increasing the stress on the underlying cartilage, which may further damage the joint.[160,164,165]

Cartilage-Derived Progenitor Cells

Similar to the tissue-derived mesenchymal cell types listed already, normal (nonarthritic) human articular cartilage also contains a tissue-specific mesenchymal stem/progenitor cell population that has been proposed for use in tissue repair applications.[166,167] These cells are often referred to as cartilage-derived chondrogenic progenitor cells (CPCs). It has been demonstrated that CPCs from healthy human articular cartilage samples can be effectively isolated using a differential adhesion assay to fibronectin.[119,166,167] The trilineage ability of CPCs to differentiate into osteogenic, adipogenic, and chondrogenic tissue has also been demonstrated in vitro[119,168,169] and in ovo.[166] These cells express MSC surface markers CD44, CD49e, CD90, CD105, CD146, and CD166.[170] Furthermore, Williams and colleagues[167] demonstrated the high telomerase activity and maintenance of telomere length in clonally isolated populations' CPCs, which is a prototypical characteristic of a MSC population.[169] CPCs from cartilage appear morphologically fibrochondrocyte-like and exhibit high colony-forming efficiency, expression of Notch1 gene, and high chondrogenic potential.[119,122,170–172]

The use of CPCs for meniscus repair and regeneration may confer benefits that expanded mature chondrocytes lack, including no terminal differentiation or dedifferentiation, improved cell quality, and enhanced potency.[171] The existence of this population within articular cartilage coupled with its phenotypic profile reduced propensity for hypertrophy, and enhanced chondrogenic capacity suggests that CPCs may have the biological repertoire necessary for cell-based regeneration and repair of the meniscus.

As is the case with BM-MSCs and SDSCs, a major challenge for using these cells for meniscus regeneration and repair is their sparse bioavailability. CPCs have been reported to compose about $1.47\% \pm 0.16\%$ of all cells from normal healthy human articular cartilage.[173] Despite their small population in cartilage, their high colony-forming capacity and proliferation rate are crucial for effective, therapeutic cell-based meniscus application. Although a current clinical model does not exist for deriving cartilage CPCs, there is the already established method of autologous chondrocyte implantation (ACI), whereby healthy chondrocytes are transferred from a non-load-bearing region of cartilage to a tissue defect.[174] Hypothetically, it should be possible to mimic this ACI method to expand and relocate CPCs isolated from non-load-bearing regions for autologous cell-based delivery for meniscal repair. This cell source is still quite new for the purposes of meniscus repair, so ongoing research is being conducted with CPCs. However, based on CPCs phenotypic and genetic profile, coupled with their hypertrophy resistance and high chondrogenic capacity, the authors believe this stem cell source could represent an ideal cell source for cell-based meniscal repair and regeneration.

Preclinical applications of cartilage-derived progenitor cells results

Notably, the newest cell type being used in the field of meniscus repair is an MSC population derived from cartilage known as CPCs. As mentioned before, these cells are reported to be highly proliferative and possess beneficial multipotentiality.[175] Perhaps most importantly, they have a high chondrogenic potential and are resistant to terminal differentiation and hypertrophy with decreased levels of hypertrophy marker, COL10A1.[119] To date, only 1 study has been published using CPCs for meniscus repair. Jayasuriya and colleagues[119] demonstrate how CPCs may be more suitable than BM-MSCs to mediate bridging and reintegration of fibrocartilage tissue tears in the meniscus using an ex vivo rat model. In this study, a radial tear was created in the inner anterior horn of a rat meniscus and cocultured the torn menisci with 1×10^5 BM-MSCs, CPCs, or no cells for 20 days. Results showed that the CPCs were able to initiate reintegration of a meniscus tissue tear in an explant culture and demonstrated for the first time that CPCs produce a paracrine effect that improves the rate of MFC proliferation that was similar, if not better, than BM-MSCs. The increased rate of proliferation and reintegration was confirmed by histology, microscopic visualization, and RT-PCR. Furthermore, CPC-treated menisci had significantly lower expression of hypertrophic marker COL10A1 mRNA levels, in comparison to the BM-MSC group. These findings suggest that CPCs from healthy human cartilage resist cellular hypertrophy and maintain high chondrogenic capacity, which are conducive for successful meniscus repair. However, because this is the only study of its kind thus far, the results are limited, and it is clear that more research needs to be done in an in vivo animal model with longer-term results.

MESENCHYMAL STEM CELL DELIVERY METHOD

Biomaterial scaffolds for meniscus tissue engineering tend to vary significantly in terms of their material composition, biomimetic properties, and 3D structure. With meniscal research expanding due to new biological advances in the basic science field, novel approaches and robust solutions for treating meniscal tears are emerging more frequently than ever. To this end, biomaterials that can be seeded or pretreated with cells and successfully retain these cells in the scaffold appear to confer the best advantages for repair. Because these biomaterials must be able to beneficially interact with the surrounding tissue (biomimetic properties), the hope is that these different meniscus scaffolds will be able to improve or replace the anatomic defect. Ideally, an effective cell-based scaffold would (1) allow for a more robust repair response through the use of an MSC source and (2) enhance stimulated migration and integration of native meniscus fibrochondrocytes into the scaffold. Various cell populations have been investigated for this role (see **Table 2**), with BM-MSCs being used most frequently as ideal choices for biomaterial engineering. Typically, this process of tissue-engineering a biomimetic scaffold involves the isolation of MSCs, which are then seeded into a biocompatible matrix or cell-carrier material that resembles the native ECM. This matrix should be able to securely house the cells to ensure that they stay in their desired and localized area when implanted into the joint. The most commonly used natural materials are type I and type II collagen-based scaffolds.[176] There are also many synthetic materials being designed, such as polyglycolic acid, poly-L-lactic acid, PCL, and other composite mixtures.[176,177] Thus, an ideal meniscal biomaterial must promote anabolic activity; namely, endogenous tissue repair, and regeneration through a biomimetic scaffold that allows for cellular attachment and growth to promote ideal tissue-scaffold integration, while resisting terminal differentiation and hypertrophy.

ACKNOWLEDGMENTS

This paper was supported by Institutional Development Award Number NIH U54GM115677 from the National Institute of General Medical Sciences (NIGMS), which funds Advance Clinical and Translational Research (Advance-CTR). This work was also supported by a grant from the Orthopaedic Research and Education Foundation (OREF) funded by the Musculoskeletal Transplant Foundation (MTF) Biologics.

REFERENCES

1. Scotti C, Hirschmann MT, Antinolfi P, et al. Meniscus repair and regeneration: review on current methods and research potential. Eur Cell Mater 2013. https://doi.org/10.22203/eCM.v026a11.

2. Sutton J. Ligaments: their nature and morphology. Bristol Med Chir J 1897; 15(58):344.

3. Huckell JR. Is meniscectomy a benign procedure? A long-term follow-up study. Can J Surg 1965;8:254–60.

4. Appel H. Late results after meniscectomy in the knee joint: a clinical and roentgenologic follow-up investigation. Acta Orthop Scand Suppl 1970;133:1–111.

5. Allen PR, Denham RA, Swan AV. Late degenerative changes after meniscectomy. Factors affecting the knee after operation. J Bone Joint Surg Br 1984; 66(5):666–71.

6. Makris EA, Hadidi P, Athanasiou KA. The knee meniscus: structure-function, pathophysiology, current repair techniques, and prospects for regeneration. Biomaterials 2011. https://doi.org/10.1016/j.biomaterials.2011.06.037.

7. Seedhom BB, Hargreaves DJ. Transmission of the load in the knee joint with special reference to the role of the menisci. Part II: experimental results, discussion and conclusions. Eng Med 1979. https://doi.org/10.1243/emed_jour_1979_008_051_02.

8. Tan GK, Cooper-White JJ. Interactions of meniscal cells with extracellular matrix molecules: towards the generation of tissue engineered menisci. Cell Adh Migr 2011. https://doi.org/10.4161/cam.5.3.14463.

9. Fox AJS, Bedi A, Rodeo SA. The basic science of human knee menisci: structure, composition, and function. Sports Health 2012. https://doi.org/10.1177/1941738111429419.

10. McDevitt C, Miller R, Sprindler K. The cells and cell matrix interaction of the meniscus. In: Mow V, Arnoczky S, Jackson D, editors. Knee meniscus: basic and clinical foundations. New York: Raven Press; 1992. p. 29–36.

11. Webber RJ, Norby DP, Malemud CJ, et al. Characterization of newly synthesized proteoglycans from rabbit menisci in organ culture. Biochem J 1984. https://doi.org/10.1042/bj2210875.

12. Fithian DC, Kelly MA, Mow VC. Material properties and structure-function relationships in the menisci. Clin Orthop Relat Res 1990. https://doi.org/10.1097/00003086-199003000-00004.

13. Athanasiou KA, Sanchez-Adams J. In: Athanasiou KA, editor. Engineering the Knee Meniscus. 1st edition. Rice University, USA: Morgan Claypool Publishers; 2009.

14. Beaufils P, Becker R, Kopf S, et al. The knee meniscus: management of traumatic tears and degenerative lesions. EFORT Open Rev 2017. https://doi.org/10.1302/2058-5241.2.160056.

15. Mordecai SC. Treatment of meniscal tears: an evidence based approach. World J Orthop 2014. https://doi.org/10.5312/wjo.v5.i3.233.

16. Jarraya M, Roemer FW, Englund M, et al. Meniscus morphology: does tear type matter? A narrative review with focus on relevance for osteoarthritis research. Semin Arthritis Rheum 2017. https://doi.org/10.1016/j.semarthrit.2016.11.005.

17. Fox AJS, Wanivenhaus F, Burge AJ, et al. The human meniscus: a review of anatomy, function, injury, and advances in treatment. Clin Anat 2015. https://doi.org/10.1002/ca.22456.

18. Logerstedt DS, Snyder-Mackler L, Ritter RC, et al. Knee pain and mobility impairments: meniscal and articular cartilage lesions. J Orthop Sports Phys Ther 2010. https://doi.org/10.2519/jospt.2010.0304.

19. Hede A, Jensen DB, Blyme P, et al. Epidemiology of meniscal lesions in the knee: 1,215 open operations in Copenhagen 1982-84. Acta Orthop 1990. https://doi.org/10.3109/17453679008993557.

20. Jones JC, Burks R, Owens BD, et al. Incidence and risk factors associated with meniscal injuries among active-duty US Military service members. J Athl Train 2012. https://doi.org/10.4085/1062-6050-47.1.67.

21. Baker BE, Peckham AC, Pupparo F, et al. Review of meniscal injury and associated sports. Am J Sports Med 1985. https://doi.org/10.1177/036354658501300101.

22. Lauder TD, Baker SP, Smith GS, et al. Sports and physical training injury hospitalizations in the Army. Am J Prev Med 2000. https://doi.org/10.1016/S0749-3797(99)00174-9.

23. Korpershoek JV, De Windt TS, Hagmeijer MH, et al. Cell-based meniscus repair and regeneration: at the brink of clinical translation?: a systematic review of preclinical studies. Orthop J Sport Med 2017. https://doi.org/10.1177/2325967117690131.
24. Englund M, Roemer FW, Hayashi D, et al. Meniscus pathology, osteoarthritis and the treatment controversy. Nat Rev Rheumatol 2012. https://doi.org/10.1038/nrrheum.2012.69.
25. McDermott ID, Amis AA. The consequences of meniscectomy. J Bone Joint Surg Br 2006. https://doi.org/10.1302/0301-620X.88B12.18140.
26. Lee SR, Kim JG, Nam SW. The tips and pitfalls of meniscus allograft transplantation. Knee Surg Relat Res 2012. https://doi.org/10.5792/ksrr.2012.24.3.137.
27. De Bruycker M, Verdonk PCM, Verdonk RC. Meniscal allograft transplantation: a meta-analysis. SICOT J 2017. https://doi.org/10.1051/sicotj/2017016.
28. Noyes FR, Barber-Westin SD. Long-term survivorship and function of meniscus transplantation. Am J Sports Med 2016. https://doi.org/10.1177/0363546516646375.
29. Rosso F, Bisicchia S, Bonasia DE, et al. Meniscal allograft transplantation: a systematic review. Am J Sports Med 2015. https://doi.org/10.1177/0363546514536021.
30. Guo W, Xu W, Wang Z, et al. Cell-free strategies for repair and regeneration of meniscus injuries through the recruitment of endogenous stem/progenitor cells. Stem Cells Int 2018.
31. Stone KR, Rodkey WG, Webber R, et al. Meniscal regeneration with copolymeric collagen scaffolds. In vitro and in vivo studies evaluated clinically, histologically, and biochemically. Am J Sports Med 1992. https://doi.org/10.1177/036354659202000202.
32. Stone KR, Steadman JR, Rodkey WG, et al. Regeneration of meniscal cartilage with use of a collagen scaffold. Analysis of preliminary data. J Bone Joint Surg Am 1997. https://doi.org/10.1042/bj1970385.
33. Zaffagnini S, Giordano G, Vascellari A, et al. Arthroscopic collagen meniscus implant results at 6 to 8 years follow up. Knee Surg Sports Traumatol Arthrosc 2007. https://doi.org/10.1007/s00167-006-0144-4.
34. Tucker B. Tissue engineering for the meniscus: a review of the literature. Open Orthop J 2012. https://doi.org/10.2174/1874325001206010348.
35. Hansen R, Choi G, Bryk E, et al. The human knee meniscus: a review with special focus on the collagen meniscal implant. J Long Term Eff Med Implants 2011. https://doi.org/10.1615/JLongTermEffMedImplants.v21.i4.60.
36. Vaquero J. Meniscus tear surgery and meniscus replacement. Muscles Ligaments Tendons J 2016. https://doi.org/10.11138/mltj/2016.6.1.071.
37. Rodkey WG, Steadman JR, Li ST. A clinical study of collagen meniscus implants to restore the injured meniscus. Clin Orthop Relat Res 1999. https://doi.org/10.1097/00003086-199910001-00027.
38. Bulgheroni P, Murena L, Ratti C, et al. Follow-up of collagen meniscus implant patients: clinical, radiological, and magnetic resonance imaging results at 5 years. Knee 2010. https://doi.org/10.1016/j.knee.2009.08.011.
39. Steadman JR, Rodkey WG. Tissue-engineered collagen meniscus implants: 5- to 6-year feasibility study results. Arthroscopy 2005. https://doi.org/10.1016/j.arthro.2005.01.006.
40. Zaffagnini S, Marcheggiani Muccioli GM, Lopomo N, et al. Prospective long-term outcomes of the medial collagen meniscus implant versus partial medial

meniscectomy: a minimum 10-year follow-up study. Am J Sports Med 2011. https://doi.org/10.1177/0363546510391179.

41. Zaffagnini S, Marcheggiani Muccioli GM, Bulgheroni P, et al. Arthroscopic collagen meniscus implantation for partial lateral meniscal defects: a 2-year minimum follow-up study. Am J Sports Med 2012. https://doi.org/10.1177/0363546512456835.

42. Wasterlain AS, Braun HJ, Harris AHS, et al. The systemic effects of platelet-rich plasma injection. Am J Sports Med 2013. https://doi.org/10.1177/0363546512466383.

43. Zhang JY, Fabricant PD, Ishmael CR, et al. Utilization of platelet-rich plasma for musculoskeletal injuries: an analysis of current treatment trends in the United States. Orthop J Sport Med 2016. https://doi.org/10.1177/2325967116676241.

44. Pujol N, Salle De Chou E, Boisrenoult P, et al. Platelet-rich plasma for open meniscal repair in young patients: any benefit? Knee Surg Sports Traumatol Arthrosc 2014. https://doi.org/10.1007/s00167-014-3417-3.

45. Blanke F, Vavken P, Haenle M, et al. Percutaneous injections of platelet rich plasma for treatment of intrasubstance meniscal lesions. Muscles Ligaments Tendons J 2015. https://doi.org/10.11138/mltj/2015.5.3.162.

46. Hutchinson ID, Rodeo SA, Perrone GS, et al. Can platelet-rich plasma enhance anterior cruciate ligament and meniscal repair? J Knee Surg 2015. https://doi.org/10.1055/s-0034-1387166.

47. Ishida K, Kuroda R, Miwa M, et al. The regenerative effects of platelet-rich plasma on meniscal cells *in vitro* and its *in vivo* application with biodegradable gelatin hydrogel. Tissue Eng 2007. https://doi.org/10.1089/ten.2006.0193.

48. Griffin JW, Hadeed MM, Werner BC, et al. Platelet-rich plasma in meniscal repair: does augmentation improve surgical outcomes? Clin Orthop Relat Res 2015. https://doi.org/10.1007/s11999-015-4170-8.

49. Zellner J, Mueller M, Berner A, et al. Role of mesenchymal stem cells in tissue engineering of meniscus. J Biomed Mater Res A 2010. https://doi.org/10.1002/jbm.a.32796.

50. Zellner J, Hierl K, Mueller M, et al. Stem cell-based tissue-engineering for treatment of meniscal tears in the avascular zone. J Biomed Mater Res B Appl Biomater 2013. https://doi.org/10.1002/jbm.b.32922.

51. Kwak HS, Nam J, Lee JH, et al. Meniscal repair in vivo using human chondrocyte-seeded PLGA mesh scaffold pretreated with platelet-rich plasma. J Tissue Eng Regen Med 2017. https://doi.org/10.1002/term.1938.

52. Zellner J, Taeger CD, Schaffer M, et al. Are applied growth factors able to mimic the positive effects of mesenchymal stem cells on the regeneration of meniscus in the avascular zone? Biomed Res Int 2014. https://doi.org/10.1155/2014/537686.

53. Sheth U, Simunovic N, Klein G, et al. Efficacy of autologous platelet-rich plasma use for orthopaedic indications: a meta-analysis. J Bone Joint Surg Am 2012. https://doi.org/10.2106/JBJS.K.00154.

54. Ionescu LC, Lee GC, Huang KL, et al. Growth factor supplementation improves native and engineered meniscus repair in vitro. Acta Biomater 2012. https://doi.org/10.1016/j.actbio.2012.06.005.

55. Forriol F. Growth factors in cartilage and meniscus repair. Injury 2009. https://doi.org/10.1016/S0020-1383(09)70005-1.

56. Font Tellado S, Balmayor ER, Van Griensven M. Strategies to engineer tendon/ligament-to-bone interface: biomaterials, cells and growth factors. Adv Drug Deliv Rev 2015. https://doi.org/10.1016/j.addr.2015.03.004.

57. Bhardwaj N, Devi D, Mandal BB. Tissue-engineered cartilage: the crossroads of biomaterials, cells and stimulating factors. Macromol Biosci 2015. https://doi.org/10.1002/mabi.201400335.

58. Fortier LA, Barker JU, Strauss EJ, et al. The role of growth factors in cartilage repair. Clin Orthop Relat Res 2011. https://doi.org/10.1007/s11999-011-1857-3.

59. Hiraide A, Yokoo N, Xin K-Q, et al. Repair of articular cartilage defect by intra-articular administration of basic fibroblast growth factor gene, using adeno-associated virus vector. Hum Gene Ther 2005. https://doi.org/10.1089/hum.2005.16.1413.

60. Kasemkijwattana C, Menetrey J, Goto H, et al. The use of growth factors, gene therapy and tissue engineering to improve meniscal healing. Mater Sci Eng C 2000. https://doi.org/10.1016/S0928-4931(00)00172-7.

61. Stewart K, Pabbruwe M, Dickinson S, et al. The effect of growth factor treatment on meniscal chondrocyte proliferation and differentiation on polyglycolic acid scaffolds. Tissue Eng 2007. https://doi.org/10.1089/ten.2006.0242.

62. Bochyńska AI, Hannink G, Verhoeven R, et al. The effect of tissue surface modification with collagenase and addition of TGF-β3 on the healing potential of meniscal tears repaired with tissue glues in vitro. J Mater Sci Mater Med 2017. https://doi.org/10.1007/s10856-016-5832-0.

63. Tarafder S, Gulko J, Sim KH, et al. Engineered healing of avascular meniscus tears by stem cell recruitment. Sci Rep 2018. https://doi.org/10.1038/s41598-018-26545-8.

64. Tanaka T, Fujii K, Kumagae Y. Comparison of biochemical characteristics of cultured fibrochondrocytes isolated from the inner and outer regions of human meniscus. Knee Surg Sports Traumatol Arthrosc 1999. https://doi.org/10.1007/s001670050125.

65. Pangborn CA, Athanasiou KA. Effects of growth factors on meniscal fibrochondrocytes. Tissue Eng 2005. https://doi.org/10.1089/ten.2005.11.1141.

66. Imler SM, Doshi AN, Levenston ME. Combined effects of growth factors and static mechanical compression on meniscus explant biosynthesis. Osteoarthr Cartil 2004. https://doi.org/10.1016/j.joca.2004.05.007.

67. Marsano A, Millward-Sadler SJ, Salter DM, et al. Differential cartilaginous tissue formation by human synovial membrane, fat pad, meniscus cells and articular chondrocytes. Osteoarthr Cartil 2007. https://doi.org/10.1016/j.joca.2006.06.009.

68. De Mulder ELW, Hannink G, Giele M, et al. Proliferation of meniscal fibrochondrocytes cultured on a new polyurethane scaffold is stimulated by TGF-β. J Biomater Appl 2013. https://doi.org/10.1177/0885328211417317.

69. Forriol F, Ripalda P, Duart J, et al. Meniscal repair possibilities using bone morphogenetic protein-7. Injury 2014. https://doi.org/10.1016/S0020-1383(14)70005-1.

70. Bhargava MM, Attia ET, Murrell GAC, et al. The effect of cytokines on the proliferation and migration of bovine meniscal cells. Am J Sports Med 1999. https://doi.org/10.1177/03635465990270051601.

71. Tumia NS, Johnstone AJ. Regional regenerative potential of meniscal cartilage exposed to recombinant insulin-like growth factor-I in vitro. J Bone Joint Surg Br 2004. https://doi.org/10.1302/0301-620X.86B7.13747.

72. Puetzer JL, Brown BN, Ballyns JJ, et al. The effect of IGF-I on anatomically shaped tissue-engineered menisci. Tissue Eng Part A 2013. https://doi.org/10.1089/ten.tea.2012.0645.

73. Acosta CA, Forriol F, Izal I, et al. In vitro healing of avascular meniscal injuries with fresh and frozen plugs treated with TGF-beta1 and IGF-1 in sheep. Int J Clin Exp Pathol 2008;1(5):426–34.
74. Petersen W, Pufe T, Stärke C, et al. The effect of locally applied vascular endothelial growth factor on meniscus healing: gross and histological findings. Arch Orthop Trauma Surg 2007. https://doi.org/10.1007/s00402-005-0024-2.
75. Hidaka C, Ibarra C, Hannafin JA, et al. Formation of vascularized meniscal tissue by combining gene therapy with tissue engineering. Tissue Eng 2002. https://doi.org/10.1089/107632702753503090.
76. Nishida T, Kubota S, Kojima S, et al. Regeneration of defects in articular cartilage in rat knee joints by CCN2 (connective tissue growth factor). J Bone Miner Res 2004. https://doi.org/10.1359/JBMR.040322.
77. Tumia NS, Johnstone AJ. Platelet derived growth factor-AB enhances knee meniscal cell activity in vitro. Knee 2009. https://doi.org/10.1016/j.knee.2008.08.008.
78. Dominici M, Le Blanc K, Mueller I, et al. Minimal criteria for defining multipotent mesenchymal stromal cells. The International Society for Cellular Therapy position statement. Cytotherapy 2006. https://doi.org/10.1080/14653240600855905.
79. He S, Nakada D, Morrison S. Mechanisms of stem cell self-renewal. Annu Rev Cell Dev Biol 2009;25:377–406.
80. Qi Y, Yang Z, Ding Q, et al. Targeted transplantation of iron oxide-labeled, adipose-derived mesenchymal stem cells in promoting meniscus regeneration following a rabbit massive meniscal defect. Exp Ther Med 2016. https://doi.org/10.3892/etm.2015.2944.
81. Ruiz-Ibán MN, Díaz-Heredia J, García-Gómez I, et al. The effect of the addition of adipose-derived mesenchymal stem cells to a meniscal repair in the avascular zone: an experimental study in rabbits. Arthroscopy 2011. https://doi.org/10.1016/j.arthro.2011.06.041.
82. Ude CC, Sulaiman SB, Min-Hwei N, et al. Cartilage regeneration by chondrogenic induced adult stem cells in osteoarthritic sheep model. PLoS One 2014. https://doi.org/10.1371/journal.pone.0098770.
83. Pak J, Lee JH, Lee SH. Regenerative repair of damaged meniscus with autologous adipose tissue-derived stem cells. Biomed Res Int 2014. https://doi.org/10.1155/2014/436029.
84. González-Fernández ML, Pérez-Castrillo S, Sánchez-Lázaro JA, et al. Assessment of regeneration in meniscal lesions by use of mesenchymal stem cells derived from equine bone marrow and adipose tissue. Am J Vet Res 2016. https://doi.org/10.2460/ajvr.77.7.779.
85. Sasaki H, Rothrauff BB, Alexander PG, et al. In vitro repair of meniscal radial tear with hydrogels seeded with adipose stem cells and TGF-β3. Am J Sports Med 2018. https://doi.org/10.1177/0363546518782973.
86. Moradi L, Vasei M, Dehghan MM, et al. Regeneration of meniscus tissue using adipose mesenchymal stem cells-chondrocytes co-culture on a hybrid scaffold: in vivo study. Biomaterials 2017. https://doi.org/10.1016/j.biomaterials.2017.02.022.
87. Toratani T, Nakase J, Numata H, et al. Scaffold-free tissue-engineered allogenic adipose-derived stem cells promote meniscus healing. Arthroscopy 2017. https://doi.org/10.1016/j.arthro.2016.07.015.
88. Kondo S, Muneta T, Nakagawa Y, et al. Transplantation of autologous synovial mesenchymal stem cells promotes meniscus regeneration in aged primates. J Orthop Res 2017. https://doi.org/10.1002/jor.23211.

89. Nakagawa Y, Muneta T, Kondo S, et al. Synovial mesenchymal stem cells promote healing after meniscal repair in microminipigs. Osteoarthr Cartil 2015. https://doi.org/10.1016/j.joca.2015.02.008.

90. Hatsushika D, Muneta T, Nakamura T, et al. Repetitive allogeneic intraarticular injections of synovial mesenchymal stem cells promote meniscus regeneration in a porcine massive meniscus defect model. Osteoarthr Cartil 2014. https://doi.org/10.1016/j.joca.2014.04.028.

91. Okuno M, Muneta T, Koga H, et al. Meniscus regeneration by syngeneic, minor mismatched, and major mismatched transplantation of synovial mesenchymal stem cells in a rat model. J Orthop Res 2014. https://doi.org/10.1002/jor.22614.

92. Hatsushika D, Muneta T, Horie M, et al. Intraarticular injection of synovial stem cells promotes meniscal regeneration in a rabbit massive meniscal defect model. J Orthop Res 2013. https://doi.org/10.1002/jor.22370.

93. Katagiri H, Muneta T, Tsuji K, et al. Transplantation of aggregates of synovial mesenchymal stem cells regenerates meniscus more effectively in a rat massive meniscal defect. Biochem Biophys Res Commun 2013. https://doi.org/10.1016/j.bbrc.2013.05.026.

94. Moriguchi Y, Tateishi K, Ando W, et al. Repair of meniscal lesions using a scaffold-free tissue-engineered construct derived from allogenic synovial MSCs in a miniature swine model. Biomaterials 2013. https://doi.org/10.1016/j.biomaterials.2012.11.039.

95. Horie M, Driscoll MD, Sampson HW, et al. Implantation of allogenic synovial stem cells promotes meniscal regeneration in a rabbit meniscal defect model. J Bone Joint Surg Am 2012. https://doi.org/10.2106/JBJS.K.00176.

96. Horie M, Sekiya I, Muneta T, et al. Intra-articular injected synovial stem cells differentiate into meniscal cells directly and promote meniscal regeneration without mobilization to distant organs in rat massive meniscal defect. Stem Cells 2009. https://doi.org/10.1634/stemcells.2008-0616.

97. Mizuno K, Muneta T, Morito T, et al. Exogenous synovial stem cells adhere to defect of meniscus and differentiate into cartilage cells. J Med Dent Sci 2008.

98. Desando G, Giavaresi G, Cavallo C, et al. Autologous bone marrow concentrate in a sheep model of osteoarthritis: new perspectives for cartilage and meniscus repair. Tissue Eng C Methods 2016. https://doi.org/10.1089/ten.tec.2016.0033.

99. Ferris DJ, Frisbie DD, Kisiday JD, et al. Clinical outcome after intra-articular administration of bone marrow derived mesenchymal stem cells in 33 horses with stifle injury. Vet Surg 2014. https://doi.org/10.1111/j.1532-950X.2014.12100.x.

100. Horie M, Choi H, Lee RH, et al. Intra-articular injection of human mesenchymal stem cells (MSCs) promote rat meniscal regeneration by being activated to express Indian hedgehog that enhances expression of type II collagen. Osteoarthr Cartil 2012. https://doi.org/10.1016/j.joca.2012.06.002.

101. Hong J, Park J-I, Kim K-H, et al. Repair of the complete radial tear of the anterior horn of the medial meniscus in rabbits: a comparison between simple pullout repair and pullout repair with human bone marrow stem cell implantation. Knee Surg Relat Res 2011;23:164–75.

102. Dutton AQ, Choong PF, Goh JC-H, et al. Enhancement of meniscal repair in the avascular zone using mesenchymal stem cells in a porcine model. J Bone Joint Surg Br 2010. https://doi.org/10.1302/0301-620X.92B1.22629.

103. Zhang H, Leng P, Zhang J. Enhanced meniscal repair by overexpression of hIGF-1 in a full-thickness model. Clin Orthop Relat Res 2009. https://doi.org/10.1007/s11999-009-0921-8.

104. Angele P, Johnstone B, Kujat R, et al. Stem cell based tissue engineering for meniscus repair. J Biomed Mater Res A 2008. https://doi.org/10.1002/jbm.a.31480.

105. Walsh CJ, Goodman D, Caplan AI, et al. Meniscus regeneration in a rabbit partial meniscectomy model. Tissue Eng 1999. https://doi.org/10.1089/ten.1999.5.327.

106. Ishimura M, Ohgushi H, Habata T, et al. Arthroscopic meniscal repair using fibrin glue. Part I: experimental study. Arthroscopy 1997. https://doi.org/10.1016/S0749-8063(97)90179-1.

107. Ding Z, Huang H. Mesenchymal stem cells in rabbit meniscus and bone marrow exhibit a similar feature but a heterogeneous multi-differentiation potential: superiority of meniscus as a cell source for meniscus repair evolutionary developmental biology and morphology. BMC Musculoskelet Disord 2015. https://doi.org/10.1186/s12891-015-0511-8.

108. Ferris D, Frisbie D, Kisiday J, et al. In vivo healing of meniscal lacerations using bone marrow-derived mesenchymal stem cells and fibrin glue. Stem Cells Int 2012. https://doi.org/10.1155/2012/691605.

109. Caminal M, Fonseca C, Peris D, et al. Use of a chronic model of articular cartilage and meniscal injury for the assessment of long-term effects after autologous mesenchymal stromal cell treatment in sheep. N Biotechnol 2014. https://doi.org/10.1016/j.nbt.2014.07.004.

110. Al Faqeh H, Nor Hamdan BMY, Chen HC, et al. The potential of intra-articular injection of chondrogenic-induced bone marrow stem cells to retard the progression of osteoarthritis in a sheep model. Exp Gerontol 2012. https://doi.org/10.1016/j.exger.2012.03.018.

111. Agung M, Ochi M, Yanada S, et al. Mobilization of bone marrow-derived mesenchymal stem cells into the injured tissues after intraarticular injection and their contribution to tissue regeneration. Knee Surg Sports Traumatol Arthrosc 2006. https://doi.org/10.1007/s00167-006-0124-8.

112. Murphy JM, Fink DJ, Hunziker EB, et al. Stem cell therapy in a caprine model of osteoarthritis. Arthritis Rheum 2003. https://doi.org/10.1002/art.11365.

113. Yuan X, Wei Y, Villasante A, et al. Stem cell delivery in tissue-specific hydrogel enabled meniscal repair in an orthotopic rat model. Biomaterials 2017. https://doi.org/10.1016/j.biomaterials.2017.04.004.

114. Zhang ZZ, Wang SJ, Zhang JY, et al. 3D-printed poly(ε-caprolactone) scaffold augmented with mesenchymal stem cells for total meniscal substitution: a 12- and 24-week animal study in a rabbit model. Am J Sports Med 2017. https://doi.org/10.1177/0363546517691513.

115. Qi Y, Chen G, Feng G. Osteoarthritis prevention and meniscus regeneration induced by transplantation of mesenchymal stem cell sheet in a rat meniscal defect model. Exp Ther Med 2016. https://doi.org/10.3892/etm.2016.3325.

116. Yamasaki T, Deie M, Shinomiya R, et al. Transplantation of meniscus regenerated by tissue engineering with a scaffold derived from a rat meniscus and mesenchymal stromal cells derived from rat bone marrow. Artif Organs 2008. https://doi.org/10.1111/j.1525-1594.2008.00580.x.

117. Izuta Y, Ochi M, Adachi N, et al. Meniscal repair using bone marrow-derived mesenchymal stem cells: experimental study using green fluorescent protein transgenic rats. Knee 2005. https://doi.org/10.1016/j.knee.2001.06.001.

118. Koch M, Achatz FP, Lang S, et al. Tissue engineering of large full-size meniscus defects by a polyurethane scaffold: accelerated regeneration by mesenchymal stromal cells. Stem Cells Int 2018. https://doi.org/10.1155/2018/8207071.

119. Jayasuriya CT, Twomey-Kozak J, Newberry J, et al. Human cartilage-derived progenitors resist terminal differentiation and require CXCR4 activation to successfully bridge meniscus tissue tears. Stem Cells 2019;37(1):102–14.
120. Friedenstein AJ, Piatetzky-Shapiro II, Petrakova KV. Osteogenesis in transplants of bone marrow cells. J Embryol Exp Morphol 1966;16(3):381–90.
121. Friedenstein AJ, Ivanov-Smolenski AA, Chajlakjan RK, et al. Origin of bone marrow stromal mechanocytes in radiochimeras and heterotopic transplants. Exp Hematol 1978;6(5):440–4.
122. Bilgen B, Jayasuriya CT, Owens BD. Current concepts in meniscus tissue engineering and repair. Adv Healthc Mater 2018. https://doi.org/10.1515/text.1. 1983.3.3.299.
123. Pittenger MF, Mackay AM, Beck SC, et al. Multilineage potential of adult human mesenchymal stem cells. Science 1999. https://doi.org/10.1126/science.284. 5411.143.
124. Alvarez-Viejo M, Menendez-Menendez Y, Blanco-Gelaz MA, et al. Quantifying mesenchymal stem cells in the mononuclear cell fraction of bone marrow samples obtained for cell therapy. Transplant Proc 2013. https://doi.org/10.1016/j. transproceed.2012.05.091.
125. Diekman BO, Rowland CR, Lennon DP, et al. Chondrogenesis of adult stem cells from adipose tissue and bone marrow: induction by growth factors and cartilage-derived matrix. Tissue Eng Part A 2010. https://doi.org/10.1089/ten. tea.2009.0398.
126. Mueller MB, Tuan RS. Functional characterization of hypertrophy in chondrogenesis of human mesenchymal stem cells. Arthritis Rheum 2008. https://doi.org/ 10.1002/art.23370.
127. Pelttari K, Winter A, Steck E, et al. Premature induction of hypertrophy during in vitro chondrogenesis of human mesenchymal stem cells correlates with calcification and vascular invasion after ectopic transplantation in SCID mice. Arthritis Rheum 2006. https://doi.org/10.1002/art.22136.
128. Chowdhury A, Bezuidenhout LW, Mulet-Sierra A, et al. Effect of interleukin-1β treatment on co-cultures of human meniscus cells and bone marrow mesenchymal stromal cells. BMC Musculoskelet Disord 2013. https://doi.org/10. 1186/1471-2474-14-216.
129. Johnstone B, Hering TM, Caplan AI, et al. In vitro chondrogenesis of bone marrow-derived mesenchymal progenitor cells. Exp Cell Res 1998. https://doi. org/10.1006/excr.1997.3858.
130. Eerola I, Salminen H, Lammi P, et al. Type X collagen, a natural component of mouse articular cartilage: association with growth, aging, and osteoarthritis. Arthritis Rheum 1998. https://doi.org/10.1002/1529-0131(199807)41:7<1287:: AID-ART20>3.0.CO;2-D.
131. Bluteau G, Labourdette L, Ronzière MC, et al. Type X collagen in rabbit and human meniscus. Osteoarthr Cartil 1999. https://doi.org/10.1053/joca.1999.0245.
132. Gao J. Immunolocalization of types I, II, and X collagen in the tibial insertion sites of the medial meniscus. Knee Surg Sports Traumatol Arthrosc 2000. https://doi.org/10.1007/s001670050013.
133. Le Graverand MPH, Ou YC, Schield-Yee T, et al. The cells of the rabbit meniscus: their arrangement, interrelationship, morphological variations and cytoarchitecture. J Anat 2001. https://doi.org/10.1017/S0021878201007671.
134. Le Graverand MPH, Sciore P, Eggerer J, et al. Formation and phenotype of cell clusters in osteoarthritic meniscus. Arthritis Rheum 2001. https://doi.org/10. 1002/1529-0131(200108)44:8<1808::AID-ART318>3.0.CO;2-B.

135. Zuk P, Zhu M, Ashjian P, et al. Human adipose tissue is a source of multipotent stem cells. Mol Biol Cell 2002;13:4279–95.

136. Frese L, Dijkman PE, Hoerstrup SP. Adipose tissue-derived stem cells in regenerative medicine. Transfus Med Hemother 2016;43(4):268–74.

137. Bourin P, Bunnell BA, Casteilla L, et al. Stromal cells from the adipose tissue-derived stromal vascular fraction and culture expanded adipose tissue-derived stromal/stem cells: a joint statement of the International Federation for Adipose Therapeutics and Science (IFATS) and the International Society for Cellular Therapy (SCT). Cytotherapy 2013. https://doi.org/10.1016/j.jcyt.2013.02.006.

138. Diekman BO, Christoforou N, Willard VP, et al. Cartilage tissue engineering using differentiated and purified induced pluripotent stem cells. Proc Natl Acad Sci U S A 2012. https://doi.org/10.1073/pnas.1210422109.

139. Hamid A, Idrus R, Saim A, et al. Characterization of human adipose-derived stem cells and expression of chondrogenic genes during induction of cartilage differentiation. Clinics 2012. https://doi.org/10.6061/clinics/2012(02)03.

140. Huang JI, Kazmi N, Durbhakula MM, et al. Chondrogenic potential of progenitor cells derived from human bone marrow and adipose tissue: a patient-matched comparison. J Orthop Res 2005. https://doi.org/10.1016/j.orthres.2005.03.018.

141. Im GI, Shin YW, Lee KB. Do adipose tissue-derived mesenchymal stem cells have the same osteogenic and chondrogenic potential as bone marrow-derived cells? Osteoarthr Cartil 2005. https://doi.org/10.1016/j.joca.2005.05.005.

142. Morito T, Muneta T, Hara K, et al. Synovial fluid-derived mesenchymal stem cells increase after intra-articular ligament injury in humans. Rheumatology 2008. https://doi.org/10.1093/rheumatology/ken114.

143. De Bari C, Dell'Accio F, Tylzanowski P, et al. Multipotent mesenchymal stem cells from adult human synovial membrane. Arthritis Rheum 2001. https://doi.org/10.1002/1529-0131(200108)44:8<1928::AID-ART331>3.0.CO;2-P.

144. Matsukura Y, Muneta T, Tsuji K, et al. Mesenchymal stem cells in synovial fluid increase after meniscus injury. Clin Orthop Relat Res 2014. https://doi.org/10.1007/s11999-013-3418-4.

145. Xie X, Zhu J, Hu X, et al. A co-culture system of rat synovial stem cells and meniscus cells promotes cell proliferation and differentiation as compared to mono-culture. Sci Rep 2018;8(1):7693.

146. Hatakeyama A, Uchida S, Utsunomiya H, et al. Isolation and characterization of synovial mesenchymal stem cell derived from hip joints: a comparative analysis with a matched control knee group. Stem Cells Int 2017. https://doi.org/10.1155/2017/9312329.

147. Zellner J, Pattappa G, Koch M, et al. Autologous mesenchymal stem cells or meniscal cells: what is the best cell source for regenerative meniscus treatment in an early osteoarthritis situation? Stem Cell Res Ther 2017. https://doi.org/10.1186/s13287-017-0678-z.

148. Sakaguchi Y, Sekiya I, Yagishita K, et al. Comparison of human stem cells derived from various mesenchymal tissues: superiority of synovium as a cell source. Arthritis Rheum 2005. https://doi.org/10.1002/art.21212.

149. Yamazaki K, Tachibana Y. Vascularized synovial flap promoting regeneration of the cryopreserved meniscal allograft: experimental study in rabbits. J Orthop Sci 2003. https://doi.org/10.1007/s007760300010.

150. Liu H, Wei X, Ding X, et al. Comparison of cellular responses of mesenchymal stem cells derived from bone marrow and synovium on combined silk scaffolds. J Biomed Mater Res A 2015. https://doi.org/10.1002/jbm.a.35154.

151. Pei M, He F, Li J, et al. Repair of large animal partial-thickness cartilage defects through intraarticular injection of matrix-rejuvenated synovium-derived stem cells. Tissue Eng Part A 2013. https://doi.org/10.1089/ten.tea.2012.0351.

152. Koay E, Athanasiou K. Development of serum-free, chemically defined conditions for human embryonic stem cell-derived fibrochondrogenesis. Tissue Eng Part A 2009;15(8):2249–57.

153. Hoben GM, Koay EJ, Athanasiou KA. Fibrochondrogenesis in two embryonic stem cell lines: effects of differentiation timelines. Stem Cells 2008. https://doi.org/10.1634/stemcells.2007-0641.

154. Brindle T, Nyland J, Johnson DL. The meniscus: review of basic principles with application to surgery and rehabilitation. J Athl Train 2001. https://doi.org/10.1093/acprof.

155. Webber RJ, Harris MG, Hough AJ. Cell culture of rabbit meniscal fibrochondrocytes: proliferative and synthetic response to growth factors and ascorbate. J Orthop Res 1985. https://doi.org/10.1002/jor.1100030104.

156. Moon MS, Kim JM, Ok IY. The normal and regenerated meniscus in rabbits. Morphologic and histologic studies. Clin Orthop Relat Res 1984.

157. Upton ML, Chen J, Guilak F, et al. Differential effects of static and dynamic compression on meniscal cell gene expression. J Orthop Res 2003. https://doi.org/10.1016/S0736-0266(03)00063-9.

158. Sweigart MA, Aufderheide AC, Athanasiou KA. Fibrochondrocytes and their use in tissue engineering of the meniscus. Tissue Eng 2003. https://doi.org/10.1016/j.ceramint.2013.05.084.

159. Mow V. Structure and function relationships of the meniscus in the knee. In: VCM, SPA, DWJ, editors. Knee meniscus: basic and clinical foundations. Raven Press; 1992. p. 37–58.

160. Mauck RL, Martinez-Diaz GJ, Yuan X, et al. Regional multilineage differentiation potential of meniscal fibrochondrocytes: implications for meniscus repair. Anat Rec 2007. https://doi.org/10.1002/ar.20419.

161. Mcdevitt CA, Webber RJ. The ultrastructure and biochemistry of meniscal cartilage. Clin Orthop Relat Res 1989. https://doi.org/10.1097/NCN.0b013e31823ea54e.

162. Adams ME, Hukins DWL. The extracellular matrix of the meniscus. In: Mow VC, Arnoczky SP, Jackson DW, editors. Knee meniscus: basic and clinical foundations. Raven Press; 1992. p. 15–28.

163. Setton LA, Guilak F, Hsu EW, et al. Biomechanical factors in tissue engineered meniscal repair. Clin Orthop Relat Res 1999. https://doi.org/10.1097/00003086-199910001-00025.

164. Baratz ME, Fu FH, Mengato R. Meniscal tears: the effect of meniscectomy and of repair on intraarticular contact areas and stress in the human knee. A preliminary report. Am J Sports Med 1986. https://doi.org/10.1177/036354658601400405.

165. Rath E, Richmond JC. The menisci: basic science and advances in treatment. Br J Sports Med 2000. https://doi.org/10.1136/bjsm.34.4.252.

166. Dowthwaite G, Bishop J, Redman S, et al. The surface of articular cartilage contains a progenitor cell population. J Cell Sci 2004;117(6):889–97.

167. Williams R, Khan IM, Richardson K, et al. Identification and clonal characterisation of a progenitor cell sub-population in normal human articular cartilage. PLoS One 2010. https://doi.org/10.1371/journal.pone.0013246.

168. Thornemo M, Tallheden T, Sjögren Jansson E, et al. Clonal populations of chondrocytes with progenitor properties identified within human articular cartilage. Cells Tissues Organs 2005. https://doi.org/10.1159/000088242.

169. Khan IM, Bishop JC, Gilbert S, et al. Clonal chondroprogenitors maintain telomerase activity and Sox9 expression during extended monolayer culture and retain chondrogenic potential. Osteoarthr Cartil 2009. https://doi.org/10.1016/j.joca.2008.08.002.
170. Jayasuriya CT, Chen Q. Potential benefits and limitations of utilizing chondroprogenitors in cell-based cartilage therapy. Connect Tissue Res 2015. https://doi.org/10.3109/03008207.2015.1040547.
171. Marcus P, De Bari C, Dell'Accio F, et al. Articular chondroprogenitor cells maintain chondrogenic potential but fail to form a functional matrix when implanted into muscles of SCID mice. Cartilage 2014. https://doi.org/10.1177/1947603514541274.
172. Koelling S, Kruegel J, Irmer M, et al. Migratory chondrogenic progenitor cells from repair tissue during the later stages of human osteoarthritis. Cell Stem Cell 2009. https://doi.org/10.1016/j.stem.2009.01.015.
173. Fellows CR, Williams R, Davies IR, et al. Characterisation of a divergent progenitor cell sub-populations in human osteoarthritic cartilage: the role of telomere erosion and replicative senescence. Sci Rep 2017. https://doi.org/10.1038/srep41421.
174. D'Angelo M, Pacifici M. Articular chondrocytes produce factors that inhibit maturation of sternal chondrocytes in serum-free agarose cultures: a TGF-β independent process. J Bone Miner Res 1997. https://doi.org/10.1359/jbmr.1997.12.9.1368.
175. DeShazo R, Mather P, Grant W, et al. Evaluation of patients with local reactions to insulin with skin tests and in vitro techniques. Diabetes Care 1987;10(3):330–6.
176. Kean CO, Brown RJ, Chapman J. The role of biomaterials in the treatment of meniscal tears. PeerJ 2017. https://doi.org/10.7717/peerj.4076.
177. Chen JP, Cheng TH. Thermo-responsive chitosan-graft-poly(N-isopropylacrylamide) injectable hydrogel for cultivation of chondrocytes and meniscus cells. Macromol Biosci 2006. https://doi.org/10.1002/mabi.200600142.

Meniscus Injuries
A Review of Rehabilitation and Return to Play

Seth L. Sherman, MD[a],*, Zachary J. DiPaolo, MD[b],
Taylor E. Ray, BS[b], Barbie M. Sachs, PT, DPT, OCS[c],
Lasun O. Oladeji, MD, MS[b]

KEYWORDS

- Meniscus repair • Rehabilitation • Return to play • Blood flow restriction

KEY POINTS

- The menisci play an important role in preserving overall joint health, thus preservation is paramount.
- Meniscus tear patterns and their associated repair techniques respond differently to physiologic loading, which has a profound influence on rehabilitation strategy.
- An ideal meniscal rehabilitation protocol should consider the tear pattern, location, size, quality of the repaired tissue, the type and strength of repair construct, and any concomitant procedures.

INTRODUCTION

There has been increased awareness of the essential role of the knee menisci in protecting the articular cartilage by assisting with shock absorption, load transmission, lubrication, and stability.[1–3] Injury to the menisci results in altered knee kinematics and increased peak contact stresses, which ultimately accelerates the risk of degenerative changes and early osteoarthritis.[4–6] Similarly, even partial meniscectomy significantly alters knee stability and joint loading, also leading to increased risk of

Conflicts of interest: The authors have no conflicts of interest.
Disclosures: S.L. Sherman is a board or committee member of ACL Study Group, American Orthopedic Society for Sports Medicine, Arthroscopy Association of North America, International Cartilage Regeneration & Joint Preservation Society, International Society of Arthroscopy, Knee Surgery, and Orthopedic Sports Medicine; is a paid consultant for and has received research support from Arthrex, Inc.; is on the editorial board of *Arthroscopy*; is a paid consultant for Ceterix Orthopedics and GLG Consulting; an unpaid consultant for Flexion Therapeutics; and is a paid consultant for JRF Ortho, Moximed, and Vericel.
a Department of Orthopaedic Surgery, Stanford University, Stanford, CA, USA; b Department of Orthopaedic Surgery, University of Missouri, 1100 Virginia Avenue, Columbia, MO 65212, USA; c Mizzou Therapy Services, University of Missouri, Columbia, MO, USA
* Corresponding author. Stanford Medicine Outpatient Center, 450 Broadway, Pavillion A, Redwood City, CA 94063.
E-mail address: dr.seth.sherman@gmail.com

Clin Sports Med 39 (2020) 165–183
https://doi.org/10.1016/j.csm.2019.08.004
0278-5919/20/© 2019 Elsevier Inc. All rights reserved.

early articular cartilage degeneration.[7,8] This information has led surgeons to a recent paradigm shift toward meniscus preservation. Between 2005 and 2011, the number of arthroscopic meniscal repairs in the United States doubled.[9] This trend is multifactorial and likely related to the improved understanding of the importance of the meniscus for overall joint health coupled with major advances in surgical technique and biologic augmentation of meniscal healing.[10–14]

As surgeons expand their indications for meniscal repair, it is critically important that they continue to analyze and advance their understanding of rehabilitation and return to play following meniscal surgery. There are numerous studies on meniscal repair techniques and their associated outcomes in the literature.[15–21] However, there is a paucity of high-quality studies evaluating rehabilitation protocols following meniscus repair. Furthermore, there is significant variation between existing postoperative rehabilitation protocols.[22–25] Despite these limitations, this article summarizes the best available evidence guiding meniscal rehabilitation progression and return-to-play decision making. In addition, it uses the current rehabilitation protocol to help highlight the scientific rationale behind rehabilitation progression and to provide a framework for safe return to activity and sport. This work recognizes inherent limitations in the existing data and discusses areas that are ripe for future collaborative investigation.

Evidence-based Considerations for Meniscus Repair Rehabilitation

Biomechanical studies have shown that the various meniscus tear patterns and their associated repair techniques respond differently when subjected to physiologic loading. For example, weight bearing across the knee helps reduce and compress vertical longitudinal and bucket-handle tears, which may improve healing rates following repair.[2] In contrast, weight bearing causes displacement and distraction of radial, root, and complex tears, which likely decreases the chances of successful healing.[26,27] As a result, accelerated rehabilitation protocols with early weight bearing and range of motion (ROM) have shown positive results in patients with vertical and more stable tear patterns.[23,28] Lind and colleagues[23] randomized 60 patients undergoing repair of unstable peripheral vertical meniscus lesions to either an accelerated or conservative postoperative rehabilitation plan. The accelerated plan consisted of 2 weeks of 0° to 90° ROM without a brace and touch-down weight bearing followed by unrestricted weight bearing and ROM. This group returned to running at 8 weeks and contact sports at 4 months. Compared with the restricted group, there were no differences in functional or subjective outcomes at 1 or 2 years. However, there is limited evidence to support these advanced protocols for more complex and unstable tear patterns.[22] Kocabey and colleagues[29] achieved positive results using a tear-specific rehabilitation protocol. Fifty-five patients undergoing a T-fix meniscal repair were stratified according to tear size. Patients with anteroposterior longitudinal meniscal tears less than 3 cm in length were full weight bearing following surgery but ROM was restricted to 0° to 90° for 3 weeks and 0° to 125° from 3 to 6 weeks. Patients with tears greater than 3 cm were immobilized in a knee brace for 3 weeks but allowed weight bearing. Patients were restricted to passive motion from 0° to 90° with a continuous passive motion (CPM) device. Between weeks 3 and 6, patients were allowed to progress to active knee flexion between 0° and 90°. In addition, patients progressed to 0° to 125° for weeks 6 to 8, after which all restrictions were terminated. Patients with complex and radial tears were further limited with respect to initial postoperative weight bearing and ROM (ie, non–weight bearing and no flexion >90° for 6 weeks). Ultimately, patients with longitudinal tears were allowed to return to sport at 3 months, whereas patients with complex and radial tears were allowed to return to sport between 4 and 5 months. The investigators reported that 96% of patients with isolated meniscus repair and 100% with combined anterior cruciate ligament (ACL) reconstruction and meniscus repair showed excellent outcomes. Given these findings, it follows that an ideal protocol must consider the tear pattern, location, and size; quality of the repaired tissue; the type and strength of repair construct; and any concomitant procedures (eg, ligament repair/construction, realignment osteotomy, cartilage restoration) that may have been performed.

The early postoperative period is crucial to protect the meniscal repair such that compression is maintained across the repair site. If the compressive forces across the repair site are lost, the odds of successful meniscal healing decrease significantly.[2,30] Two main factors are at play with regard to compression at the repair site: (1) the strength and security of the fixation at the time of surgery, and (2) the weight bearing status postoperatively. The quality of the repair construct is under the control of the surgeon and every attempt should be made at anatomic reduction and fixation of the torn meniscus in order to optimize its healing potential and to restore normal knee biomechanics.[31] There has been an evolution of fixation strategies to assist surgeons in achieving this goal. A myriad of all-inside, inside-out, outside-in, and novel suture passers and fixation devices are available for most tear patterns, including meniscal root and ramp lesions. Having a broad arsenal for meniscal repair can assist surgeons in achieving the goal of anatomic reduction and strong time-zero meniscus fixation. In addition, the weight-bearing status is determined both by surgeon preference and patient compliance. Early weight bearing can be helpful to provide compression and reduction in more stable tear patterns, and these patients should be allowed to weight bear as tolerated (WBAT) immediately following surgery.[32] In contrast, weight bearing can create distractive forces for unstable tear patterns, specifically radial, complex, and posterior root tears, and thus these patients should be made non–weight bearing for a period of several weeks (**Fig. 1**).[2,33,34]

It is also important to consider the axial alignment of the patient before advancing weight-bearing status. Previous work has shown that patients with varus deformity are at higher risk of developing atraumatic medial meniscus tears.[35] Therefore,

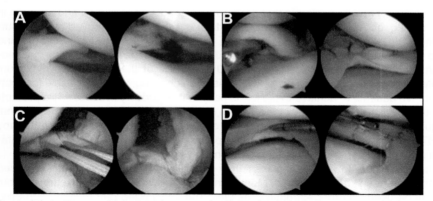

Fig. 1. (*A*) A 17-year-old boy with a complex lateral meniscus flap tear treated with an all-inside repair. This patient was limited to foot-flat 0% weight bearing for 6 weeks. (*B*) A 14-year-old female dancer who sustained a noncontact injury and presented with a bucket-handle medial meniscus tear that was treated with a hybrid all-inside and inside-out repair. This patient was allowed to WBAT immediately after surgery. (*C*) A lateral meniscus transosseous posterior root repair in a patient who was limited to foot-flat 0% weight bearing for 6 weeks. (*D*) A horizontal cleavage tear treated with all-inside circumferential stitch. This patient was allowed to WBAT immediately after surgery.

patients with varus malalignment undergoing rehabilitation following a medial meniscus repair may benefit from a more conservation approach to progressive weight bearing. The same principles should be applied to those with valgus alignment undergoing a lateral meniscus repair because of the increased compressive loads in the lateral compartment.[2] These select patients may also benefit from a medial or lateral unloader brace when initiating weight bearing postoperatively to reduce loads across the meniscus repair within the compartment at risk.[36,37]

In addition to the postoperative weight-bearing status, knee ROM also needs to be carefully considered. It has been shown that immobilization following meniscal repair is detrimental to meniscal healing.[38-41] Protected early ROM is important for healing and to reduce the risk of postsurgical arthrofibrosis. However, it is imperative to avoid deep flexion given that cadaveric studies have shown greater femorotibial contact pressures in higher degrees of knee flexion as opposed to full extension or low degrees of knee flexion.[42-44] The progression toward high knee flexion angles during weight bearing leads to higher peak contact pressures, which may be detrimental to meniscal healing, particularly following radial and root repairs.[27] However, these restrictions may not be required following fixation of more stable tear patterns (ie, vertical longitudinal tears).[44-46] Extrapolating data from the knee cartilage restoration and repair literature, it seems that early gravity-assisted ROM (even past 90°) and/or use of CPM are likely safe and beneficial in the early postsurgical period.[47,48] Progression to loaded deep-flexion activities should be avoided until meniscus healing is well underway (ie, 3 months) because of the increased loads and translation experienced by the menisci in higher degrees of knee flexion.[49-51]

Blood Flow Restriction Therapy: A Novel Approach to Quadriceps Atrophy

It is well known that knee pain and effusion can lead to quadriceps dysfunction and atrophy; this is particularly true in the setting of a meniscal tear, both preoperatively and postoperatively.[52-55] Furthermore, there is likely a correlation between the length of time a patient has a meniscal tear (ie, longer time with painful effusion) and the amount of quadriceps dysfunction and/or atrophy (ie, longer duration of quadriceps avoidance). It has been shown that the return of quadriceps function and strength in the setting of ACL injury and reconstruction is related to improved patient outcomes.[56,57] However, it can be difficult to restore quadriceps muscle strength and size while protecting a meniscal repair. The American College of Sports Medicine recommends a resistance training load of 70% to 85% of the 1-repetition maximum (1RM) to promote muscle hypertrophy.[58] It is often challenging or impossible for postoperative patients to achieve these loads early in the recovery process while protecting the meniscus, particularly in the setting of complex tear patterns and repairs that require early limitations in weight bearing and ROM. Blood flow restriction therapy (BFRT) has become a growing part of the preoperative and postoperative rehabilitation regimen to combat this difficult problem.

During a blood flow restriction session, a specialized blood pressure cuff is placed on the patient's extremity (**Fig. 2**). Most commonly, this is the operative extremity, but it may be used on other extremities as well. The specialized cuff measures the patient's blood pressure and sets the cuff pressure at a specific level to prevent venous outflow from the patient's limb, which ultimately results in the development of an anaerobic environment with subsequent release of growth factors. It is the release of these growth factors that promotes muscle hypertrophy.[59-61] The beauty of BFRT is that it can stimulate an anaerobic environment using loads much less than the traditional 70% to 85% of 1RM, thus minimizing stresses to the meniscal repair. Most studies on BFR use loads near 30% of 1RM, with results showing significant

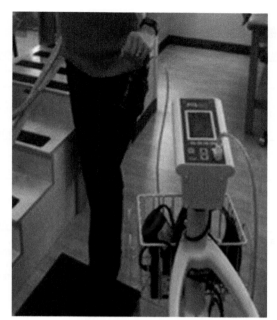

Fig. 2. A patient undergoing a therapy session while wearing the blood flow restriction tourniquet.

increases in both muscle hypertrophy and strength.[62] Although there are scant data on the use of BFR following meniscal repair, there are encouraging studies in the ACL reconstruction literature proving the safety and efficacy of BFRT.[59,63] According to a recent meta-analysis, strength and muscle hypertrophy were significantly greater in the groups performing exercise with BFR 2 to 3 d/wk compared with those exercising 4 to 5 d/wk.[64]

In our practice, our physical therapists are certified in BFRT and use it in select patients with complex repairs requiring prolonged weight-bearing limitations. We also use this in our athletic population following standard or complex repairs to accelerate the return of quadriceps function and to help facilitate earlier return to sport. We are actively collecting prospective data on several populations using BFR for rehabilitation following ACL reconstruction (randomized controlled trial enrolling), meniscus repair, and cartilage restoration; and should have data on its efficacy for early quadriceps return and functional outcomes in the near future.

MENISCAL REPAIR REHABILITATION

This article focuses on isolated meniscal repair in patients with otherwise normal knees. Our guidelines for rehabilitation following meniscal repair are divided into 4 phases. They can be referenced in **Tables 1–4**.

Phase I, Postinjury Phase, Protected Motion

Following an isolated meniscal repair, the immediate postoperative period should focus on minimizing effusion, pain control, as well as the return of quadriceps function (see **Table 1**). Cryotherapy and compression are used until effusion is controlled. A transcutaneous electrical nerve stimulation unit may be indicated to reduce narcotic

Table 1
Meniscus rehabilitation protocol, phase I

Phase I: Immediate Postoperative/Postinjury Phase (Protected Motion)	
Frequency	Rehabilitation appointments begin within 10–14 d of surgery and continue 2–3 times per week
Rehabilitation Goals	• Protect healing of repaired tissues • Reduce pain and swelling in the knee, foot, and ankle • Restore full knee extension • Restore quadriceps and surrounding muscle activation
Precautions	• Maximum protection of inflamed joint • No running, jumping, plyometric activity • Modified weight bearing with assistive device
Inflammation Control	• TENS • Cryotherapy • Compression (garment/bandage) • Elevation with straight knee (extra support under ankle)

ROM Interventions	• Patellar mobility (superior/inferior/medial)
	• Full passive terminal extension equal to contralateral limb
	  ○ Seated or supine low-level long-duration stretch
	  ○ Emphasize hamstring/gastrocnemius soft tissue mobility
	  ○ Long sitting gastrocnemius stretch
	• Flexion progression per guidelines
	  ○ Gravity-assisted knee flexion/CPM
	  ○ Therapist assisted without overpressure
	  ○ Stationary bike (high seat, no or low resistance)
	• Assisted heel slides (supine or wall with towel/belt)

Therapeutic Exercises	• Core stabilization
	  ○ Supine core activation
	• Hip strengthening
	  ○ Straight leg raises (extension/abduction/adduction)
	  ○ Clam shells (within flexion restrictions)
	• Quadriceps recruitment progression without patellofemoral pain
	  ○ Isometric quadriceps sets
	  ○ Prone TKE (only if WBAT)
	  ○ Short-arc quadriceps (with physician approval)
	  ○ Straight leg raise
	• Gait (with weight-bearing approval)
	  ○ Weight shifting
	  ○ Marching
	  ○ Step over/hurdle walking
	  ○ Retroversion/side stepping
	• Double-limb balance (with weight-bearing approval)

Cardiovascular Exercises	None at this time
Requirements for Progression	• Full active knee extension (equal to contralateral side) • Normal gait without compensation (hip hiking, adequate extension during midstance) • No active effusion (negative or trace Brush test) • Normal patellar mobility (superior, inferior, medial) • Ability to complete 20 straight leg raises without extensor lag • Physician clearance to WBAT, brace, and crutches

Abbreviations: TENS, transcutaneous electrical nerve stimulation; TKE, terminal knee extension.

Table 2
Meniscus rehabilitation protocol, phase II

Phase II: Intermediate Phase (Low Impact)	
Frequency	Rehabilitation appointments continue 1–3 times per week
Rehabilitation Goals	• Restore full knee ROM (within guidelines on face sheet) • Restore normal weight-bearing kinematics • Restore normal balance on the operative/injured limb • Normalize gait pattern without assistive device • Return to light work/moderately heavy labor (eg, truck driving) • Return to recreational sports (swimming, cycling, walking, linear jogging 2 times per week)
Precautions	• Clearance required for running, jumping, plyometric activity • Full weight bearing (with the exception of weight bearing past 90° with closed chain exercises)

ROM Interventions	• Maintain knee extension
	• Progress flexion per restrictions
	  ○ Upright/recumbent bike
	  ○ Manual interventions
	• Aquatic therapy as needed

Therapeutic Exercises	• Neutral spine/core stabilization
	  ○ Plank progression (side/prone)
	• Emphasize posterior kinetic chain (hamstrings, gluteals, anterior core, gastrocnemius)
	• Closed chain exercises
	  ○ Double-limb activity (equal weight bearing, knees stay behind toes, patella in line with second toe, stable trunk, no pain through motion)
	    ■ Leg press
	    ■ Squat progression
	    ■ RDL/deadlift
	    ■ Bridge progression
	    ■ Heel raises
	    ■ Side stepping (with/without resistance)
	    ■ Split squat/lunge
	  ○ Single-limb activity (no pelvic drop)
	    ■ RDL
	    ■ Squat progression
	    ■ Bridge progression
	    ■ Balance progression
	    ■ Heel raises
	    ■ Step-ups forward/lateral
	    ■ 4-way resisted hip with single-leg stance (flexion/extension/abduction/adduction)
	    ■ Hip hikes
	Open Chain Exercises
	  ○ Hamstring curls
	  ○ Straight leg raises with quadriceps activated
	  ○ Short-arc quadriceps (unweighted)
	  ○ Long-arc quadriceps (unweighted)
	Begin applying dual-task modifiers during exercise (cognitive/visual/balance)
	  ○ Spelling, verbalizing days of the week backward, reciting alphabet, counting, memory recall, and so forth

(continued on next page)

Table 2 (*continued*)	
Phase II: Intermediate Phase (Low Impact)	
Cardiovascular Exercises	Swimming (without frog kicking)
	Stationary/level-surface biking without resistance
	Elliptical without or minimal resistance
Requirements for Progression	• Ability to reciprocally ascend/descend 1 flight of stairs without compensation
	• Soreness lasting no longer than 24 h after activity
	• Performs squat to 75° without pain and symmetric weight bearing
	• Good understanding and self-correction of exercise techniques
	• Single-leg stance for 30 s without loss of balance
	• Return-to-work functional testing (per discretion of physician)
	• Return to linear running testing (per discretion of physician)
	○ Modified return-to-sport testing at 3 mo
	▪ Isokinetic testing
	• ≥70% quadriceps/quadriceps strength
	• ≥70% hamstring/hamstring strength
	• Lateral step-down: no more than mild dynamic valgus

Abbreviation: RDL, Romanian deadlift.

requirements and for muscle stimulation. Aspiration of postsurgical hemarthrosis is indicated at the first postoperative visit if there is swelling that is causing increased pain, difficulty with ROM, or excessive quadriceps atrophy. All meniscal repair patients begin rehabilitation with a hinged knee brace locked in extension for sleeping and ambulation. Crutches should be used until the patients is able to WBAT without pain or antalgic gait. The brace is removed for hygiene and for ROM exercises. The purpose of the hinged knee brace is 3-fold. First, it provides rotational control of the patient's extremity; this is important because most acute meniscal injuries occur as the result of combined rotational and flexion forces.[65] Second, it allows early protected weight bearing despite relative quadriceps weakness caused by pain, effusion, and shutdown. Third, as quadriceps activation returns, the brace can be set to only permit flexion to a specific degree, further protecting the meniscus repair from deep-flexion weight bearing.

Stable tear patterns (ie, vertical longitudinal, bucket handle, horizontal) are typically allowed to WBAT in a hinged knee brace locked in extension for the first 4 weeks.[23,25] The brace can be unlocked to allow full flexion with adequate quadriceps control after that time, and discontinued no sooner than 6 weeks postoperatively. Complex meniscus repairs, including radial, root, and flap tears, with poor tissue quality are protected with foot-flat 0% weight bearing for 4 weeks in a hinged knee brace locked in extension. These patients can typically progress to WBAT in the hinged brace after 4 weeks. The brace can be unlocked to 90° with quadriceps control, typically by 6 weeks postoperatively, and discontinued shortly thereafter.

Patients should begin early ROM shortly after surgery. In general, ROM is either gravity assisted using the nonoperative limb in the seated position or with a CPM machine. ROM exercises can be performed without the hinged knee brace in a protected environment. However, the brace should be reapplied for sleeping, ambulation, and any other transfers until adequate quadriceps control is attained. In general, there are no restrictions on non–weight-bearing ROM following meniscus repair. The goal

Table 3
Meniscus rehabilitation protocol, phase III

	Phase III: Minimal Protection Phase (Linear)
Frequency	Rehabilitation appointments continue 1–3 times per week
Rehabilitation Goals	• Maintain full knee ROM • Restore normal weight-bearing kinematics • Restore stability during single-limb activities • Restore proprioception of the lower limb • Restore normal running gait • Return to work/heavy labor (eg, construction) • Return to competitive cycling, recreational sports (tennis, racquetball, skiing, jogging 5 times per week)
Precautions	• No pivoting, cutting activities • No plyometrics

Therapeutic Exercises	• Strength/endurance (continue phase II exercises with progressions to the following)
	  ○ Quadriceps
	    ■ Split squat/lunge
	    ■ Lateral step-down
	    ■ Single-leg squat
	    ■ Squat progression (including beyond 75° as indicated)
	  ○ Hamstrings/gluteals
	    ■ Single-leg RDL
	  ○ Integrated
	    ■ Lateral/posterior kinetic chain strengthening
	• Multiplanar balance/stability training
	  ○ Push/pull
	  ○ Controlled rotational
	  ○ Uneven/unstable surface progression
	• Low-velocity, low-amplitude agility drills
	  ○ Forward/backward skipping
	  ○ Side shuffle
	  ○ Skaters/carioca/crossovers
	  ○ Forward/backward jog
	  ○ Shallow double-limb jump landings
	• Integrated dual-task activities
	  ○ Cognitive
	  ○ Visual
	  ○ Balance

Cardiovascular Exercises	• Swimming (all strokes, pain free) • Stationary biking with resistance • Elliptical trainer with moderate resistance • Treadmill/walking (incline/decline) • Jogging/deep water running (linear only, no cutting/pivoting/hopping) • Stair stepper

Requirements for Progression	• <2 out of 10 pain with weight-bearing exercise
	• Cleared to hop/run/jog per physician discretion (not before 3 mo for reconstruction/repair, or 6 wk for arthroscopy or nonoperative knee injury)
	• Good single-leg balance without dynamic valgus
	• Normal jogging gait pattern
	• Modified return-to-sport testing
	  ○ Isokinetic testing
	    ■ ≥75% quadriceps/quadriceps strength
	    ■ ≥75% hamstring/hamstring strength
	• Lateral step-down: no more than trace dynamic valgus

Table 4
Meniscus rehabilitation protocol, phase IV

Phase IV: Return to Activity Phase (High Impact)		
Frequency	Rehabilitation appointments continue 1–2 times per week	
Rehabilitation Goals	• Progression through running/agility interval program • Normal double-leg and single-leg landing control without side-to-side differences or compensations • Return to recreational contact sports • Return to competitive/elite sports (soccer, football, rugby, wrestling, gymnastics, hockey, basketball, track and field events, running)	
Precautions	• No pain allowed during any strength or plyometric activity • Soreness lasting >24 h requires 1 d of rest, repeat last routine at next training day	

Therapeutic Exercises	• Strength/endurance (continued from phase III with inclusion of the following)
	  ○ Deadlift
	  ○ Squat
	  ○ Dynamic posterior kinetic chain progression
	  ○ Hip strengthening (prevention of hip adduction at landing and stance)
	• Plyometrics/agility/jumping progression
	  ○ Double limb to single limb
	  ○ Uniplanar to multiplanar
	  ○ Hopping to plyometric progression (emphasize appropriate mechanics with landing)
	  ○ Skipping/side shuffle/skaters/carioca/crossovers/agility ladder
	• Power
	  ○ Higher amplitude double-leg and single-leg landing drills
	  ○ Uniplanar to multiplanar
	• Neuromuscular Reeducation
	  ○ Unanticipated movement control drills, cutting/pivoting
	  ○ Balance and proprioceptive drills
	• Core strength and stabilization (prevent frontal plane trunk lean during landing and single-leg stance)
	• Sport-specific training	

Cardiovascular Exercises	• Interval running program • Swimming • Biking • Elliptical/stair climber • Row machine	

Requirements for Return to Sport	• 0 out of 10 pain with all activity
	• ACL-RSI Questionnaire ≥65%
	• No active effusion (negative brush test)
	• Quadriceps girth within 1.5 cm bilaterally
	• Return-to-sport testing
	  ○ ROM equal or within 2° of contralateral limb
	  ○ Isokinetic testing
	    ■ ≥90% quadriceps/quadriceps ratio
	    ■ ≥90% hamstring/hamstring ratio
	    ■ ≥66% hamstring/quadriceps ratio
	  ○ Y balance testing
	    ■ Anterior reach within 4 cm bilaterally
	    ■ Composite score ≥90% bilaterally
	  ○ Lateral step-down (no dynamic valgus)
	  ○ Hop testing (≥90% contralateral limb)
	    ■ 5-0-5 test
	    ■ Single hop
	    ■ Triple hop
	    ■ Triple crossover hop
	    ■ 6 m hop	

is gravity-assisted ROM at or past 90° by 4 weeks and 120° by 6 weeks. In the case of tenuous repair or poor tissue quality, ROM may be held for 1 to 2 weeks at minimal increased risk of postsurgical stiffness. Weight-bearing ROM is not initiated until after 4 weeks for stable patterns and after 6 weeks for complex tears. As discussed earlier, deep squatting past 90° is limited for 3 months following meniscus repair to reduce risk of undue stress on the repair site in deeper flexion.[23,25,66,67]

Early focus is on edema control, patella mobilization, regaining full terminal passive extension or hyperextension (hamstring stretching), foot/ankle pumps, calf stretching, and quadriceps isometrics. Progression of quadriceps activation from isometrics to short-arc quadriceps to straight leg raise should be implemented in the immediate postoperative period without any detrimental effects on meniscal healing. Early quadriceps activation can help minimize effusion, allow an earlier return to weight bearing, and potentially lead to better overall functional outcomes.[68,69] As previously stated, BFR therapy can be used during the period of protection to maximize quadriceps return without compromising the integrity of the repair construct. Core stabilization and hip strengthening exercises are also safely implemented in phase I.

Phase II, Low Impact; and Phase III, Linear

Criteria to progress into phase II (see **Table 2**) include full active knee extension, normal gait, no effusion, normal patella mobility, and ability to complete 20 straight leg raises without extensor lag. Patients should be able to WBAT without an assist device in this phase. A compression sleeve or unloader brace may be used, as indicated. As discussed earlier, the timing of progression into this phase is variable and dependent on the type of tear, quality of the repair, and functional progression of the individual patient. For example, patients should not progress past painful effusion or terminal extension ROM loss just because they have passed time criteria. Advancing weight bearing under these conditions creates a vicious feedback cycle that increases the risk of worsening pain and swelling. This cycle exacerbates the lack of quadriceps control and the inability to achieve full knee extension. Most stable tear patterns enter phase II by 6 weeks. Unstable patterns may take 6 to 8 weeks or longer to initiate phase II rehabilitation. Certain patients achieve knee homeostasis (ie, no effusion, full ROM) sooner than others and thus are able to pass through each phase more quickly.

The length of phases II to IV is highly variable and not as time dependent as the phase I period of protection. In the later phases of rehabilitation, patients progress at their own pace from one phase to the next based on performance measures. Emphasizing a time-dependent rehabilitation protocol is counterproductive and potentially harmful to the repaired meniscus because the patient may not have adequate ROM, strength, or proprioceptive control to progress to the next phase.

Phase II of the rehabilitation process emphasizes neutral spine, core stabilization, posterior chain strengthening (hamstring, gluteus, gastrocnemius), and double-limb/single-limb closed chain activities, and progression toward pain-free open chain exercises (ie, hamstring curls, weighted SLR), swimming, stationary bike, and elliptical. Criteria for progression into phase III (see **Table 3**) include ability to reciprocally ascend/descend 1 flight of stairs without compensation, squat to 75° without pain or asymmetry, and single-leg stance for 30 seconds without balance loss. Phase III focuses on strength and endurance training; multiplanar balance/stability training; low-velocity, low-amplitude agility drills; and integrated dual-task activities. Patients progress on the treadmill toward jogging, deep water running, and/or use of stair stepper at this time. Consideration for initiation of linear jogging/running include lateral step-down test with no more than mild dynamic valgus (no pain) and isokinetic testing showing greater than 70% side-to-side quadriceps/quadriceps and hamstring/hamstring strength. Low-demand patients with Tegner activity goal levels of 0 to 3 may not choose to progress toward jogging/running and may return to their sedentary or medium-demand occupations during this phase, likely by 3 to 4 months after surgery. Patients with Tegner activity goals of 4 to 5 (recreational sports, competitive cycling, jogging) should complete phase III before returning to their normal activities. Return to this level of activity may take 4 to 6 months or longer. Athletes and heavier laborers progress into phase III to IV before clearing for higher-level activities and sport.

Phase IV, Return to Activity (High Impact)

Progression to phase IV (see **Table 4**) is reserved for those patients with Tegner activity goal levels of 6 to 10. Criteria for progression into this phase include pain level less than 2 for all prior activities, good single-leg balance, normal jogging pattern, lateral step-down with no pain and at most trace valgus, and isokinetic side-to-side testing greater than 80%. These criteria are important because athletes who return to play before achieving functional stability and strength are more likely to encounter a poor outcome.[70] The final phase of the rehabilitation process builds on prior phases and focuses on functional strength/endurance, plyometrics/agility, power, neuromuscular reeducation, and sport-specific training.

Patients undergo return-to-play functional evaluation (**Box 1**) at the completion of phase IV. This evaluation includes subjective outcome scores and confidence measures (ie, ACL–Return to Sport after Injury Scale questionnaire) and a battery of objective functional tests supervised by an independent athletic trainer or physical therapist objective testing. The athlete should have a visual analog scale of 0 to 2 with all activities without the presence of an effusion. Furthermore, quadriceps girth of the repaired extremity should be within 1.5 cm of the noninjured extremity. During the return-to-sport testing, ROM must be within 2° of the contralateral extremity. Isokinetic testing must also reveal a quadriceps/quadriceps and hamstring/hamstring ratio of at least 90%. The hamstring/quadriceps ratio should be at least 66%. Y balance testing is performed and the athlete must have an anterior reach within 4 cm bilaterally and a composite score of at least 90% bilaterally. Lateral step-down and automated drop vertical jump test should show no evidence of dynamic valgus, asymmetry, or pain. Triple-hop tests should be greater than 90% of the opposite limb. Ultimately, the benefit of this approach is that it places an objective score on the patient's performance that can be followed over time to evaluate the appropriate timing for clearance to return to play.

Box 1
Return-to-sport functional evaluation

Subjective assessment

1. SANE score: if 100% is normal, what percentage of normal is your knee?
   a. A score less than 90% indicates evaluation failure

2. Baseline visual analog scale (VAS): please rate your baseline pain on a scale from 0 to 10, with 0 being no pain and 10 being the worst imaginable pain
   a. A score of 2 out of 10 or greater on any of the physical assessments below indicates evaluation failure

3. ACL–Return to Sport after Injury Scale questionnaire: a psychological and functional readiness test (a score of <65 indicates evaluation failure)

Physical assessment

1. Full knee motion compared with other side
   a. Loss of knee extension by more than 2° indicates evaluation failure

2. No or trace effusion using modified brush test

3. Less than 1 cm difference in quadriceps girth at 15 cm above joint line

4. Biodex strength testing: Biodex testing is performed for 5 repetitions at 90°/s, 10 repetitions at 180°, and 15 repetitions at 300°/s
   a. Less than 90% average of all 3 testing speeds for quadriceps/quadriceps and hamstring/hamstring ratios or less than 66% average of all 3 testing speeds for hamstring/quadriceps ratios indicates evaluation failure

5. Assessment of single-leg step-down on 20-cm (8-inch) step for 3 repetitions
   a. Pain reported greater than 2 out of 10 and/or balance loss and more than mild dynamic knee valgus indicates evaluation failure

6. Y balance test
   a. Composite reach of at least 90% of leg length
   b. Difference of uninvolved to involved anterior reach length of 4 cm or less

7. Kinect-drop jump test (measure knee/ankle separation ratio for 3 trials)
   a. An average of less than 0.65 knee ankle separation at initial contact or pain greater than 2 out of 10 indicates evaluation failure

8. Single-leg hop tests (3 trials each test per leg)
   a. Single-leg hop for distance
   b. Triple hop for distance
   c. Crossover triple hop for distance
   d. Meter timed hop test
   e. Less than 90% average of all 4 hop tests involved to uninvolved or VAS pain greater than 2 out of 10 indicates evaluation failure

However, there are no well-established guidelines in the meniscal repair literature guiding return to play.[71] Most of the recommendations discussed earlier have evolved from the literature following ACL reconstruction. Following clearance to return, athletes should progress from individual and noncontact drills to contact drills, team practice, and eventually full game play. During this progression, the athletes should be able to perform sport-specific tasks with adequate strength, speed, and coordination in the noncompetition environment before being fully released to sport. It is important to counsel the patients on the potential risk of reinjury and to emphasize the importance of a maintenance advanced functional training program to be performed on a regular basis. These programs allow the athletes to build on the gains they have made since surgery and, it is hoped, to prevent a recurrent meniscus tear or ligamentous injury to the same or contralateral extremity.[72]

Ultimately, time to return to play is highly variable and based on patient-specific and sport-specific factors in addition to the type of meniscus repair that was performed. In general, patients with noncomplex meniscus tears and low-risk sports (ie, running, cycling, swimming) may be able to return to sport as early as 3 to 4 months, provided they meet the necessary criteria and pass the return-to-play functional evaluation. Alternatively, patients with complex meniscal tears who play high-risk sports (ie, soccer, basketball, football) may not be able to return to sport until 6 to 8 months. Again, the emphasis on return to play is not time dependent; it is predicated on the patient's ability to perform sport-specific tasks with solid neuromuscular and proprioceptive control as well as sufficient speed and strength.

Table 5
Outcomes and return to sport following meniscal repair

Study	N	Technique	Follow-up	RTS (%)	Time to RTS (Isolated Meniscus)
Logan et al,[74] 2009	42 (45 repairs)	Inside out	8.5 y	81	5.6 mo (isolated repairs)
Stein et al,[76] 2010	26	Inside out	8.8 y	94.4	Not listed
Vanderhave et al,[75] 2011	45 (49 knees)	Inside out	27 mo	88.9	5.56 mo (isolated repairs)
Hirtler et al,[77] 2015	37	All inside	24.7 wk	100	27 wk
Tucciarone et al,[78] 2012	20	All inside	24 mo	90	Not listed
Alvarez-Diaz et al,[73] 2016	29	All inside	6 y	89.6	4.3 mo

Abbreviation: RTS, return to sport.

OUTCOMES FOLLOWING MENISCAL REPAIR AND RETURN TO PLAY

Outcomes of meniscal repair and return-to-sport data are summarized in **Table 5**. Overall, patients typically experience high levels of success following meniscal repair. Most studies report a mean return to play in the range of 4 to 6 months; however, complex tears may require more time for return.[73–75] Eberbach and colleagues[72] performed a systemic review of 28 studies and found that mixed-level athletes returned to their preinjury levels of sport in 90% of cases, whereas professional athletes returned in 86% of cases. Willinger and colleagues[71] recently presented the results of a study that included young athletes with traumatic meniscus tears treated with arthroscopic repair. The 30 patients included in this study underwent MRI at the following time points: preoperatively and 6, 12, and 26 weeks after surgery. By the final study visit at 6 months, 100% of participants had returned to sport but only 44.8% had returned to their preinjury level of sport. Note that, despite this high level of return to activity, only 55.9% of those included in the study showed complete healing on MRI. Although most patients experience good outcomes and return to sport within 6 months, in most cases the meniscus is still healing during this period. These findings further reinforce the importance of counseling patients on the potential risk of reinjury and possibility of future surgical intervention.

SUMMARY

Given the critically important role of the knee menisci, there has been a growing trend toward meniscal preservation. Along with improvements in meniscal repair techniques and technology, there have been similar advances in concepts surrounding meniscal repair rehabilitation and return to play. Rehabilitation and return-to-sport considerations following meniscal repair are multifactorial and must be patient specific. Biomechanical and clinical data support the use of accelerated rehabilitation protocols for vertical longitudinal and horizontal cleavage tear patterns treated with stable fixation. Caution is needed when considering accelerated rehabilitation for radial, root, and complex meniscal repairs. BFRT is an innovative way to promote muscle hypertrophy without increased stress at the repair site. However, there remains a paucity of data specific to meniscus repair. There are few established guidelines or clear criteria to guide return to play following meniscal repair. Using best-evidence time-based and criteria-based progression allows safe and successful return to play in most cases.

REFERENCES

1. Shimomura K, Hamamoto S, Hart DA, et al. Meniscal repair and regeneration: current strategies and future perspectives. J Clin Orthop Trauma 2018;9(3): 247–53.
2. Cavanaugh JT. Rehabilitation of meniscal injury and surgery. J Knee Surg 2014; 27(6):459–78.
3. Blake MH, Johnson DL. Knee meniscus injuries: common problems and solutions. Clin Sports Med 2018;37(2):293–306.
4. Koenig JH, Ranawat AS, Umans HR, et al. Meniscal root tears: diagnosis and treatment. Arthroscopy 2009;25(9):1025–32.
5. Kopf S, Colvin AC, Muriuki M, et al. Meniscal root suturing techniques: implications for root fixation. Am J Sports Med 2011;39(10):2141–6.
6. Kim JG, Lee YS, Bae TS, et al. Tibiofemoral contact mechanics following posterior root of medial meniscus tear, repair, meniscectomy, and allograft transplantation. Knee Surg Sports Traumatol Arthrosc 2013;21(9):2121–5.
7. Thorlund JB, Holsgaard-Larsen A, Creaby MW, et al. Changes in knee joint load indices from before to 12 months after arthroscopic partial meniscectomy: a prospective cohort study. Osteoarthritis Cartilage 2016;24(7):1153–9.
8. Bedi A, Kelly NH, Baad M, et al. Dynamic contact mechanics of the medial meniscus as a function of radial tear, repair, and partial meniscectomy. J Bone Joint Surg Am 2010;92(6):1398–408.
9. Abrams GD, Frank RM, Gupta AK, et al. Trends in meniscus repair and meniscectomy in the United States, 2005-2011. Am J Sports Med 2013;41(10):2333–9.
10. Cox JS, Nye CE, Schaefer WW, et al. The degenerative effects of partial and total resection of the medial meniscus in dogs' knees. Clin Orthop Relat Res 1975;(109):178–83.
11. Fairbank JC, Pynsent PB, van Poortvliet JA, et al. Mechanical factors in the incidence of knee pain in adolescents and young adults. J Bone Joint Surg Br 1984; 66(5):685–93.
12. Lee SJ, Aadalen KJ, Malaviya P, et al. Tibiofemoral contact mechanics after serial medial meniscectomies in the human cadaveric knee. Am J Sports Med 2006; 34(8):1334–44.
13. Harner CD, Mauro CS, Lesniak BP, et al. Biomechanical consequences of a tear of the posterior root of the medial meniscus. Surgical technique. J Bone Joint Surg Am 2009;91(Suppl 2):257–70.
14. LaPrade CM, Jansson KS, Dornan G, et al. Altered tibiofemoral contact mechanics due to lateral meniscus posterior horn root avulsions and radial tears can be restored with in situ pull-out suture repairs. J Bone Joint Surg Am 2014; 96(6):471–9.
15. Woodmass JM, Johnson JD, Wu IT, et al. Horizontal cleavage meniscus tear treated with all-inside circumferential compression stitches. Arthrosc Tech 2017;6(4):e1329–33.
16. Saliman JD. The circumferential compression stitch for meniscus repair. Arthrosc Tech 2013;2(3):e257–64.
17. Brooks KR. Vertical lasso and horizontal lasso sutures for repair of horizontal cleavage and horizontal oblique meniscal tears: surgical technique and indications. Arthrosc Tech 2017;6(5):e1767–73.
18. Fillingham YA, Riboh JC, Erickson BJ, et al. Inside-out versus all-inside repair of isolated meniscal tears: an updated systematic review. Am J Sports Med 2017; 45(1):234–42.

19. Samuelsen BT, Johnson NR, Hevesi M, et al. Comparative outcomes of all-inside versus inside-out repair of bucket-handle meniscal tears: a propensity-matched analysis. Orthop J Sports Med 2018;6(6). 2325967118779045.

20. Kang DG, Park YJ, Yu JH, et al. A systematic review and meta-analysis of arthroscopic meniscus repair in young patients: comparison of all-inside and inside-out suture techniques. Knee Surg Relat Res 2019;31(1):1–11.

21. Elmallah R, Jones LC, Malloch L, et al. A meta-analysis of arthroscopic meniscal repair: inside-out versus outside-in versus all-inside techniques. J Knee Surg 2019;32(8):750–7.

22. O'Donnell K, Freedman KB, Tjoumakaris FP. Rehabilitation protocols after isolated meniscal repair: a systematic review. Am J Sports Med 2017;45(7): 1687–97.

23. Lind M, Nielsen T, Fauno P, et al. Free rehabilitation is safe after isolated meniscus repair: a prospective randomized trial comparing free with restricted rehabilitation regimens. Am J Sports Med 2013;41(12):2753–8.

24. Perkins B, Gronbeck KR, Yue RA, et al. Similar failure rate in immediate postoperative weight bearing versus protected weight bearing following meniscal repair on peripheral, vertical meniscal tears. Knee Surg Sports Traumatol Arthrosc 2018;26(8):2245–50.

25. VanderHave KL, Perkins C, Le M. Weightbearing versus nonweightbearing after meniscus repair. Sports Health 2015;7(5):399–402.

26. Richards DP, Barber FA, Herbert MA. Compressive loads in longitudinal lateral meniscus tears: a biomechanical study in porcine knees. Arthroscopy 2005; 21(12):1452–6.

27. Starke C, Kopf S, Lippisch R, et al. Tensile forces on repaired medial meniscal root tears. Arthroscopy 2013;29(2):205–12.

28. Suganuma J, Mochizuki R, Yamaguchi K, et al. Cam impingement of the posterior femoral condyle in medial meniscal tears. Arthroscopy 2010;26(2):173–83.

29. Kocabey Y, Nyland J, Isbell WM, et al. Patient outcomes following T-Fix meniscal repair and a modifiable, progressive rehabilitation program, a retrospective study. Arch Orthop Trauma Surg 2004;124(9):592–6.

30. Spang RC Iii, Nasr MC, Mohamadi A, et al. Rehabilitation following meniscal repair: a systematic review. BMJ Open Sport Exerc Med 2018;4(1):e000212.

31. LaPrade CM, Foad A, Smith SD, et al. Biomechanical consequences of a nonanatomic posterior medial meniscal root repair. Am J Sports Med 2015;43(4): 912–20.

32. Barber FA. Accelerated rehabilitation for meniscus repairs. Arthroscopy 1994; 10(2):206–10.

33. Starke C, Kopf S, Grobel KH, et al. Tensile forces at the porcine anterior meniscal horn attachment. J Orthop Res 2009;27(12):1619–24.

34. Abraham AC, Villegas DF, Kaufman KR, et al. Internal pressure of human meniscal root attachments during loading. J Orthop Res 2013;31(10):1507–13.

35. Habata T, Ishimura M, Ohgushi H, et al. Axial alignment of the lower limb in patients with isolated meniscal tear. J Orthop Sci 1998;3(2):85–9.

36. Kalra M, Bakker R, Tomescu SS, et al. The effect of unloader knee braces on medial meniscal strain. Prosthet Orthot Int 2018;43(2):132–9.

37. Tomescu S, Bakker R, Wasserstein D, et al. Dynamically tensioned ACL functional knee braces reduce ACL and meniscal strain. Knee Surg Sports Traumatol Arthrosc 2018;26(2):526–33.

38. Dowdy PA, Miniaci A, Arnoczky SP, et al. The effect of cast immobilization on meniscal healing. An experimental study in the dog. Am J Sports Med 1995;23(6): 721–8.

39. de Albornoz PM, Forriol F. The meniscal healing process. Muscles Ligaments Tendons J 2012;2(1):10–8.

40. Guisasola I, Vaquero J, Forriol F. Knee immobilization on meniscal healing after suture: an experimental study in sheep. Clin Orthop Relat Res 2002;(395): 227–33.

41. Zhang ZN, Tu KY, Xu YK, et al. Treatment of longitudinal injuries in avascular area of meniscus in dogs by trephination. Arthroscopy 1988;4(3):151–9.

42. Becker R, Wirz D, Wolf C, et al. Measurement of meniscofemoral contact pressure after repair of bucket-handle tears with biodegradable implants. Arch Orthop Trauma Surg 2005;125(4):254–60.

43. Flanigan DC, Lin F, Koh JL, et al. Articular contact pressures of meniscal repair techniques at various knee flexion angles. Orthopedics 2010;33(7):475.

44. Lin DL, Ruh SS, Jones HL, et al. Does high knee flexion cause separation of meniscal repairs? Am J Sports Med 2013;41(9):2143–50.

45. Marchetti DC, Phelps BM, Dahl KD, et al. A contact pressure analysis comparing an all-inside and inside-out surgical repair technique for bucket-handle medial meniscus tears. Arthroscopy 2017;33(10):1840–8.

46. Volpe EP, Turpen JB. Thymus: primary site of lymphopoiesis. Ann Immunol (Paris) 1976;127(6):833–40.

47. Howard JS, Mattacola CG, Romine SE, et al. Continuous passive motion, early weight bearing, and active motion following knee articular cartilage repair: evidence for clinical practice. Cartilage 2010;1(4):276–86.

48. Fazalare JA, Griesser MJ, Siston RA, et al. The use of continuous passive motion following knee cartilage defect surgery: a systematic review. Orthopedics 2010; 33(12):878.

49. Fox AJ, Bedi A, Rodeo SA. The basic science of human knee menisci: structure, composition, and function. Sports Health 2012;4(4):340–51.

50. Walker PS, Erkman MJ. The role of the menisci in force transmission across the knee. Clin Orthop Relat Res 1975;(109):184–92.

51. Brantigan OC, Voshell AF. The mechanics of the ligaments and menisci of the knee joint. J Bone Joint Surg Am 1941;23(1):44–66.

52. Akima H, Furukawa T. Atrophy of thigh muscles after meniscal lesions and arthroscopic partial menisectomy. Knee Surg Sports Traumatol Arthrosc 2005;13(8): 632–7.

53. Hassan AA, el-Sewedy SM, Minatogawa Y, et al. In vitro effect of dimethoate on the activity of tryptophan pyrrolase in rat liver. J Environ Sci Health B 1991;26(3): 333–8.

54. Moffet H, Richards CL, Malouin F, et al. Impact of knee extensor strength deficits on stair ascent performance in patients after medial menisectomy. Scand J Rehabil Med 1993;25(2):63–71.

55. Palmieri-Smith RM, Villwock M, Downie B, et al. Pain and effusion and quadriceps activation and strength. J Athl Train 2013;48(2):186–91.

56. Eitzen I, Grindem H, Nilstad A, et al. Quantifying quadriceps muscle strength in patients with acl injury, focal cartilage lesions, and degenerative meniscus tears: differences and clinical implications. Orthop J Sports Med 2016;4(10). 2325967116667717.

57. Eitzen I, Eitzen TJ, Holm I, et al. Anterior cruciate ligament-deficient potential copers and noncopers reveal different isokinetic quadriceps strength profiles in the early stage after injury. Am J Sports Med 2010;38(3):586–93.

58. American College of Sports M. American College of Sports Medicine position stand. Progression models in resistance training for healthy adults. Med Sci Sports Exerc 2009;41(3):687–708.

59. Takarada Y, Takazawa H, Ishii N. Applications of vascular occlusion diminish disuse atrophy of knee extensor muscles. Med Sci Sports Exerc 2000;32(12):2035–9.

60. Day B. Personalized blood flow restriction therapy: how, when and where can it accelerate rehabilitation after surgery? Arthroscopy 2018;34(8):2511–3.

61. DePhillipo NN, Kennedy MI, Aman ZS, et al. The role of blood flow restriction therapy following knee surgery: expert opinion. Arthroscopy 2018;34(8):2506–10.

62. Takarada Y, Takazawa H, Sato Y, et al. Effects of resistance exercise combined with moderate vascular occlusion on muscular function in humans. J Appl Physiol (1985) 2000;88(6):2097–106.

63. Ohta H, Kurosawa H, Ikeda H, et al. Low-load resistance muscular training with moderate restriction of blood flow after anterior cruciate ligament reconstruction. Acta Orthop Scand 2003;74(1):62–8.

64. Loenneke JP, Wilson JM, Marin PJ, et al. Low intensity blood flow restriction training: a meta-analysis. Eur J Appl Physiol 2012;112(5):1849–59.

65. Cavanaugh JT, Killian SE. Rehabilitation following meniscal repair. Curr Rev Musculoskelet Med 2012;5(1):46–58.

66. Kozlowski EJ, Barcia AM, Tokish JM. Meniscus repair: the role of accelerated rehabilitation in return to sport. Sports Med Arthrosc Rev 2012;20(2):121–6.

67. Brelin AM, Rue JP. Return to play following meniscus surgery. Clin Sports Med 2016;35(4):669–78.

68. Stevens-Lapsley JE, Balter JE, Wolfe P, et al. Early neuromuscular electrical stimulation to improve quadriceps muscle strength after total knee arthroplasty: a randomized controlled trial. Phys Ther 2012;92(2):210–26.

69. Thomas AC, Stevens-Lapsley JE. Importance of attenuating quadriceps activation deficits after total knee arthroplasty. Exerc Sport Sci Rev 2012;40(2):95–101.

70. Myer GD, Paterno MV, Ford KR, et al. Rehabilitation after anterior cruciate ligament reconstruction: criteria-based progression through the return-to-sport phase. J Orthop Sports Phys Ther 2006;36(6):385–402.

71. Willinger L, Herbst E, Diermeier T, et al. High short-term return to sports rate despite an ongoing healing process after acute meniscus repair in young athletes. Knee Surg Sports Traumatol Arthrosc 2019;27(1):215–22.

72. Eberbach H, Zwingmann J, Hohloch L, et al. Sport-specific outcomes after isolated meniscal repair: a systematic review. Knee Surg Sports Traumatol Arthrosc 2018;26(3):762–71.

73. Alvarez-Diaz P, Alentorn-Geli E, Llobet F, et al. Return to play after all-inside meniscal repair in competitive football players: a minimum 5-year follow-up. Knee Surg Sports Traumatol Arthrosc 2016;24(6):1997–2001.

74. Logan M, Watts M, Owen J, et al. Meniscal repair in the elite athlete: results of 45 repairs with a minimum 5-year follow-up. Am J Sports Med 2009;37(6):1131–4.

75. Vanderhave KL, Moravek JE, Sekiya JK, et al. Meniscus tears in the young athlete: results of arthroscopic repair. J Pediatr Orthop 2011;31(5):496–500.

76. Stein T, Mehling AP, Welsch F, et al. Long-term outcome after arthroscopic meniscal repair versus arthroscopic partial meniscectomy for traumatic meniscal tears. Am J Sports Med 2010;38(8):1542–8.

77. Hirtler L, Unger J, Weninger P. Acute and chronic menisco-capsular separation in the young athlete: diagnosis, treatment and results in thirty seven consecutive patients. Int Orthop 2015;39(5):967–74.
78. Tucciarone A, Godente L, Fabbrini R, et al. Meniscal tear repaired with Fast-Fix sutures: clinical results in stable versus ACL-deficient knees. Arch Orthop Trauma Surg 2012;132(3):349–56.

Return to Play Following Meniscal Repair

Taylor J. Wiley, MD[a],*, Nicholas J. Lemme, MD[a,1], Stephen Marcaccio, MD[a,1], Steven Bokshan, MD[a,1], Paul D. Fadale, MD[a,1], Cory Edgar, MD, PhD[b], Brett D. Owens, MD[a,1]

KEYWORDS

- Meniscus • Repair • Return to play • Sports • Athlete

KEY POINTS

- Meniscal repair can be performed in an attempt to preserve meniscal tissue in situations whereby there is viable tissue with satisfactory healing potential, because partial or total meniscectomy has been shown to increase knee cartilage degeneration in younger athletes.
- The decision of when the athlete can RTP should become a shared decision-making process including all parties of interest, and ultimately, these decisions will be individualized to each athlete.
- Timing of return to play is dependent on many factors including the type of tear sustained, presence of concomitant injuries and the type of repair performed, postoperative rehab protocol, time of season and type of sport played.
- RTP rates following meniscal repairs in athletes are reassuring with 80% to 95% of athletes returning to play with the average RTP time being 4 to 6 months.

INTRODUCTION AND EPIDEMIOLOGY

The knee menisci are semicircular, fibrocartilaginous structures that serve several important roles in normal knee function, including load transmission, shock absorption, and secondary stabilization of the knee.[1] The vascular supply of the meniscus has been well studied, with the vascularized peripheral 30% known as the red-red zone and the relatively avascular inner aspects known as the red-white and white-white zones. Tears of the meniscus are common knee injuries in the young, athletic

Disclosure Statement: T.J. Wiley, N. Lemme, S. Marcaccio, S. Bokshan, and P.D. Fadale report no relevant disclosures. C. Edgar reports B.D. Owens reports consulting for Mitek, Conmed/MTF, and Vericel.
[a] Department of Orthopedics, Brown University, Providence, RI, USA; [b] Department of Orthopedic Surgery, UConn Health, 263 Farmington Avenue, Farmington, CT 06030, USA
[1] Present address: 1 Kettle Point Avenue, East Providence, RI 02914.
* Corresponding author. 1 Kettle Point Avenue, East Providence, RI 02914.
E-mail address: twiley@universityorthopedics.com

population and are particularly prevalent in contact and pivoting sports.[1] The overall incidence of meniscus tears requiring surgery is 60 to 70 per 100,000 person-years.[2] Ultimately, the decision to pursue surgery for a meniscus tear is complex and multifactorial. Although there may be incentive to manage these injuries without surgery for an in-season athlete, the presence of persistent pain and inability to return to a high athletic level may ultimately push toward operative management.[3]

With operative management, significant effort should be made to preserve viable meniscal tissue.[4] Isolated meniscectomy should be reserved for scenarios in which there is nonviable tissue or there is a nonsatisfactory healing potential, because this may ultimately require an additional surgery and further delay of return to play (RTP).[4] It is essential for the surgeon to manage expectations of both the patient and the athletic training staff with regard to meniscal surgery. Recent studies have shown that return to play times vary dramatically based on the surgical procedure performed and range from as little as 7 to 9 weeks with isolated meniscectomy to 5.6 months with meniscal repair.[5] Both the patient and the athletic training staff must be aware of these expected recovery times and for the potential to take a shorter or longer time depending on the specific athlete.

The authors present a review of the factors influencing RTP following meniscus repair surgery. Rehabilitation protocols following meniscus repair surgery are discussed followed by RTP timing, outcomes, and future considerations.

MENISCAL REPAIR IN THE ATHLETE

Preservation and restoration of meniscal function and normal knee kinematics are of utmost importance in athletes sustaining knee injuries. If not managed appropriately, meniscal injuries in athletes can devastate careers and may accelerate the rate of degenerative changes of the knee joint.[6] Managing meniscal injuries in athletes can be extremely difficult given the significant pressure from the athlete, coaches, parents, and athletic trainers to get the athlete back to play as soon as possible. Physicians must have a sophisticated understanding of the implications of each treatment type, the type of sports played by the athlete, the natural history of these injuries, and milestones that must be met before RTP. Understanding these principles will allow the provider to balance rapid RTP with the risk of premature return and subsequent failed repair or reinjury. The decision of when the athlete can RTP should become a shared decision-making process including all parties of interest, and ultimately, these decisions will be individualized to each athlete, depending on their circumstances.

Sports medicine physicians are performing meniscal repairs more frequently as the indications for this intervention have expanded over time and may be preferred in athletes because it restores the native anatomy of knee.[7,8] In comparison, meniscectomy raises concerns for associated increased contact forces about the tibiofemoral joint, with potentially increased pain, worse patient outcome measures, and more rapid degeneration of the knee joint when compared with meniscal repair.[9,10] Meniscal repair, however, requires more extensive rehabilitation and results in a longer time out of play.

MENISCAL REPAIR REHABILITATION

Rehabilitation protocols following meniscal repair vary widely.[11] The significant variability in rehabilitation protocols may stem from the multitude of factors contributing to meniscal healing. When developing a rehabilitation plan, tear location (peripheral vs central) and pattern (longitudinal, radial, complex) should be considered. In addition, many other factors (tear chronicity, concomitant injuries, alignment, tissue quality, surgical technique) may impact physical therapy protocols and clinical outcomes, further contributing to the heterogeneity in protocols across the literature. An individualized approach to the patient's recovery, while following general rehabilitation guidelines, should be established between the surgeon and physical therapist.[12]

Following meniscal repair, 2 general approaches to postoperative rehabilitation exist: protective versus accelerated. The more traditional protective protocols recommend non-weight-bearing while limiting knee flexion to 90° for the first 6 weeks postoperatively, with deep knee flexion avoided for 4 to 6 months.[12] Early protocols recommended immobilization in full extension for 6 weeks.[13,14]

Over time, more aggressive accelerated rehabilitation protocols allowing earlier weight-bearing and unrestricted range of motion (ROM) have been developed, challenging the dogma of the traditional protective approach.[15–17] Multiple biomechanical studies have lent support to the tenets of an accelerated rehabilitation approach. A cadaveric study by Ganley and colleagues[18] demonstrated that loading of a posteromedial meniscal tear did not significantly distort the repair, whereas a cadaveric study by Lin and colleagues[19] found that compression rather than repair gapping occurs in longitudinal posteromedial tears during knee flexion. A more recent study by McCulloch and colleagues[20] also found compressive forces across longitudinal medial meniscal tears during simulated gait. Barber[15] has shown this to be safe and effective with no difference in healing rates or patient outcomes in patients undergoing accelerated rehabilitation. Furthermore, Shelbourne and colleagues[16] demonstrated that athletes undergoing accelerated rehabilitation were able to RTP twice as fast as athletes undergoing the standardized protocol (10 weeks vs 20 weeks), without any differences in failure rates or functional performance on RTP. In addition, a metaanalysis by O'Donnell and colleagues[21] demonstrated that early ROM and immediate postoperative weight-bearing have no detrimental effects on clinical success after isolated meniscus repair.

All varieties of meniscal tears may not be amenable to an accelerated rehabilitation protocol. Radial tears present 1 example, because axial loading through complete radial tears leads to circumferential hoop stresses, which create distraction at the tear site.[22] Weight-bearing in 90° of knee flexion results in a 4-fold increase in posterior horn meniscal pressures compared with weight-bearing in full extension, lending evidence to the practice of avoiding deep knee flexion after complex pattern repairs.[23]

Rehabilitation Phases

The phases of physical therapy following meniscal repair can generally be divided into protective, restorative, and return to activity/sports preparation phases. Although 1 suggested timeline is outlined in this article, the timing should be tailored to each patient based on their progression through rehabilitation.

A typical protective phase spans the first 6 postoperative weeks and is usually the most time-driven phase of rehabilitation to allow an adequate period of meniscal healing. The early protective phase (0–3 weeks) includes a focus on pain/edema control, early patellar mobilization, maintenance of terminal knee extension, and quadriceps neuromuscular training. Peripheral longitudinal tears may be advanced from toe-touch weight-bearing in extension to full weight-bearing in extension over the first 6 weeks, whereas more complex or radial repairs may be held at partial weight-bearing longer. For simple peripheral repairs, ROM may progress rapidly through goals of 0° to 90° by the end of week 1 to 0° to 135° by week 4. ROMprogression is slower for complex posterior tears, limiting flexion to 70° up to week 3, 90° at week

4, and 120° at week 5. Hamstring strengthening should be avoided because of the posterior attachments of the semimembranosus and popliteus to the medial and lateral menisci, respectively. A normalized gait pattern free of bracing is the goal at 6 weeks.[12]

Criteria for progression to the restorative phase of rehabilitation include full passive ROM, no effusion, and neuromuscular control of the quadriceps. The typical timeframe of this phase includes weeks 6 to 12 postoperatively. The focus of the restoration phase is closed kinetic chain strengthening, including squatting above 90° flexion, lunges, and step-ups. Hamstring strengthening can be initiated in this phase. Another key component of the restoration phase is proprioceptive and single leg balance training.[12]

At approximately 12 to 16 weeks, a return to activity phase of rehabilitation begins once the patient demonstrates full active ROM and adequate single leg dynamic knee control. The focus during return to activity is increasing neuromuscular control and building strength, with isokinetic exercises permitted. A graduated return to jogging is typically permitted for peripheral tears during this phase once the patient has appropriate strength, has good frontal and sagittal plane control, and performs low-level agility exercises without pain. In complex repairs, surgeons may choose to refrain from a return to jogging program for 16 to 24 weeks at their discretion.[12]

Kozlowski and colleagues[24] described a return to sport rehabilitation program following the basic therapy principles of progression from low to high loads, slow to fast motions, stable to unstable platforms, uniplanar to multiplanar motions, and concentrating to distracted performances. The investigators provided a set of baseline criteria for initiation of the return to sport phase, which included absence of effusion, full active ROM, 70% operative leg strength versus contralateral, and Lysholm and SANE subjective scores greater than 75 points.

RETURN TO PLAY

It is important that the athlete be appropriately counseled preoperatively regarding the extensive rehabilitation period to manage the athlete's expectations regarding time to RTP. Although no evidence-based definitive RTP criteria have been established, certain principles can be followed (**Box 1**). Allowing the athlete to RTP should be an informed, shared decision between the physician, the athlete, and the athletic trainer or physical therapist supervising the athlete's rehabilitation. The athlete should be assessed for full, symmetric, pain-free ROM at the knee, with no obvious strength discrepancies, including ability to perform single leg squat. The athlete's psychological readiness to RTP should also be considered. Coordination with the athletic trainer

---

Box 1
Return-to-play criteria

- Full, painless knee ROM that is symmetric to the uninjured limb
- No reactive effusions with sport-specific activities
- Return of normalized running mechanics
- Appropriate neuromuscular coordination demonstrated by the ability to perform regular and single leg jumps, agility ladder drills, lateral hops, and change in direction/cutting drills
- Greater than 90% of strength regained for knee extension, flexion, and single-leg press
- Psychologically ready for return demonstrated by lack of apprehension with sport-specific activities

or physical therapist supervising the athlete's rehabilitation protocol helps ensure the athlete is able to perform sport-specific activities without apprehension. Finally, the athlete must demonstrate normal running mechanics and sufficient neuromuscular control when performing dynamic sport-specific activities before returning to play. The authors do not currently recommend using repeat imaging or second-look arthroscopy to evaluate healing to determine if a player is ready to RTP. Studies have demonstrated that the use of MRI is limited, because it is difficult to determine the degree of healing, and incomplete healing may not be correlated with a decrease in function or an increased risk of retear.[25,26] Willinger and colleagues[27] demonstrated reassuring RTP rates in 30 athletes despite incomplete healing in 56% of menisci 6 months after meniscal repair. Despite incomplete healing, 100% of the athletes were able to RTP without functional impairments. Although second-look arthroscopy may be indicated if one is concerned with reinjury or persistent pain, it is not recommended in an asymptomatic athlete because of the potential risks and costs.[28–30]

RETURN-TO-PLAY CONSIDERATIONS

Several factors may influence healing and increase the risk of reinjury following meniscal repair. These factors include tear type, rim width/zone of tear, medial versus lateral meniscus tear, and the presence of concomitant injuries.[31–36] Although there is a paucity of data showing how these tear characteristics affect RTP and performance, it is important to consider them when discussing RTP with athletes and managing their expectations regarding risk of failure and the possible need for further procedures down the road. In a study of isolated arthroscopic meniscal repair in patients less than 18 years old, Krych and colleagues[33] observed significant differences in rim width and tear complexity among successfully repaired menisci and failed repairs, with tears having rim widths greater than 3 mm being significantly more likely to fail. Complex tears and bucket-handle tears were more likely to fail compared with simple tears, with each accounting for 41% of all failures. Regarding isolated medial versus lateral meniscus repair, the data regarding the relative risk of failure are conflicting. Lyman and colleagues[34] retrospectively reviewed 9529 patients who had a meniscal repair over a 7-year study period and demonstrated a decreased risk of failure requiring subsequent meniscectomy for lateral meniscal repair compared with medial. Conversely, Tuckman and colleagues[37] demonstrated repairs of the medial meniscus to have a 20.3% failure rate compared with 44.8% in the lateral meniscus. Such conflicting data likely suggest that no significant difference exist; however, further research elucidating any difference is needed.

Concomitant meniscal injuries in the presence of acute anterior cruciate ligament (ACL) rupture is extremely common with studies demonstrating up to 80% ACL ruptures to have associated meniscal tears.[32,38,39] The current standard of care in the active population is to repair these injuries simultaneously. Biomechanical data have demonstrated the forces about the meniscus to increase up to 200% in the ACL deficient knee, suggesting an increased rate of failure following meniscal repair in an ACL deficient knee.[40] Studies to date have supported this finding, demonstrating decreased rates of failure following meniscal repair if performed simultaneously with ACL reconstruction (ACLR).[35,36,41–43] In a matched-cohort population study, Wasserstein and colleagues[36] compared the need for reoperation in a total of 1332 patients with isolated meniscal tears undergoing meniscal repair only versus those with concomitant ACL injuries undergoing simultaneous meniscal repair and ACL. The investigators demonstrated a 42% relative risk reduction of reoperation in those undergoing simultaneous ACLR and meniscal repair versus patients undergoing meniscal repair alone. There have been multiple hypotheses for these observed differences, including possible biological augmentation secondary to bone marrow stimulation at the time of bony tunnel drilling, similar to microfracture techniques.[44] In athletes with these concomitant injuries, it is important to counsel the athlete to expect longer times to RTP than those with isolated meniscus injury, and this delayed return may contribute to improved meniscal healing rates. A recent systematic review showed a mean RTP at 5.6 months for isolated meniscal repair versus 11.8 months in athletes requiring concurrent ACLR.[5]

MENISCAL REPAIR OUTCOMES

Meniscal repair can be performed in an attempt to preserve meniscal tissue in situations whereby there is viable tissue with satisfactory healing potential, because partial or total meniscectomy has been shown to increase knee cartilage degeneration in younger athletes.[45,46] Multiple repair techniques exist, including the inside-out, all-inside, and open repair, with the inside out technique remaining the gold standard for repair.[47] Logan and colleagues[48] evaluated 42 elite athletes who underwent meniscal repairs using an inside-out technique and reported that 81% of patients returned to their main sport at a similar level at a mean time of 10.4 months. This timing reflects the fact that there was a high level of concomitant ACLR within this study population. This study also demonstrated an overall failure rate of 24%, with the vast majority being from medial meniscus repair.[48] Alvarez-Diaz and colleagues[47] evaluated 29 elite athletes who underwent meniscal repair (14 meniscal repair alone, 15 with associated ACLR) using an all-inside technique, reporting that 89.6% returned to the same level of sport, and those who underwent a meniscal repair alone returned at a mean time of 4.3 months, with a 6.7% failure rate. Tucciarone and colleagues[49] evaluated 20 patients with isolated meniscal tears who underwent an all-inside repair, reporting 90% return to sport at 2-year follow-up. Meniscal repair can provide excellent results for athletes with goals of returning to sport; however, the physician must set appropriate expectations with the patient regarding recovery time and postoperative rehabilitation.

MENISCAL REPAIR VERSUS PARTIAL MENISCECTOMY

In comparison to meniscal repair, isolated meniscectomy has been performed in situations whereby there is nonviable meniscal tissue or nonsatisfactory healing potential. Nawabi and colleagues[50] evaluated 90 elite soccer players who underwent isolated partial lateral or medial meniscectomy and reported that 100% of patients returned to previous level of sport at an average of 5 to 7 weeks, but noted that the time for return to sport was significantly longer in patients undergoing partial lateral meniscectomy when compared with those undergoing medial meniscectomy (7 weeks vs 5 weeks, $P<.01$). Furthermore, it should be noted that 69% of players who underwent partial lateral meniscectomy experienced adverse events, including persistent effusions and lateral joint line pain, in comparison to only 8% of these events experienced in the medial meniscectomy group.[50] Furthermore, 7% of the partial lateral meniscectomy patients required subsequent arthroscopic surgery, whereas no patients in the partial medial meniscectomy group required further intervention. Kim and colleagues[10] evaluated 56 athletes who underwent partial lateral or medial meniscectomy and reported a significantly faster return to sport in those undergoing partial lateral meniscectomy (61 vs 79 days, $P = .017$). Osti and colleagues[51] evaluated 41 athletes who underwent isolated partial lateral meniscectomy and reported 98% return to sport at a mean time of 55 days, with elite athletes averaging a shorter return to sport time than recreational athletes. Athletes should be counseled that partial meniscectomy can provide an opportunity for more rapid return to sport than meniscal repair, but there is significant risk of future cartilage degeneration.[52]

COMPLICATIONS

Although the results of both partial meniscectomy and meniscal repair are consistently good to excellent, complication rates can vary based on treatment type and level of athlete. Complications include significant knee pain that delays RTP, failure of meniscal repair that requires reoperation, or failure of meniscal repair or partial meniscectomy requiring further meniscal excision. In a systematic review, Eberbach and colleagues[53] evaluated sport-specific outcomes after meniscal repair in patients ranging from recreational athletes to professional athletes. In their review of 27 studies and 637 patients, the pooled failure rate was 21%; however, there was a significantly lower failure rate among professional athletes when compared with mixed-level athletes (9% vs 22%, respectively). Although partial meniscectomy generally produces good to excellent results with low complication rates, several studies have reported persistent knee pain requiring athletes to decrease their activity level.[9,54–56] Furthermore, rapid chondrolysis has been reported after partial lateral meniscectomy in active patients, a rare but serious complication that can severely debilitate athletes with goals of returning to sport.[57] Although rare, physicians must counsel their patients about the possible complications of sustained debilitating knee pain and the potential necessity of reoperation, regardless of surgical treatment.

CONTROVERSIES

Meniscal injuries in young and athletically active patients present a challenge in terms of treatment, rehabilitation, and return to sports. The surgeon must balance the importance of preserving meniscal tissue with the patient's needs for rapid return to sport. Paxton and colleagues[58] highlighted the importance of meniscal preservation in a systematic review that compared meniscal repair and partial meniscectomy in both short- and long-term outcomes. This study evaluated more than 1000 patients and found that although partial meniscectomy had a lower reoperation rate at short-term follow-up, patients undergoing meniscal repair recorded significantly high functional scores at long-term follow-up. These results were supported by additional systematic reviews.[59,60] Despite excellent long-term results, meniscal repair typically requires a longer rehabilitation period and is a more technically challenging procedure than partial meniscectomy; therefore, partial meniscectomy is frequently preferred by patients and surgeons to allow earlier return to sports. Furthermore, partial meniscectomy has generally demonstrated excellent short-term results with low complications rates, making this procedure attractive to athletes with short-term career goals (professional athlete at end of career).[61] Physicians must counsel their athletic patients on the role of the menisci in preservation of knee joint biomechanics, because several studies have shown that removal of meniscal tissue in patients with high functional demands can accelerate degeneration of the articular cartilage and decrease both athletic performance level and career lengths.[54,55] Therefore, it is paramount that physicians counsel patients to achieve an understanding of individual athletic goals when counseling on appropriate treatment of meniscal injury.

RETURN TO PLAY AND PERFORMANCE FOLLOWING MENISCAL REPAIR

RTP rates following meniscal repairs in athletes are reassuring with 80% to 95% of athletes returning to play (**Table 1**).[47–49,62–64] Furthermore, studies to date have

Table 1
Rates of return to play

Authors, Year	Journal	Sport	Level of Play	% RTP	Time to RTP	Performance on RTP	Additional Findings
Alvarez-Diaz et al,[47] 2016	Arthroscopy	Soccer	Professional	89.6	4.2 mo	Same level of play	
Logan et al,[48] 2009	Am J Sports Med	Not specified	Professional	81.0	5.6 mo (isolated MR), 11.8 mo (ACLR + MR)	Same level of play	83.3% w/simultaneous ACLR
Pujol et al,[63] 2013	Knee Surg Sports Traumatol Arthrosc	Not specified	Not specified	95	10 mo	Same level	
Tucciarone et al,[49] 2012	Arch Orthop Trauma Surg	Soccer, football, basketball	Professional	90	Not specified	Same level	
Vanderhave et al,[64] 2011	J Pediatr Orthop	Not specified	Not specified	89	5.56 mo (MR) vs 8.23 mo (MR + ACLR)	Same level	69% with simultaneous ACLR
Griffin et al,[62] 2015	Clin Orthop Relat Res	Not specified	Not specified	80	Not specified	Not specified	15 repairs augmented with PRP (no significant difference in RTP with PRP use)
Nakayama et al,[65] 2017	Asia Pac J Sports Med Arthrosc Rehabil Technol	Not specified	Not specified	80.4	5.5 mo (medial meniscus) vs 6.8 mo (lateral meniscus)	Not specified	

Abbreviation: PRP, platelet rich plasma.

demonstrated that athletes undergoing isolated meniscal repairs can expect to RTP around 4 to 6 months.[47–49,62–64] Understandably, athletes with concomitant ACLR should expect longer RTP times, with most studies demonstrating athletes returning to play at 8 to 12 months because the timing is limited by the ACLR.[47–49,62–64] Specific data regarding performance upon RTP are sparse. A recent metaanalysis focusing on sport-specific outcomes following meniscal repair demonstrated improved functional outcome scores with the Tegner activity ratings increasing from a means score of 3.5 preoperatively to 6.2 (*P*<.01) postoperatively in 664 patients pooled from 28 studies.[53] Unfortunately, data looking at differences in RTP rates and performance outcomes for specific sports are currently lacking. It is likely that RTP rates and performance vary significantly between sports because of the differences in demands and sport-specific activity requirements. The authors encourage further research to further investigate these differences.

REFERENCES

1. Poulsen MR, Johnson DL. Meniscal injuries in the young, athletically active patient. Phys Sportsmed 2011;39:123–30.

2. Brelin AM, Rue JP. Return to play following meniscus surgery. Clin Sports Med 2016;35:669–78.

3. McCarty EC, Marx RG, Wickiewicz TL. Meniscal tears in the athlete. Operative and nonoperative management. Phys Med Rehabil Clin N Am 2000;11(4):867–80.

4. Greis PE, Holmstrom MC, Bardana DD, et al. Meniscal injury II: management. J Am Acad Orthop Surg 2002;10:177–87.

5. Lee YS, Lee OS, Lee SH. Return to sports after athletes undergo meniscal surgery: a systematic review. Clin J Sport Med 2019;29(1):29–36.

6. Aune KT, Andrews JR, Dugas JR, et al. Return to play after partial lateral meniscectomy in National Football League athletes. Am J Sports Med 2014;42(8): 1865–72.

7. Abrams GD, Frank RM, Gupta AK, et al. Trends in meniscus repair and meniscectomy in the United States, 2005-2011. Am J Sports Med 2013. https://doi.org/10.1177/0363546513495641.

8. Kawata M, Sasabuchi Y, Taketomi S, et al. Annual trends in arthroscopic meniscus surgery: analysis of a national database in Japan. PLoS One 2018. https://doi.org/10.1371/journal.pone.0194854.

9. Jorgensen U, Sonne-Holm S, Lauridsen F, et al. Long-term follow-up of meniscectomy in athletes. A prospective longitudinal study. J Bone Joint Surg Br 2018. https://doi.org/10.1302/0301-620x.69b1.3818740.

10. Kim SG, Nagao M, Kamata K, et al. Return to sport after arthroscopic meniscectomy on stable knees. BMC Sports Sci Med Rehabil 2013. https://doi.org/10.1186/2052-1847-5-23.

11. DeFroda SF, Bokshan SL, Boulos A, et al. Variability of online available physical therapy protocols from academic orthopedic surgery programs for arthroscopic meniscus repair. Phys Sportsmed 2018;46(3):355–60.

12. Lennon OM, Totlis T. Rehabilitation and return to play following meniscal repair. Oper Tech Sports Med 2017;25(3):194–207.

13. Rosenberg TD, Scott SM, Coward DB, et al. Arthroscopic meniscal repair evaluated with repeat arthroscopy. Arthroscopy 1986;2(1):14–20.

14. Mooney M, Rosenberg TD. Meniscus repair: zone-specific technique. Sports Med Arthrosc Rev 1993;1:136–44.

15. Barber FA. Accelerated rehabilitation for meniscus repairs. Arthroscopy 1994;10: 206–10.
16. Shelbourne KD, Patel DV, Adsit WS, et al. Rehabilitation after meniscal repair. Clin Sports Med 1996;15:595–612.
17. Lind M, Nielsen T, Faunø P, et al. Free rehabilitation is safe after isolated meniscus repair: a prospective randomized trial comparing free with restricted rehabilitation regimens. Am J Sports Med 2013;41:2753–8.
18. Ganley T, Arnold C, McKernan D, et al. The impact of loading on deformation about posteromedial meniscal tears. Orthopedics 2000;23:597–601.
19. Lin DL, Ruh SS, Jones HL, et al. Does high knee flexion cause separation of meniscal repairs? Am J Sports Med 2013;41:2143–50.
20. McCulloch P, Jones H, Hamilton K, et al. Does simulated walking cause gapping of meniscal repairs? J Exp Orthop 2016;3:11.
21. O'Donnell K, Freedman KB, Tjoumakaris FP. Rehabilitation protocols after isolated meniscal repair. Am J Sports Med 2017;45(7):1687–97.
22. Stärke C, Kopf S, Petersen W, et al. Meniscal repair. Arthroscopy 2009;25(9): 1033–44.
23. Becker R, Wirz D, Wolf C, et al. Measurement of meniscofemoral contact pressure after repair of bucket-handle tears with biodegradable implants. Arch Orthop Trauma Surg 2005;125:254–60.
24. Kozlowski EJ, Barcia AM, Tokish JM. Meniscus repair: the role of accelerated rehabilitation in return to sport. Sports Med Arthrosc Rev 2012;20(2):121–6.
25. Barber BR, McNally EG. Meniscal injuries and imaging the postoperative meniscus. Radiol Clin North Am 2013. https://doi.org/10.1016/j.rcl.2012.10.008.
26. Vance K, Meredick R, Schweitzer ME, et al. Magnetic resonance imaging of the postoperative meniscus. Arthroscopy 2009. https://doi.org/10.1016/j.arthro.2008. 08.013.
27. Willinger L, Herbst E, Diermeier T, et al. High short-term return to sports rate despite an ongoing healing process after acute meniscus repair in young athletes. Knee Surg Sports Traumatol Arthrosc 2019;27(1):215–22.
28. McCarty EC, Marx RG, DeHaven KE. Meniscus repair: considerations in treatment and update of clinical results. Clin Orthop Relat Res 2002;(402):122–34.
29. Morgan CD, Wojtys EM, Casscells CD, et al. Arthroscopic meniscal repair evaluated by second-look arthroscopy. Am J Sports Med 1991;19(6):632–7.
30. Tachibana Y, Sakaguchi K, Goto T, et al. Repair integrity evaluated by second-look arthroscopy after arthroscopic meniscal repair with the FasT-Fix during anterior cruciate ligament reconstruction. Am J Sports Med 2010. https://doi.org/10. 1177/0363546509356977.
31. Scott GA, Jolly BL, Henning CE. Posterior incision and arthroscopic intra-articular repair of the meniscus: examination of factors affecting healing. J Bone Joint Surg Am 1986;68(6):847–60.
32. Kilcoyne KG, Dickens JF, Haniuk E, et al. Epidemiology of meniscal injury associated with ACL tears in young athletes. Orthopedics 2012. https://doi.org/10. 3928/01477447-20120222-07.
33. Krych AJ, Mcintosh AL, Voll AE, et al. Arthroscopic repair of isolated meniscal tears in patients 18 years and younger. Am J Sports Med 2008;1283–9. https:// doi.org/10.1177/0363546508314411.
34. Lyman S, Hidaka C, Valdez AS, et al. Risk factors for meniscectomy after meniscal repair. Am J Sports Med 2013. https://doi.org/10.1177/0363546513503444.

35. Tenuta JJ, Arciero RA. Arthroscopic evaluation of meniscal repairs: factors that effect healing. Am J Sports Med 1994. https://doi.org/10.1177/036354659402200611.
36. Wasserstein D, Dwyer T, Gandhi R, et al. A matched-cohort population study of reoperation after meniscal repair with and without concomitant anterior cruciate ligament reconstruction. Am J Sports Med 2013. https://doi.org/10.1177/0363546512471134.
37. Tuckman DV, Bravman JT, Lee SS, et al. Outcomes of meniscal repair: minimum of 2-year follow-up. Bull Hosp Jt Dis 2006;63(3-4):100–4.
38. Binfield PM, Maffulli N, King JB. Patterns of meniscal tears associated with anterior cruciate ligament lesions in athletes. Injury 1993. https://doi.org/10.1016/0020-1383(93)90038-8.
39. Millett PJ, Willis AA, Warren RF. Associated injuries in pediatric and adolescent anterior cruciate ligament tears: does a delay in treatment increase the risk of meniscal tear? Arthroscopy 2002. https://doi.org/10.1053/jars.2002.36114.
40. Allen CR, Wong EK, Livesay GA, et al. Importance of the medial meniscus in the anterior cruciate ligament-deficient knee. J Orthop Res 2000. https://doi.org/10.1002/jor.1100180116.
41. Gill SS, Diduch DR. Outcomes after meniscal repair using the Meniscus Arrow in knees undergoing concurrent anterior cruciate ligament reconstruction. Arthroscopy 2002. https://doi.org/10.1053/jars.2002.29897.
42. Haas AL, Schepsis AA, Hornstein J, et al. Meniscal repair using the FasT-Fix all-inside meniscal repair device. Arthroscopy 2005. https://doi.org/10.1016/j.arthro.2004.10.012.
43. Melton JTK, Murray JR, Karim A, et al. Meniscal repair in anterior cruciate ligament reconstruction: a long-term outcome study. Knee Surg Sports Traumatol Arthrosc 2011. https://doi.org/10.1007/s00167-011-1501-5.
44. Freedman KB, Nho SJ, Cole BJ. Marrow stimulating technique to augment meniscus repair. Arthroscopy 2003. https://doi.org/10.1016/S0749-8063(03)00695-9.
45. DeHaven KE, Bronstein RD. Arthroscopic medial meniscal repair in the athlete. Clin Sports Med 1997;16(1):69–86.
46. Ishida K, Kuroda R, Sakai H, et al. Rapid chondrolysis after arthroscopic partial lateral meniscectomy in athletes: a case report. Knee Surg Sports Traumatol Arthrosc 2006;14(12):1266–9.
47. Alvarez-Diaz P, Alentorn-Geli E, Llobet F, et al. Return to play after all-inside meniscal repair in competitive football players: a minimum 5-year follow-up. Knee Surg Sports Traumatol Arthrosc 2016;24(6):1997–2001.
48. Logan M, Watts M, Owen J, et al. Meniscal repair in the elite athlete results of 45 repairs with a minimum 5-year follow-up. Am J Sports Med 2009. https://doi.org/10.1177/0363546508330138.
49. Tucciarone A, Godente L, Fabbrini R, et al. Meniscal tear repaired with fast-fix sutures: clinical results in stable versus ACL-deficient knees. Arch Orthop Trauma Surg 2012. https://doi.org/10.1007/s00402-011-1391-5.
50. Nawabi DH, Cro S, Hamid IP, et al. Return to play after lateral meniscectomy compared with medial meniscectomy in elite professional soccer players. Am J Sports Med 2014;42(9):2193–8.
51. Osti L, Liu SH, Raskin A, et al. Partial lateral meniscectomy in athletes. Arthroscopy 1994;10(4):424–30.

52. Lee SJ, Aadalen KJ, Malaviya P, et al. Tibiofemoral contact mechanics after serial medial meniscectomies in the human cadaveric knee. Am J Sports Med 2006; 34(8):1334–44.
53. Eberbach H, Zwingmann J, Hohloch L, et al. Sport-specific outcomes after isolated meniscal repair: a systematic review. Knee Surg Sports Traumatol Arthrosc 2018. https://doi.org/10.1007/s00167-017-4463-4.
54. Bonneux I, Vandekerckhove B. Arthroscopic partial lateral meniscectomy long-term results in athletes. Acta Orthop Belg 2002;68(4):356–61.
55. Brophy RH, Gill CS, Lyman S, et al. Effect of anterior cruciate ligament reconstruction and meniscectomy on length of career in National Football League athletes. Am J Sports Med 2009;37(11):2102–7.
56. Mariani PP, Garofalo R, Margheritini F. Chondrolysis after partial lateral meniscectomy in athletes. Knee Surg Sports Traumatol Arthrosc 2008;16(6):574–80.
57. Alford JW, Lewis P, Kang RW, et al. Rapid progression of chondral disease in the lateral compartment of the knee following meniscectomy. Arthroscopy 2005; 21(12):1505–9.
58. Paxton ES, Stock MV, Brophy RH. Meniscal repair versus partial meniscectomy: a systematic review comparing reoperation rates and clinical outcomes. Arthroscopy 2011;27(9):1275–88.
59. Stein T, Mehling AP, Welsch F, et al. Long-term outcome after arthroscopic meniscal repair versus arthroscopic partial meniscectomy for traumatic meniscal tears. Am J Sports Med 2010. https://doi.org/10.1177/0363546510364052.
60. Xu C, Zhao J. A meta-analysis comparing meniscal repair with meniscectomy in the treatment of meniscal tears: the more meniscus, the better outcome? Knee Surg Sports Traumatol Arthrosc 2015;23(1):164–70.
61. Hoshikawa Y, Kurosawa H, Fukubayashi T, et al. The prognosis of meniscectomy in athletes. The simple meniscus lesions without ligamentous instabilities. Am J Sports Med 1983;11(1):8–13.
62. Griffin JW, Hadeed MM, Werner BC, et al. Platelet-rich plasma in meniscal repair: does augmentation improve surgical outcomes? Clin Orthop Relat Res 2015. https://doi.org/10.1007/s11999-015-4170-8.
63. Pujol N, Bohu Y, Boisrenoult P, et al. Clinical outcomes of open meniscal repair of horizontal meniscal tears in young patients. Knee Surg Sports Traumatol Arthrosc 2013. https://doi.org/10.1007/s00167-012-2099-y.
64. Vanderhave KL, Moravek JE, Sekiya JK, et al. Meniscus tears in the young athlete: results of arthroscopic repair. J Pediatr Orthop 2011. https://doi.org/10.1097/BPO.0b013e31821ffb8.
65. Nakayama H, Kanto R, Kambara S, et al. Clinical outcome of meniscus repair for isolated meniscus tear in athletes. Asia-Pacific J Sport Med Arthrosc Rehabil Technol 2017;10:4–7.

Degenerative Meniscus Tear in Older Athletes

Brian R. Wolf, MD, MS[a,b,*], Trevor R. Gulbrandsen, MD[c]

KEYWORDS

- Meniscus tear • Degenerative meniscus • Older athlete • Partial meniscectomy
- Meniscal injury

KEY POINTS

- The older athlete is part of an active and healthier population with a strong desire for return to sport.
- Managing patient expectations is a crucial part of initial and continuing evaluation and treatment in this population. Understanding patients' expected clinical outcome and desired return to play should direct the treatment modality.
- With higher activity, unstable meniscal flaps and horizontal tears may be more symptomatic.
- Retain as much viable meniscus as possible if surgery is done.
- If history, physical examination, and imaging demonstrate a symptomatic meniscal tear in an older athlete with minimal arthritis changes present, then the treating surgeon need not exclude these patients from possible arthroscopic treatment solely due to age.

INTRODUCTION

The meniscus is necessary for joint stability, load transmission during weight bearing, and for maintaining the health of articular cartilage. It should be preserved whenever possible, as several studies have demonstrated that the overall longevity of the knee joint heavily relies on the integrity of the menisci.[1–8]

A meniscal tear is a very common diagnosis. Baker and colleagues[9] reported the incidence of isolated meniscal injury resulting in meniscectomy as 61 per 100,000 in

Disclosure Statement: The authors have no conflicts of interest related to the issues discussed.
[a] Department of Orthopedic Surgery, University of Iowa Sports Medicine, University of Iowa Hospitals and Clinics, 160-D OSMR, 2701 Priarie Meadow Drive, Iowa City, IA 52242, USA;
[b] Department of Orthopedics and Rehabilitation, University of Iowa Hospitals and Clinics, University of Iowa Athletics, 160-D OSMR, 2701 Priarie Meadow Drive, Iowa City, IA 52242, USA;
[c] Department of Orthopedic Surgery, University of Iowa Hospitals and Clinics, 200 Hawkins Drive, Iowa City, IA 52242, USA
* Corresponding author. University of Iowa Sports Medicine, 160-D OSMR, 2701 Priarie Meadow Drive, Iowa City, IA 52242.
E-mail address: brian-wolf@uiowa.edu

Clin Sports Med 39 (2020) 197–209
https://doi.org/10.1016/j.csm.2019.08.005
0278-5919/20/Published by Elsevier Inc.
sportsmed.theclinics.com

the general population. Arthroscopic partial meniscectomy has been reported as the most frequent procedure performed by orthopedic surgeons in the United States, with 50% of those performed in patients aged 45 years or older.[10]

Degenerative meniscal tears are the most common type of meniscal lesions, consisting of nearly 30% of all tears with a peak incidence in patients aged 41 to 70 years.[11] Englund and colleagues[12] reported that 32% of asymptomatic patients aged 50 to 59 years and 56% of patients aged 60 to 90 years had a meniscal tear demonstrated on MRI. In addition, it has been reported that with increasing age, there was an increase in prevalence of meniscal damage in both men and women. These tears may be caused by trauma; however, they commonly have an insidious onset and are associated with complex, multiple tear patterns.[13] Although associated ligamentous injury is common in the younger population, isolated medial meniscus injury is more common in older population.[14,15]

The role of operative management of a degenerative meniscus injury is highly debated. Most of the literature has concluded that operative management is not superior to physical therapy with the treatment of degenerative meniscal tears. However, most of this literature is weakened by moderate-quality studies with small sample sizes.[16,17] Although nonoperative management with physical therapy can be indicated and beneficial, symptomatic degenerative meniscus patients with mechanical symptoms often fail and can be treated arthroscopically.

Although degenerative meniscal tears have been extensively studied in the general population, to the author's knowledge, there are no studies on degenerative meniscal tears strictly in older athletes. However, this is a unique population by having higher risk of meniscal injury due to the participation in sports along with the added risk of degenerative changes to the meniscus.[18,19] In addition, with higher activity, unstable flaps and horizontal tears may be more symptomatic with an increased risk of persistent symptoms (**Fig. 1**). As such, the authors review current literature and their approach to symptomatic meniscal tear in an older athlete.

DIAGNOSTIC WORKUP

There are many acute and chronic causes for knee pain. The physician should be critical with history and physical to further explore the specific cause. In the older athlete, determining meniscal injury versus osteoarthritis of the knee is essential. Wang and colleagues[20] found a 40% concomitant prevalence of degenerative meniscal tear and osteoarthritis determined by arthroscopy.

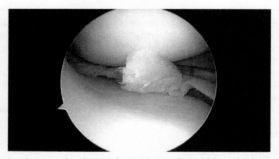

Fig. 1. Medial meniscal parrot beak tear from the undersurface of a horizontal tear in a 53-year-old runner with persistent pain and mechanical symptoms.

The typical symptoms of osteoarthritis include the following:

- Diffuse knee pain that is worse with prolonged ambulation
- Diffuse knee swelling that is worse with prolonged ambulation
- Pain at night or rest
- Knee stiffness

The typical symptoms of meniscal tears include the following:

- Localized pain to the lateral or medial side at the joint line
- Mechanical symptoms (locking, catching, clicking, popping)
- Delayed or intermittent swelling

The contralateral knee should be examined first for comparison. Both knees should be inspected for signs of infection or trauma. Joint line tenderness, locking, palpable clicking, positive McMurray test, positive Apley compression test, and Thessaly test suggest meniscal injury. Although acute meniscal and ligamentous tears usually consist of joint effusion, degenerative tears rarely do unless there is a large displaced meniscus fragment in the joint. Range of motion may be decreased in displaced meniscal tears; however, the patient may also have full active and passive range of motion.

The authors have found that the 2 most valuable physical examination findings include positive McMurray test and joint line tenderness. A positive McMurray test has a sensitivity of 32% to 34% and a specificity of 78% to 86%. Joint line tenderness has sensitivity ranges of 63% to 87%; however specificity ranges only from 30% to 50%.[21,22]

The physician should be aware that there are overlapping symptoms and findings. Although meniscal injuries are commonly associated with mechanical symptoms, osteoarthritis, patellofemoral syndrome, and loose bodies can also present with clicking, grinding, or popping. Osteoarthritis is a progressive and insidious process with no inciting event. However, Drosos and Pozo found that one-third (28.8%) of the patients with meniscal tears could not identify any specific event or incident that resulted in an injury.[13] This is especially true with degenerative tears. It is common for patients with osteoarthritis to have increased pain and limitation with ambulation; however, Lange and colleagues[23] found that meniscal tears also result in decreased walking endurance and balance performance.

Radiographic knee series should be obtained to further evaluate for knee pathology, especially osteoarthritis. This includes weight-bearing anteroposterior (AP), lateral, and skyline view. Rosenberg projection views can also be beneficial to compare and further analyze the contralateral knee (**Fig. 2**).

MRI is a valuable noninvasive tool and is the current gold standard for soft tissue imaging of the knee (**Fig. 3**). However, the medical specialist should also be aware that meniscal abnormalities demonstrated on MRI are not always significant.[24–26] With advances in MRI over the years, it is common to find asymptomatic meniscal tears in the older population. One study demonstrated 26% of those with meniscal tears were asymptomatic.[12] Brunner and colleagues[27] and Kaplan and colleagues[28] separately found a 20% prevalence of asymptomatic meniscal tears in professional and collegiate athletes. Shellock and colleagues[29] performed a small study with asymptomatic marathon runners (8 men, 15 women; average age: 40 years; average number of years training: 10; average training distance per week: 41 miles) who regularly compete in 26-mile, 50-mile, or 100-mile marathon races. They reported a 9% prevalence rate of meniscal tears. Subanalysis found a 6% prevalence rate in those younger than 45 years and 14% in those aged 45 years or older. More recently, Beals

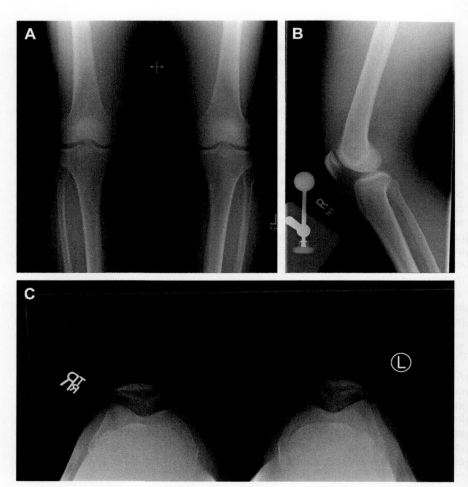

Fig. 2. Radiographs. (*A*) Rosenberg, (*B*) right lateral, and (*C*) skyline view of a 53-year-old patient with limited sport play and running due to persistent medial joint pain of the right knee. On examination the patient had significant joint line tenderness and a positive McMurray sign. Radiographs demonstrate mild narrowing of medial compartment of both knees. The patient's left knee was asymptomatic with excellent function.

and colleagues[30] performed a systematic review on the incidence of asymptomatic meniscus pathology in athletes. This study consisted of 14 articles and included 295 athletes (208 men, 87 women; age range: 14–66 years, mean: 31.2 years). They reported an overall prevalence of intrasubstance meniscal damage (grade 1 and 2 on MRI) to be 27.2% (105/386), whereas 3.9% (15/386) of knees had a tear (grade 3 and 4 on MRI).

MRI should not be used without insight in the patient's history and physical examination.[31] Ercin and colleagues[32] found better specificity, positive predictive value, negative predictive value, and diagnostic accuracy with an experienced practitioner than MRI in diagnosing medial meniscal tears. They concluded that a thorough physical examination from an experienced physician is sufficient for diagnosis. Therefore,

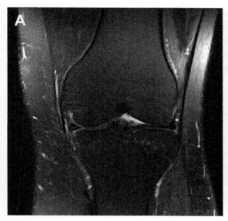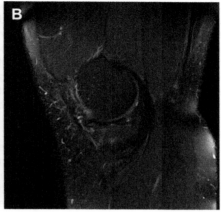

Fig. 3. (*A*) Sagittal and (*B*) coronal T2-weighted MRI. Complex tear of the body and posterior horn of the medial meniscus. Patient is a competitive racquetball player who developed insidious catching and locking that did not improve with physical therapy.

knowing the symptoms and performing a thorough physical examination is key to diagnosis and in determining the optimal treatment for degenerative meniscal tears.

TREATMENT AND DECISION-MAKING

Nonsurgical management of degenerative meniscal tears is an initial treatment option that is typically indicated for patients with full range of motion and no mechanical symptoms. Nonsurgical therapy generally includes rest, activity modification, icing, elevation, nonsteroidal antiinflammatories, short-term offloading, and physical therapy. Although several studies have demonstrated mild to moderate clinical improvement in pain, swelling, and overall knee function with dedicated physical therapy programs,[33–36] there has been limited research that describes the best methods or protocol for conservative treatment. In a study by Kise and colleagues,[36] both arthroscopic partial meniscectomy and supervised exercise therapy provided improvement in clinical outcomes; however, the exercise therapy had positive effects over partial meniscectomy in improving thigh muscle strength. Stensrud and colleagues[37] published a case series of patients with knee pain and degenerative meniscal tears demonstrated on MRI. Twenty patients (aged 38–58 years) underwent 12 weeks of formal strength and neuromuscular training that consisted of plyometrics and single-leg exercises on varying surfaces. Sixteen of the twenty symptomatic patients showed clinical improvement in Knee Injury and Osteoarthritis Outcome Score (KOOS), quality of life, and pain subscales. At 1-year follow-up, this clinical improvement was sustained, and surgery had not been performed in any of the 20 patients.

The traditional indications for surgical management of a meniscal tear include a history of mechanical symptoms including locking, catching, popping, joint line pain, and failure of conservative, nonoperative management.[38,39] Nevertheless, indication for operative management of symptomatic degenerative meniscal tears in the adult population is controversial and has been debated over the years.[39–41] There have been several studies recently published, which have called operative management of the degenerative meniscus tear into question. Thorlund and colleagues[42] recently published a systematic review and meta-analysis that evaluated the benefit of arthroscopy. Nine studies were included in their criteria, and after further analysis they concluded that arthroscopy was associated with harm and should not be recommended for older patients with or without signs of osteoarthritis. However, the studies' inclusion criteria are inconsistent with several nonrelevant, poorly designed studies, including only 5 related to degenerative meniscal tears. In addition, other current, relevant, and valid studies were excluded from the analysis and conclusions. In December 2015, Bollen described the biases in this study stating that "the evidence that arthroscopic intervention for 'knee pain' is of no benefit would seem to be thin at best."[40]

Conversely, there have been several studies showing the beneficial outcomes associated with arthroscopic partial meniscectomy in patients with symptomatic meniscal tears. In 1991, Aichroth and colleagues[43,44] published the classic study showing the promising outcomes in discomfort and function with patients who underwent arthroscopic debridement. More recently, Gauffin studied 150 older patients (aged 45–64 years; mean: 54 ± 5 years) with symptomatic meniscal tears after undergoing physiotherapy. The patients were randomized into 2 groups, a nonsurgical group that continued a formal physiotherapy exercise program and the surgical group that received the same physiotherapy exercise program but also underwent knee arthroscopy within 4 weeks of presentation, in which significant meniscal injuries were resected. This study reported significantly lower pain at 12 months in the patients who underwent meniscectomy. In addition, they found a significantly larger improvement in KOOS (pain) in the surgical group. It was concluded that partial meniscectomy had substantial benefits when added to physiotherapy programs.[33]

El Ghazaly found similar results with their study of 70 patients (age: 18–67 years, mean: 39.87 years) with unstable meniscal tears. All patients underwent physical therapy 3 times a week for 8 weeks. Those who were unsatisfied and symptomatic were offered arthroscopic partial meniscectomy. Overall this study reported improvement in pain and swelling after physical therapy, yet these were not statistically significant and many of the patients continued to experience limited range of motion of the knee. After arthroscopic partial meniscectomy there was significant improvement with pain, swelling, and overall function of the knee, including in those patients with mild osteoarthritis.[34]

Yim and colleagues[16] performed a randomized controlled trial to investigate operative versus nonoperative management of degenerative meniscal tears. They randomized 102 patients, aged 43 to 62 years, with symptomatic degenerative horizontal medial meniscal tears into an operative group (arthroscopic meniscectomy) and a nonoperative group (physical therapy/strengthening exercises). At 2-year follow-up, they found no difference in functional or clinical outcome scores. Furthermore, there was no significant difference in progression of Kellgren-Lawrence grade demonstrated on radiographs. Nonetheless, this study did not specify how many patients were athletic patients looking to return to sports and exercise. On further analysis the patient demographics in this study included a majority being overweight (meniscectomy group: mean body mass index [BMI] = 25; nonoperative group: mean BMI = 26.4).

Katz and Losina[35] performed a multicenter, randomized controlled trail comparing standardized physical therapy with arthroscopic partial meniscectomy with postoperative physical therapy in patients with meniscal tears and mild to moderate osteoarthritis. This study found that both groups experienced improvement in the Western Ontario and McMaster Universities Osteoarthritis Index physical function score with no significance at 6- or 12-month follow-up. However, at 6 months, 30% (51) of the patients originally assigned to the standardized physical therapy group crossed over and elected to undergo arthroscopic partial meniscectomy (in discretion of the patient and the surgeon). Only 6% (9) of the patients initially assigned to the surgical group ultimately did not undergo arthroscopic operative management. This large cross-over group provides insight into the possibility that many were not satisfied with their results from physical therapy and therefore underwent additional treatment. Furthermore, this result emphasizes the importance of clearly defining patient expectations.

As previously mentioned, the studies are abundant with varying conclusions on the optimal treatment of degenerative meniscal tears. Two recent reviews further determined that even with plenty of studies, we still cannot definitely conclude the optimal treatment of degenerative meniscal tears at this time.[45] This lack of conclusion in the literature provides increased demand for the surgeon to make decisions on a patient-specific basis. Managing patient expectations is a crucial part of the initial visit. Understanding the patient's expected clinical outcome and desired return to play should direct the treatment modality.

Age has often been a deterrent from operative management. It is common for medical specialists to regard patients aged 50 to 70 years with a meniscus tear, normal radiographs, and no osteoarthritis as a nonoperative candidate. However, through their practice the authors have found these patients to potentially achieve great clinical and functional outcomes, if appropriately indicated. If the examination and imaging demonstrate meniscal tear and the patient remains symptomatic, we should not exclude these patients solely due to age. We must remember that the main goal of operative management of meniscal tears is to decrease pain, prevent early arthrosis, and ultimately provide the patient the opportunity to potentially return to preinjury function and level of activity.

Meniscus Repair Versus Meniscectomy

Meniscus repair is appropriate in the peripheral, unstable, vertical meniscal tears in the vascular zone of the meniscus, whereas most degenerative tears and tears located in avascular zones of the meniscus should be managed with partial meniscectomy.[46] However, with further understanding of tear patterns and proper techniques, indications for meniscal repairs have expanded over the last 10 years to include older patients and more complex tear patterns.[47] Generally, it has been found that complex degenerative tears have limited ability and potential to heal and are usually not appropriate for operative meniscal repair.[11]

THE AUTHORS' PREFERRED SURGICAL TECHNIQUE

The patient is positioned supine on the operating table. Pneumatic tourniquet and a side post or leg holder are used on the ipsilateral thigh. After induction of general anesthesia, the joint is evaluated for stability and range of motion. Standard anterior portals are established with a 15 blade. A standard lateral arthroscopic portal is first established followed by a superomedial outflow portal. A 30-degree arthroscope is used. The location of the medial portal is determined using needle localization. Portal location is crucial to allow appropriate instrumentation of the involved meniscus without damaging the surrounding articular cartilage. In general, degenerative medial tears require a lower, inferior portal to allow direct access to the posterior medial joint space that can be tight and difficult to instrument. By contrast, when treating lateral meniscus tears the medial portal is placed more superior and proximal to allow instruments in the medial portal to go over the tibial spines while entering the lateral compartment. Typically, the lateral compartment opens more than medial and can be easier to instrument.

Diagnostic arthroscopy should always be the first step that is performed. The meniscal injury is then identified. A handheld meniscus biter and motorized shaver are commonly used to perform meniscal debridement. There are a variety of meniscus trimming instruments including straight, up-biting, side-biting, and others to assist with tears in different locations. It is prudent that the meniscal debris is than irrigated or suctioned out of the knee after debridement is complete (**Fig. 4**). Once meniscectomy is complete, the surgeon can also treat concurrent synovitis or chondral defects. Synovectomy and chondroplasty by removing unstable cartilage flaps can be performed.

One key factor for partial meniscectomy is to only debride what is deemed nonviable damaged meniscus tissue. *It is prudent to save as much viable meniscus as possible while also contouring the remaining meniscus to a smooth edge and not leaving tissue behind that looks to be at risk for further future tearing* (**Fig. 5**). This is critical with older athletes who undergo partial meniscectomy. We must remember that the meniscus is necessary for joint stability, load transmission during weight bearing, and the health of articular cartilage.[1–8]

One pitfall of arthroscopy is the risk of iatrogenic cartilage damage. This is especially true with narrow and tight medial compartments, which often can limit the ability to fully visualize and treat the posterior horn of the medial meniscus. In addition, in the older patient with a degenerative meniscus tear the articular cartilage can be especially friable and easy to damage with instruments. Over the last 10 years, percutaneous trephination of the medial collateral ligament (MCL) to allow further opening of the medial compartment has been shown to be safe without untoward results.[48] However, the surgeon should not expect to do MCL trephination on every case, and this method should be determined on a case-by-case basis during arthroscopic examination. MCL trephination is done by first identifying the junction of the body and the posterior horn of the medial meniscus. An 18-gauge spinal needle is inserted percutaneously through the medial knee skin at a level proximal to the meniscus. Gentle valgus force is applied. The spinal needle tip is then used to create numerous punctures in the deep MCL, starting at the posterior aspect of the ligament and extending anteriorly as needed. Trephination is done until the MCL subtly relaxes and visualization of the posterior medial meniscus is improved to allow access. There is no need for postoperative bracing with MCL trephination, and it has been found that patients do not have significantly increased laxity.[48–50]

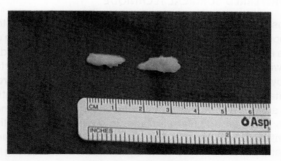

Fig. 4. Meniscal fragments removed during arthroscopic partial meniscectomy.

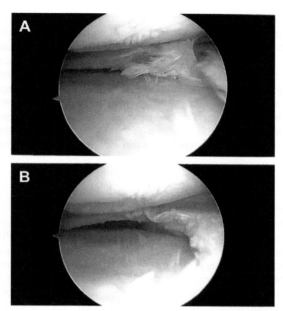

Fig. 5. (*A*) Injured degenerative medial meniscus visualized during diagnostic arthroscopy. Medial femoral condyle chondromalacia is present. (*B*) Medial meniscus postdebridement. Outer rim (Cooper 1 and 2) is preserved.

REHABILITATION

For the general population, partial meniscectomy has the benefit of providing only minor daily life modifications in the postoperative course. Postoperatively the patient can begin weight bearing as tolerated with no restrictions of range of motion.

Physical therapy typically begins within 1 to 2 weeks of surgery. However, the older athlete may desire to decline formal physical therapy. The patient should then be instructed to begin home exercises, including quad sets, straight leg raises, and 4 hip sways. Before their next follow-up they can eventually transition to light weight, higher repetition, closed kinetic chain exercises in the gym. The elliptical or bike can be utilized with gradual transition to higher-impact activities. Icing and nonsteroidal antiinflammatory drugs may be used for swelling, which is commonly associated with the increased activity.

At 6 to 8 weeks postoperative the patient should be evaluated. If they are progressing as expected, at this point they can return to full activity as tolerated if they have not done so already.

The older athlete population may have a strong desire for return to sporting activity compared with less active, but similar age patients. Fortunately, return to play does not need to be extensively delayed. Yeh and colleagues[15] reported that those in the National Basketball Association with medial meniscal tears missed 43.8 ± 35.7 days of play. Of the reported 128 players with meniscal injuries, 19.4% (25 players) did not return to play. Nevertheless, for those who did, on returning to competition, there was no change in Player Efficacy Rating from their preinjury status. In addition, the mean number of seasons further completed was 4.1 ± 3.7 seasons.

The patient should be instructed on the increased risk of knee osteoarthritis with meniscal injuries. Meniscus deficiency leads to less shock absorption capacity, a 2- to 3-fold decrease in stress reduction, increased friction, decreased proprioception and stability, and an increase in contact forces on the articular cartilage. This ultimately leads to degenerative changes in the knee.[51–54] This is especially true for the older athlete. The type of sport is an important factor for return to sport and subsequent risk of osteoarthritis. A study that investigated 2000 former elite international athletes demonstrated increased risk of progression of osteoarthritis with team and power athletes. In addition, there was a high risk of knee disability among those who participated in team sports, reflecting the increased demand and risk of certain sports.[55–57]

SUMMARY

Degenerative meniscal tears often have an insidious onset and are associated with complex, multiple tear patterns. Older athletes with meniscus tears often fail conservative treatment due to persistent pain and mechanical symptoms, often exacerbated by sports. There are studies that support both conservative and surgical management of meniscal tears. Nevertheless, degenerative meniscal tears with persistent symptoms from degenerative meniscus including locking and catching can be successfully treated with arthroscopic partial meniscectomy. Patient expectations should be clearly defined and age should not necessarily be a contraindication for partial meniscectomy. During arthroscopic treatment the surgeon should try to salvage viable meniscus while removing nonviable and nonfunctional torn tissue. Overall, it has been found that patients tolerate arthroscopic partial meniscectomy well with a relatively quick return to athletic activities.

REFERENCES

1. Ahmed AM, Burke DL. In-vitro measurement of static pressure distribution in synovial joints–Part I: tibial surface of the knee. J Biomech Eng 1983;105(3):216–25.
2. Burr DB, Radin EL. Meniscal function and the importance of meniscal regeneration in preventing late medical compartment osteoarthrosis. Clin Orthop Relat Res 1982;(171):121–6.
3. Fairbank TJ. Knee joint changes after meniscectomy. J Bone Joint Surg Br 1948; 30B(4):664–70.
4. Kettelkamp DB, Jacobs AW. Tibiofemoral contact area–determination and implications. J Bone Joint Surg Am 1972;54(2):349–56.
5. Kurosawa H, Fukubayashi T, Nakajima H. Load-bearing mode of the knee joint: physical behavior of the knee joint with or without menisci. Clin Orthop Relat Res 1980;(149):283–90.
6. Seedhom BB. Loadbearing function of the menisci. Physiotherapy 1976; 62(7):223.
7. Shrive NG, O'Connor JJ, Goodfellow JW. Load-bearing in the knee joint. Clin Orthop Relat Res 1978;(131):279–87.
8. Walker PS, Erkman MJ. The role of the menisci in force transmission across the knee. Clin Orthop Relat Res 1975;(109):184–92.
9. Baker BE, Peckham AC, Pupparo F, et al. Review of meniscal injury and associated sports. Am J Sports Med 1985;13(1):1–4.
10. Hall MJ, Lawrence L. Ambulatory sur- gery in the United States, 1996. Advance data from vital and health statistics. No. 300. Hyattsville (MD): National Center for Health Statistics; 1998 (DHHS publication no. (PHS) 98-1250.).

11. Schepsis AA, Busconi BD. Sports medicine. Lower extremity. Philadelphia: Lippincott Williams & Wilkins; 2006.

12. Englund M, Guermazi A, Gale D, et al. Incidental meniscal findings on knee MRI in middle-aged and elderly persons. N Engl J Med 2008;359(11):1108–15.

13. Drosos GI, Pozo JL. The causes and mechanisms of meniscal injuries in the sporting and non-sporting environment in an unselected population. Knee 2004;11(2):143–9.

14. Ridley TJ, McCarthy MA, Bollier MJ, et al. Age differences in the prevalence of isolated medial and lateral meniscal tears in surgically treated patients. Iowa Orthop J 2017;37:91–4.

15. Yeh PC, Starkey C, Lombardo S, et al. Epidemiology of isolated meniscal injury and its effect on performance in athletes from the National Basketball Association. Am J Sports Med 2012;40(3):589–94.

16. Yim JH, Seon JK, Song EK, et al. A comparative study of meniscectomy and nonoperative treatment for degenerative horizontal tears of the medial meniscus. Am J Sports Med 2013;41(7):1565–70.

17. Hohmann E, Glatt V, Tetsworth K, et al. Arthroscopic partial meniscectomy versus physical therapy for degenerative meniscus lesions: how robust is the current evidence? A critical systematic review and qualitative synthesis. Arthroscopy 2018; 34(9):2699–708.

18. Fox AJ, Wanivenhaus F, Burge AJ, et al. The human meniscus: a review of anatomy, function, injury, and advances in treatment. Clin Anat 2015;28(2):269–87.

19. Wolf BR, Amendola A. Impact of osteoarthritis on sports careers. Clin Sports Med 2005;24(1):187–98.

20. Wang DW, Cai X, Liu YJ, et al. Meniscus injury in osteoarthritis of knee joints: under arthroscopy. Zhonghua Yi Xue Za Zhi 2005;85(34):2425–7.

21. Couture JF, Al-Juhani W, Forsythe ME, et al. Joint line fullness and meniscal pathology. Sports Health 2012;4:47–50.

22. Galli M, Ciriello V, Menghi A, et al. Joint line tenderness and McMurray tests for the detection of meniscal lesions: what is their real diagnostic value? Arch Phys Med Rehabil 2013;94:1126–31.

23. Lange AK, Fiatarone Singh MA, Smith RM, et al. Degenerative meniscus tears and mobility impairment in women with knee osteoarthritis. Osteoarthritis Cartilage 2007;15(6):701–8.

24. Boden SD, Davis DO, Dina TS, et al. A prospective and blinded investigation of magnetic resonance imaging of the knee. Abnormal findings in asymptomatic subjects. Clin Orthop Relat Res 1992;(282):177–85.

25. Crues JV 3rd, Mink J, Levy TL, et al. Meniscal tears of the knee: accuracy of MR imaging. Radiology 1987;164(2):445–8.

26. LaPrade RF, Burnett QM 2nd, Veenstra MA, et al. The prevalence of abnormal magnetic resonance imaging findings in asymptomatic knees. With correlation of magnetic resonance imaging to arthroscopic findings in symptomatic knees. Am J Sports Med 1994;22(6):739–45.

27. Brunner MC, Flower SP, Evancho AM, et al. MRI of the athletic knee. Findings in asymptomatic professional basketball and collegiate football players. Invest Radiol 1989;24(1):72–5.

28. Kaplan LD, Schurhoff MR, Selesnick H, et al. Magnetic resonance imaging of the knee in asymptomatic professional basketball players. Arthroscopy 2005;21(5): 557–61.

29. Shellock FG, Deutsch AL, Mink JH, et al. Do asymptomatic marathon runners have an increased prevalence of meniscal abnormalities? An MR study of the knee in 23 volunteers. AJR Am J Roentgenol 1991;157(6):1239–41.

30. Beals CT, Magnussen RA, Graham WC, et al. The prevalence of meniscal pathology in asymptomatic athletes. Sports Med 2016;46(10):1517–24.

31. Sherman SL, Gulbrandsen TR, Lewis HA, et al. Overuse of magnetic resonance imaging in the diagnosis and treatment of moderate to severe osteoarthritis. Iowa Orthop J 2018;38:33–7.

32. Ercin E, Kaya I, Sungur I, et al. History, clinical findings, magnetic resonance imaging, and arthroscopic correlation in meniscal lesions. Knee Surg Sports Traumatol Arthrosc 2012;20:851–6.

33. Gauffin H, Tagesson S, Meunier A, et al. Knee arthroscopic surgery is beneficial to middle-aged patients with meniscal symptoms: a prospective randomised single blinded study. Osteoarthritis Cartilage 2014;22:1808–16.

34. El Ghazaly S, Rahman AAA, Yusry AH, et al. Arthroscopic partial meniscectomy is superior to physical rehabilitation in the management of symptomatic unstable meniscal tears. Int Orthop 2015;39:769–75.

35. Katz JN, Losina E. Surgery versus physical therapy for meniscal tear and osteoarthritis. N Engl J Med 2013;369(7):677–8.

36. Kise NJ, Risberg MA, Stensrud S, et al. Exercise therapy versus arthroscopic partial meniscectomy for degenerative meniscal tear in middle aged patients: Randomised controlled trial with two year follow-up. BMJ 2016;354:i3740.

37. Stensrud S, Roos EM, Risberg MA. A 12-week exercise therapy program in middle-aged patients with degenerative meniscus tears: a case series with 1-year follow-up. J Orthop Sports Phys Ther 2012;42(11):919–31.

38. Conaghan PG, Dickson J, Grant RL. Guideline develop- ment group. Care and management of osteoarthritis in adults: Summary of NICE guidance. BMJ 2008;336:502–3.

39. Krych AJ, Carey JL, Marx RG, et al. Does arthroscopic knee surgery work? Arthroscopy 2014;30:544–5.

40. Bollen SR. Is arthroscopy of the knee completely useless? Meta-analysis–a reviewer's nightmare. Bone Joint J 2015;97:1591–2.

41. Elattrache N, Lattermann C, Hannon M, et al. New England Journal of Medicine evaluating the usefulness of meniscectomy is flawed. Arthroscopy 2014;30: 542–3.

42. Thorlund JB, Juhl CB, Roos EM, et al. Arthroscopic surgery for degenerative knee: Systematic review and meta-analysis of benefits and harms. BMJ 2015; 350:h2747.

43. Aichroth PM, Patel DV, Moyes ST. A prospective review of arthroscopic debridement for degenerative joint disease of the knee. Int Orthop 1991;15(4):351–5.

44. Buchbinder R. Meniscectomy in patients with knee osteoarthritis and a meniscal tear? N Engl J Med 2013;368:1740–1.

45. Ha AY, Shalvoy RM, Voisinet A, et al. Controversial role of arthroscopic meniscectomy of the knee: a review. World J Orthop 2016;7:287–92.

46. Brophy RH, Matava M. Surgical options for meniscal replacement. J Am Acad Orthop Surg 2012;20:265–72.

47. Woodmass JM, LaPrade RF, Sgaglione NA, et al. Meniscal repair: reconsidering indications, techniques, and biologic augmentation. J Bone Joint Surg Am 2017; 99(14):1222–31.

48. Hinton MA. Percutaneous partial medial collateral ligament release (PPMCLR) does not result in residual medial collateral laxity (MCL). Orthop J Sports Med 2015;3(7 suppl 2). 2325967115S00117.

49. Atoun E, Debbi R, Lubovsky O, et al. Arthroscopic trans-portal deep medial collateral ligament pie-crusting release. Arthrosc Tech 2013;2(1):e41–3.

50. Li X, Selby RM, Newman A, et al. Needle assisted arthroscopic clysis of the medial collateral ligament of the knee: a simple technique to improve exposure in arthroscopic knee surgery. Orthop Rev (Pavia) 2013;5(4):e38.

51. Alhalki MM, Howell SM, Hull ML. How three methods for fixing a medial meniscal autograft affect tibial contact mechanics. Am J Sports Med 1999;27:320–8.

52. Frizziero A, Ferrari R, Giannotti E, et al. The meniscus tear: state of the art of rehabilitation protocols related to surgical procedures. Muscles Ligaments Tendons J 2012;2:295–301.

53. Makris EA, Hadidi P, Athanasiou KA. The knee meniscus: structure-function, pathophysiology, current repair techniques, and prospects for regeneration. Biomaterials 2011;32:7411–31.

54. Voloshin AS, Wosk J. Shock absorption of meniscectomized and painful knees: a comparative in vivo study. J Biomed Eng 1983;5:157–61.

55. Kujala UM, Kaprio J, Sarna S. Osteoarthritis of weight bearing joints of lower limbs in former elite male athletes. Br Med J 1994;308(6923):231–4.

56. Kujala UM, Kettunen J, Paananen H, et al. Knee osteoarthritis in former runners, soccer players, weight lifters, and shooters. Arthritis Rheum 1995;38(4):539–46.

57. Kettunen JA, Kujala UM, Kaprio J, et al. Lower-limb function among former elite male athletes. Am J Sports Med 2001;29(1):2–8.

Role of Alignment and Osteotomy in Meniscal Injuries

Pablo Eduardo Gelber, MD, PhD[a,b,]*, Bjorn Barenius, MD[c],
Simone Perelli, MD[a,1]

KEYWORDS

- Alignment • Osteotomy • Meniscus • Meniscectomy • Varus • Valgus

KEY POINTS

- The menisci and lower limb alignment are intrinsically linked in the distribution of forces across the knee joint.
- Lower limb alignment should be assessed in each case of meniscal injury.
- When meniscus tears undergo repair surgery, several factors should be considered to determine whether a concomitant osteotomy is necessary.
- The most relevant factors to take into consideration are concomitant cartilage injuries, whether the meniscal injury is traumatic or degenerative, the meniscal tear pattern, and anterior cruciate ligament status.

INTRODUCTION

The menisci and lower limb alignment both play a crucial role in load transmission across the knee joint. The meniscus distributes the mechanical load by increasing the contact surface area, sharing the weight bearing across the articular surfaces.[1] Any loss of functional meniscal tissue alters this function and contributes to

Disclosure Statement: The authors of the current study certify that they have no affiliations with or involvement in any organization or entity with any financial interest (such as honoraria; educational grants; participation in speakers' bureaus; membership, employment, consultancies, stock ownership, or other equity interest; and expert testimony or patent-licensing arrangements), or nonfinancial interest (such as personal or professional relationships, affiliations, knowledge or beliefs) in the subject matter or materials discussed in this article.
[a] ICATME-Hospital Universitari Dexeus, Universitat Autònoma de Barcelona, Barcelona, Spain;
[b] Hospital de la Santa Creu i Sant Pau, Universitat Autònoma de Barcelona, Barcelona, Spain;
[c] Department of Clinical Science and Education, Södersjukhuset, Karolinska Intitutet, Solnavägen 1, Solna, Stockholm 17177, Sweden
[1] Present address: Sabino de Arana 5, 2nd floor. Barcelona 08028, Spain.
* Corresponding author. Department of Orthopaedic Surgery, Hospital de la Santa Creu i Sant Pau, Universitat Autònoma de Barcelona, C/Sant Quintí, 89, Barcelona 08041, Spain.
E-mail address: personal@drgelber.com

Clin Sports Med 39 (2020) 211–221
https://doi.org/10.1016/j.csm.2019.08.006
0278-5919/20/© 2019 Elsevier Inc. All rights reserved.

compartmental instability. Similarly, varus or valgus malalignment contributes to knee overload by altering the load distribution across the knee.[2] As meniscal pathology is commonly combined with malalignment, both aspects should be assessed when evaluating meniscal injury. This study reviews and analyzes the most important aspects to be considered in this scenario and highlights indications for isolated and combined treatments.

BIOMECHANICS OF THE MENISCI

The menisci distribute the load across the knee and also stabilize the joint during motion. However, because of the anatomic differences of the medial and lateral compartments, the biomechanical properties of the medial and lateral menisci differ. Although the medial compartments have a concave form, the lateral tibial plateau is smaller and more convex. The corresponding menisci are shaped to conform to these differences. Due to the convex shape of the lateral tibial plateau, this compartment is less congruent and the lateral meniscus transfers a greater load during weight bearing.[3] As a result, any amount of meniscal tissue resection decreases the contact area and increases the peak loads transmitted to the tibial plateau.[4] In a normally aligned knee, the lateral and medial compartments carry 42% and 58%, respectively, of the total load. However, due to its shock absorber property, the menisci transfer only 70% of the total load to the tibial plateau.

BIOMECHANICS OF LOWER LIMB ALIGNMENT

The most relevant aspects of lower limb alignment in relation to the meniscus are those that comprise the coronal plane. Most studies in the literature have assessed alignment in osteoarthritis (OA) and only a few have done so in healthy young individuals. Bellemans and colleagues[5] assessed lower limb alignment in healthy young adults without knee problems. They found a mean hip-knee-ankle (HKA) angle of 1.9° of varus (SD ±2.4) in men and an angle of 0.81° (SD ±2.1) in women. Sixty-six percent of men and 80% of women had an HKA between 3° of varus and 3° of valgus. A varus alignment of more than 3° was observed in approximately 32% of men and 17% of women. Conversely, valgus alignment of more than 3° was only seen in 2% to 3% of cases.

The aim of osteotomy is to shift the load to the nonaffected compartment. The contact pressure in the unloaded compartment depends on the degree of alignment correction and whether a varus or a valgus osteotomy is being performed. In any case, a 7° varus or valgus osteotomy could unload the affected compartment by up to 70%, matching that of the meniscus shock absorber effect.[6,7]

DEALING WITH A PROBLEM OF THE MENISCUS OR ALIGNMENT?

As meniscus function and knee alignment are closely related, they must both be assessed when either of the 2 conditions is diagnosed. For the medial compartment, alignment is of paramount importance. There is an ongoing debate in the literature regarding OA progression and the effect of alignment. Sharma and colleagues[8] found OA progression correlated with alignment, with significantly higher functional deterioration over 18 months when malalignment was greater than 5° either in varus or valgus. Thorlund and colleagues[9] also reported that the load transfer changes after meniscectomy. They found knee load indices increased 12 months after arthroscopic partial meniscectomy (APM), indicating compartment overload. Alignment also has been implicated in OA progression after meniscus resection. Covall and Wasilewski[10] found less joint space narrowing more than 5 years after medial meniscectomy in patients with a preoperative tibiofemoral valgus of more than 4°. Burks and colleagues[11] found more joint space narrowing 15 years after partial medial meniscectomy for varus with less than 0° in HKA as the cutoff. In contrast, in a regression analysis of 500 patients more than 10 years after APM, Chatain and colleagues[12] did not identify alignment as a significant factor in OA progression.

Varus alignment is also a risk factor for medial meniscus posterior root tear (MMPRT).[13] Hwang and colleagues[13] compared MMPRT with other meniscus injuries and found a mean of 4.5° (SD ±3.4) of varus in the MMPRT group and 2.4° (SD ±2.7) of varus in the group with other meniscal injuries.

Meniscal repair can also be influenced by lower limb alignment. Due to the mobility of the menisci and to the role of the menisci in load transmission, it seems logical that varus or valgus alignment might respectively affect the healing potential of a medial or lateral meniscus repair. Surprisingly, no studies have addressed this aspect in detail. Since the adoption of a more comprehensive approach to root repair and meniscus transplantation in recent years, our understanding of the influence of alignment on meniscus injuries has evolved. The etiology of posterior root injury differs between the lateral and medial menisci. The more mobile lateral meniscus posterior root is frequently injured in a traumatic event in a younger person, usually when an anterior cruciate ligament (ACL) injury occurs.[14] In these circumstances, Okoroha and colleagues[15] reported that malalignment might be a risk factor for a lateral meniscus posterior root tear (LMPRT). With a varus angle of more than 3°, they found a 5.2-fold increase of LMPRT. They also observed that a posterior tibial slope of more than 12° was related to a 5.4-fold increase of this LMPRT. These findings highlight the stabilizing effect of the lateral meniscus as a secondary constraint to anterior tibial translation and the internal rotational force in an ACL injury. In contrast, the more tethered medial meniscus posterior root injury is most often part of a degenerative process, with varus malalignment, overweight, OA, and gender being the most common risk factors.[14]

MEDIAL AND LATERAL MENISCUS IN VARUS AND VALGUS ALIGNED KNEES

Several investigators have reported clinical correlations between alignment and OA.[16,17] However, the deleterious effect on the articular cartilage due to malalignment and meniscus injuries has been little studied, and the influence of alignment on the outcome after meniscectomy is controversial. Although some believe that malalignment compromises the result of meniscectomy,[18] others have stated that the lower limb axis does not affect the outcomes.[12] One of the main reasons for this controversy is that preoperative alignment was not considered in many long-term studies after meniscectomy, and therefore, it was not assessed as an independent risk factor influencing clinical outcomes or osteoarthritis progression.

The effect of meniscectomy on postoperative alignment has been better studied. Findings have revealed an increase in valgus alignment after lateral meniscectomy[19] and also after medial meniscectomy.[20] It seems that the deformity produced by the meniscectomy is influenced by the amount of resected meniscal tissue, but not by the preoperative alignment.[20] The study with the longest follow-up to date, 40 years, analyzed the tibiofemoral angle modification after meniscectomy and showed that a meniscectomy led to malalignment in the corresponding tibiofemoral compartment.[21] However, this effect was more pronounced after a medial meniscectomy leading to a varus knee than after a lateral meniscectomy leading to a valgus knee. The tibiofemoral angle, the magnitude of malalignment, and the range of motion were strongly correlated with both Ahlback and Kellgren and Laurence scores. Be that as it may, patient-reported outcome measures did not correlate with the degree of OA.[21] In fact, long-term follow-up after arthroscopic partial medial or lateral meniscectomy showed progressive degenerative radiographic changes, with small or no significant negative effects on knee function. One possible explanation is that body mass index (BMI) and degenerative meniscal tears are stronger risk factors for these degenerative changes than the degree of malalignment.[22] It is generally accepted that cartilage deterioration is more frequently observed after lateral meniscectomy than after medial meniscectomy. This higher deleterious effect on the articular cartilage after lateral meniscectomy could be due to the convexity of the lateral tibial plateau being compensated with a larger meniscus covering more area than in the medial compartment.[22] Finite elements analysis supports these concepts, showing that the maximum stresses and strains occurred on the medial tibial cartilage after medial meniscectomy only in a varus knee. Conversely, the drop from before to after in the contact stresses and strains was higher in the lateral cartilage after lateral meniscectomy regardless of whether the lower limb had a valgus or varus alignment.[23]

The increase in peak contact stress after loss of meniscal tissue is directly related to the amount of tissue resection.[4] The volume of removed meniscal tissue should also therefore be considered at the time of the surgery, given that it affects long-term radiological and clinical outcomes both in the medial and lateral compartments[11] (**Box 1**).

Brophy and colleagues[24] studied different factors in patients with reconstructed ACL. They found that varus alignment was associated with articular cartilage status in the medial compartment but not in the lateral compartment. Medial cartilage status was also correlated with BMI, whereas lateral compartment chondral injuries were significantly associated with age.[24] For both compartments, they observed a relevant association with meniscal status. Patients with previous partial meniscectomy showed higher rates of degenerative changes than patients with previous meniscal repair or no previous meniscal surgery.[24] In view of these observations, in an ACL reconstructed knee,

---

- Varus deformity is an independent risk factor for the development of medial osteoarthritis
- The combination of medial meniscectomy and varus alignment could increase the risk of cartilage degeneration
- Valgus deformity is a risk factor only for lateral OA when it is associated with advanced age or previous meniscectomy. In such patients, the association of medial meniscectomy and varus malalignment could increase the risk of cartilage degeneration.

Box 1
Known facts between meniscectomy and malalignment

- Varus and valgus alignment tend to increase after medial and lateral meniscectomy, respectively.
- This increment is more pronounced in the medial compartment.
- The cartilage deterioration is more pronounced in the lateral compartment.
- The deformity after surgery is more related to the amount of resected meniscal tissue rather than to the degree of preoperative alignment.
- The deformity after surgery does not correlate with functional outcomes.

Although a correlation between alignment correction and the healing capacity of a meniscal repair has not yet been clearly demonstrated, some studies have found a high percentage of posteromedial root tears healed following a medial valgus osteotomy.[25]

INDICATIONS FOR ISOLATED OR COMBINED TREATMENT

Osteotomy is a load-shifting procedure with well-documented favorable outcomes even in subjects with a high activity level. To achieve optimal surgical results, appropriate patient selection is mandatory. First, it is crucial to acknowledge the factors that negatively affect the results of an osteotomy (**Table 1**).

There is no clear consensus or scientific data on which to base a specific cutoff value of alignment to perform a varus or valgus osteotomy around the knee, perhaps because the severity of the symptoms does not always correlate with the degree of deformity. For varus malalignment, for example, it has been demonstrated that patients with a mild degree of preoperative deformity (3° to 5°) have the same baseline characteristic and the same postoperative outcomes as patients with a higher degree of preoperative deformity.[26] In some scenarios, differences as small as 2° between the mechanical axis of the 2 lower limbs could justify an osteotomy. This could be the case if

- Meniscal repair, large meniscal resection, or articular cartilage treatment is to be performed.
- The difference in the chondral status between the affected compartment (International Cartilage Repair Society [ICRS] grade 3–4) and the nonaffected compartment (ICRS 0–1) is clearly evident.

The precise characteristics of the meniscus tear also must be considered when determining the best surgical technique in each case. In cases of malalignment associated with meniscal injuries, it first should be elucidated whether the pain originates in the meniscal injury or in the malalignment. Two crucial parameters to consider are as follows:

- Whether the meniscal lesion is traumatic or degenerative
- The pattern of the meniscal tear.

Table 1	
Contraindications and prognostic factors that worsen the results after a knee osteotomy	
Avoid Valgus Osteotomy if:	**Avoid Varus Osteotomy if[33]:**
Severe medial OA[27]	Extreme valgus deformity with tibial subluxation
Patellofemoral OA[28]	Gross knee instability
Lateral OA[28]	Tricompartmental OA
Range of motion deficits[29]	Flexion contracture >15°
Lateral tibial thrust[29]	Severe patellofemoral OA, high BMI, rheumatoid arthritis, age >65 y, and severe lateral compartment bone loss also should be excluded
BMI to determine whether to perform HTO or not is controversial[32]	

Abbreviations: BMI, body mass index; HTO, high tibial osteotomy; OA, osteoarthritis.

Traumatic or Degenerative Meniscal Tear

There is now a certain consensus concerning treatment of degenerative meniscus in middle-aged patients, but it is not exempt of controversy.[27,28] Several investigators have suggested that a degenerative meniscal lesion may be an early sign of knee OA rather than a separate clinical problem requiring meniscal intervention.[19] However, it is difficult to discriminate between symptoms caused by a meniscus tear and symptoms of early-stage OA.[27] Certainly, in case of symptomatic *degenerative* meniscal lesions associated with malalignment and cartilage degeneration, an osteotomy at the time of partial meniscectomy is suggested. However, if cartilage degeneration is absent, an isolated meniscectomy is still the gold standard.

> - Osteotomy is needed in concomitant cartilage degeneration
> - Isolated meniscectomy otherwise

In the case of traumatic meniscal tears with no cartilage changes in a malaligned knee, the treatment of choice is an isolated meniscal procedure. It is of utmost importance in this overloaded compartment to try to perform a meniscal repair rather than a meniscectomy. If symptoms do not improve after a large meniscectomy of a traumatic injury, an osteotomy could then be performed in a second-stage surgery. In this case, a concomitant meniscal transplantation also should be considered in young patients.[29]

When a traumatic meniscal injury is associated with articular chondral injuries in a malaligned knee, the origin of pain can be difficult to identify. In these cases, a combined osteotomy is preferred, especially if the lesion requires a meniscectomy. This viewpoint is based on the fact that symptoms from cartilage injuries can worsen after a meniscectomy and a load-shifting procedure will likely improve both sources of pain.

> - Isolated meniscal resection or preferably meniscal repair if there is no deterioration of cartilage
> - Osteotomy at index surgery if cartilage injury is present
> - Osteotomy in a second stage if symptoms do not subside

Meniscal Tear Pattern

The presence of an MMPRT or complete radial tear of the posterior horn leads to a loss of the hoop stress mechanism, thus predisposing to OA changes.[30] These lesions are frequently accompanied by meniscal extrusion that is also correlated with OA progression.[31] Surprisingly, although meniscal extrusion does not seem to correlate with the degree of mechanical axis malalignment,[32] a recent study showed that it is correlated with the medial proximal tibial angle (MPTA).[33] This suggests that patients with a combination of low MPTA and meniscal extrusion could be appropriate candidates for early intervention with a high tibial osteotomy, supporting the concept of performing an osteotomy when facing a root tear or a complete radial tear with any degree of deformity. This view is also reinforced by the correlation between alignment correction and the previously discussed healing capacity of a meniscal repair.[25]

> Perform a concomitant valgus osteotomy in cases of an MMPRT or complete radial tear in the posterior horn of the medial meniscus.

The same can also be applied to the lateral femorotibial compartment in a valgus aligned knee.

> Perform a concomitant varus osteotomy in cases of an LMPRT or complete radial tear in the posterior horn of the lateral meniscus (**Fig. 1**).

It goes without saying that age and chondral status also must be taken into account. In any case, the degree of deformity should not influence the final decision. When a meniscal extrusion is present in combination with a varus or valgus alignment, it must be determined whether or not the extrusion is due to a hoop tension injury of the meniscus. If this is the case, the rationale has already been pointed out. If not, it can be assumed that the meniscal rim is already degenerated and is no longer functioning as a shock absorber. A combination of osteotomy and meniscectomy of the

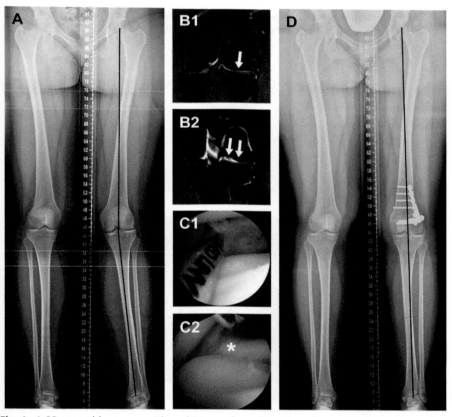

Fig. 1. A 23-year-old woman with no history of previous surgeries presenting with a valgus knee and LMPRT in her left knee. (*A*) Long standing radiograph showing a mechanical axis of 6° of valgus. (*B*) Coronal MRIs showed no joint space narrowing or cartilage damage (*B1, arrow*) and the LMPRT (*B2, double arrow*). (*C*) Arthroscopic views where the posterior root of the lateral meniscus is being repaired (*C1*), and once the root has been reattached (*C2, asterisk*). (*D*) Postoperative long standing radiograph after the distal varus osteotomy and repair of the LMPRT showing a corrected mechanical axis of 0°.

more unstable meniscal flap is then suggested. This is even more important if the deformity is due to a low MPTA, as previously discussed.

Other Specific Cases

Discoid lateral meniscus in association with a constitutional valgus alignment. In patients younger than 20 years, a lateral meniscectomy of a torn discoid lateral meniscus leads to a significantly higher valgus deformity than in large nondiscoid lateral meniscectomy.[34] A *prophylactic* varus osteotomy should therefore be considered in this subgroup of patients when a wide meniscectomy is necessary.

Obesity is likely to have both biomechanical and biochemical links to osteoarthritis, and a recent study demonstrated that it modulates changes in the gene expression of meniscal tears.[35] In cases of malalignment associated with meniscal lesions in the obese, therefore, we should theoretically opt for alignment correction to avoid early OA. On the other hand, it should be kept in mind that obesity is a risk factor for nonunion. Nonunion also should be taken into account in the presence of other risk factors, such as smoking, diabetes, or vasculopathy.

ACL deficient knees are suitable for osteotomy if associated with unicompartmental OA, and even without combining ACL reconstruction, osteotomy provides good

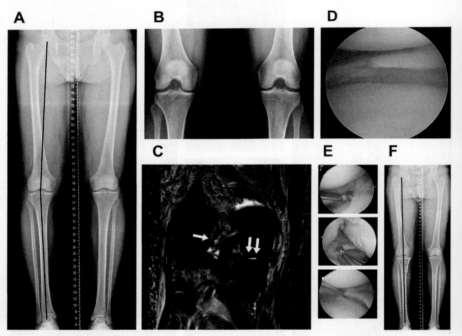

Fig. 2. A 30-year-old man with mild varus, ACL injury and complete radial tear of the medial meniscus in the right knee. (*A*) Long standing radiograph showing a mechanical axis of 5° of varus. (*B*) Weight-bearing posteroanterior radiograph at 30° of knee flexion shows no joint space narrowing. (*C*) Coronal MRI showing ACL tear (*arrow*) and complete radial tear of the posterior horn of the medial meniscus, with no evident articular cartilage injury (*double arrow*). (*D*) Arthroscopic view confirming the complete radial tear of the posterior horn of the medial meniscus with a healthy cartilage. (*E*) Three arthroscopic views of the large meniscal resection performed. (*F*) Postoperative long standing radiograph after the high tibial valgus osteotomy and ACL reconstruction showing a corrected mechanical axis of 0°.

outcomes.[36] The opposite scenario is more challenging. Considering the increased incidence of medial compartment chondrosis at the time of revision ACL surgery in patients with varus malalignment and deficient medial meniscus, varus knees undergoing large medial meniscal resections at the time of ACL reconstruction have the potential to benefit from a high tibial osteotomy to reduce the risk of medial OA[24] (**Fig. 2**). As this is a more prophylactic indication, other variables, such as BMI and the patient's daily activities, also should be considered.

SUMMARY

Meniscus injury together with alterations in lower limb alignment is commonly observed in clinical practice. Several factors must be considered for correct diagnosis and to choose the best treatment option. To obtain a clear, complete picture of each meniscal condition, lower limb alignment should be systematically assessed in all patients. A tailored approach considering the previously detailed, most relevant aspects for each patient is then recommended.

REFERENCES

1. Thompson WO, Thaete FL, Fu FH, et al. Tibial meniscal dynamics using three-dimensional reconstruction of magnetic resonance images. Am J Sports Med 1991;19:210–6.
2. Ding CH, Martel-Pelletier J, Pelletier JP, et al. Knee meniscal extrusion in a largely non-osteoarthritic cohort: association with greater loss of cartilage volume. Arthritis Res Ther 2007;9:R21.
3. Walker PS, Hajek JV. The load-bearing area in the knee joint. J Biomech 1972;5: 581–9.
4. Baratz ME, Fu FH, Mengato R. Meniscal tears: The effect of meniscectomy and of repair on intrarticular contact areas and stress in the human knee. A preliminary report. Am J Sports Med 1986;14:270–5.
5. Bellemans J, Colyn W, Vandenneucker H, et al. The Chitranjan Ranawat award: is neutral mechanical alignment normal for all patients? The concept of constitutional varus. Clin Orthop Relat Res 2012;470:45–53.
6. Trad Z, Barkaoui A, Chafra M, et al. Finite element analysis of the effect of high tibial osteotomy correction angle on articular cartilage loading. Proc Inst Mech Eng H 2018;232:553–64.
7. Wylie JD, Scheiderer B, Obopilwe E, et al. The effect of lateral opening wedge distal femoral varus osteotomy on tibiofemoral contact mechanics through knee flexion. Am J Sports Med 2018;46:3237–44.
8. Sharma L, Song J, Felson DT, et al. The role of knee alignment in disease progression and functional decline in knee osteoarthritis. JAMA 2001;286:188–95.
9. Thorlund JB, Holsgaard-Larsen A, Creaby MW, et al. Changes in knee joint load indices from before to 12 months after arthroscopic partial meniscectomy: a prospective cohort study. Osteoarthritis Cartilage 2016;24:1153–9.
10. Covall DJ, Wasilewski SA. Roentgenographic changes after arthroscopic meniscectomy: five-year follow-up in patients more than 45 years old. Arthroscopy 1992;8:242–6.
11. Burks RT, Metcalf MH, Metcalf MW. Fifteen-year follow-up of arthroscopic partial meniscectomy. Arthroscopy 1997;13:673–9.
12. Chatain F, Adeleine P, Chambat P, et al. A comparative study of medial versus lateral arthroscopic partial meniscectomy on stable knees: 10-year minimum follow-up. Arthroscopy 2003;19:842–9.

13. Hwang BY, Kim SJ, Lee SW, et al. Risk factors for medial meniscus posterior root tear. Am J Sports Med 2012;40:1606–10.

14. Koo JH, Choi SH, Lee Sa, et al. Comparison of medial and lateral meniscus root tears. PLoS One 2015;10:e0141021.

15. Okoroha KR, Patel RB, Kadri O, et al. Abnormal tibial alignment is a risk factor for lateral meniscus posterior root tears in patients with anterior cruciate ligament ruptures. Knee Surg Sports Traumatol Arthrosc 2018. https://doi.org/10.1007/s00167-018-5271-4.

16. Brouwer GM, Tol AWV, Bergink AP, et al. Association between valgus and varus alignment and the development and progression of radiographic osteoarthritis of the knee. Arthritis Rheum 2007;56:1204–11.

17. Cerejo R, Dunlop DD, Cahue S, et al. The influence of alignment on risk of knee osteoarthritis progression according to baseline stage of disease. Arthritis Rheum 2002;46:2632–6.

18. Hulet C, Menetrey J, Beaufils P, et al. Clinical and radiographic results of arthroscopic partial lateral meniscectomies in stable knees with a minimum follow up of 20 years. Knee Surg Sports Traumatol Arthrosc 2015;23:225–31.

19. Hoser C, Fink C, Brown C, et al. Long term results of arthroscopic partial lateral meniscectomy in knees without associated damage. J Bone Joint Surg Br 2001; 83:513–6.

20. Kyoung HY, Sang HL, Dae KB, et al. Does varus alignment increase after medial meniscectomy? Knee Surg Sports Traumatol Arthrosc 2013;21:2131–6.

21. Pengas IP, Nash W, Khan W, et al. Coronal knee alignment 40 years after total meniscectomy in adolescents: a prospective cohort study. Open Orthop J 2017;11: 424–31.

22. Longo UG, Ciuffreda M, Candela V, et al. Knee osteoarthritis after arthroscopic partial meniscectomy: prevalence and progression of radiographic changes after 5 to 12 years compared with contralateral knee. J Knee Surg 2018. https://doi.org/10.1055/s-0038-1646926.

23. Yang N, Nayeb-Hashemi H, Canavan P. The combined effect of frontal plane tibiofemoral knee angle and meniscectomy on the cartilage contact stresses and strains. Ann Biomed Eng 2009;37:2360–72.

24. Brophy RH, Haas AK, Huston LJ, et al. Association of meniscal status, lower extremity alignment, and body mass index with chondrosis at revision anterior cruciate ligament reconstruction. Am J Sports Med 2015;43:1616–22.

25. Nha KW, Lee YS, Hwang DH, et al. Second-look arthroscopic findings after open-wedge high tibia osteotomy focusing on the posterior root tears of the medial meniscus. Arthroscopy 2013;29:226–31.

26. Na YG, Lee BK, Hwang DH, et al. Can osteoarthritic patients with mild varus deformity be indicated for high tibial osteotomy? Knee 2018;25:856–65.

27. Beaufils P, Becker R, Kopf S, et al. The knee meniscus: management of traumatic tears and degenerative lesions. EFORT Open Rev 2017;11(2):195–203.

28. Beaufils P, Becker R, Kopf S, et al. Surgical management of degenerative meniscus lesions: the 2016 ESSKA meniscus consensus. Joints 2017;5:59–69.

29. Gelber PE, Verdonk P, Getgood AM, et al. Meniscal transplantation: state of the art. J Isakos 2017;2:229–49.

30. Allaire R, Muriuki M, Gilbertson L, et al. Biomechanical consequences of a tear of the posterior root of the medial meniscus. Similar to total meniscectomy. J Bone Joint Surg Am 2008;90:1922–31.

31. Emmanuel K, Quinn E, Niu J, et al. Quantitative measures of meniscus extrusion predict incident radiographic knee osteoarthritis—data from the Osteoarthritis Initiative. Osteoarthritis Cartilage 2016;24:262–9.

32. Erquicia J, Gelber PE, Cardona-Munoz JI, et al. There is no relation between mild malalignment and meniscal extrusion in trauma emergency patients. Injury 2012; 43:68–72.

33. Goto N, Okasaki K, Akiyama T, et al. Alignment factors affecting the medial meniscus extrusion increases the risk of osteoarthritis development. Knee Surg Sports Traumatol Arthrosc 2018. https://doi.org/10.1007/s00167-018-5286-7.

34. Wang J, Xiong J, Xu Z, et al. Short-term effects of discoid lateral meniscectomy on the axial alignment of the lower limb in adolescents. J Bone Joint Surg Am 2015;97:201–7.

35. Rai MF, Patra D, Sandell LJ, et al. Transcriptome analysis of injured human meniscus reveals a distinct phenotype of meniscus degeneration with aging. Arthritis Rheum 2013;65:2090–101.

36. Marriott K, Birmingham TB, Pinto R, et al. Gait biomechanics after combined HTO-ACL reconstruction versus HTO alone: a matched cohort study. J Orthop Res 2018. https://doi.org/10.1002/jor.24157.

Moving?

Make sure your subscription moves with you!

To notify us of your new address, find your **Clinics Account Number** (located on your mailing label above your name), and contact customer service at:

Email: journalscustomerservice-usa@elsevier.com

800-654-2452 (subscribers in the U.S. & Canada)
314-447-8871 (subscribers outside of the U.S. & Canada)

Fax number: 314-447-8029

Elsevier Health Sciences Division
Subscription Customer Service
3251 Riverport Lane
Maryland Heights, MO 63043

*To ensure uninterrupted delivery of your subscription, please notify us at least 4 weeks in advance of move.

Moving?

Printed and bound by CPI Group (UK) Ltd, Croydon, CR0 4YY

08/05/2025

01864691-0004